PHYSICAL DISABILITY

BOOKS IN LIBRARY AND INFORMATION SCIENCE
A Series of Monographs and Textbooks
EDITOR
ALLEN KENT
*School of Library and Information Science
University of Pittsburgh
Pittsburgh, Pennsylvania*

ADVISORY BOARD

C. David Batty
University of Maryland

Julie H. Bichteler
The University of Texas at Austin

Anindya Bose
University of Denver

Scott Bruntjen
Pittsburgh Regional Library Center

Eric de Grolier
Paris, France

Tom Featheringham
New Jersey Institute of Technology

Maurice J. Freedman
Columbia University

Thomas J. Galvin
University of Pittsburgh

Edward J. Kazlauskas
University of Southern California

Chai Kim
University of Rhode Island

Irving M. Klempner
State University of New York at Albany

Boaz Lazinger
Jerusalem, Israel

John A. McCrossan
University of South Florida

Paul E. Peters
Columbia University

Allan D. Pratt
The University of Arizona

Gary R. Purcell
The University of Tennessee

Tefko Saracevic
Case Western Reserve University

Thomas P. Slavens
The University of Michigan

Roy B. Stokes
The University of British Columbia

K. Subramanyam
Drexel University

Jean M. Tague
The University of Western Ontario

PREFACE

This book is intended as a guide to the literature for professionals who work with physically disabled individuals. Rehabilitation literature has grown rapidly in recent years as a result of political activity of disabled individuals and federal legislation, such as the Rehabilitation Act of 1973 (P.L. 93-112). Unfortunately bibliographic control of rehabilitation literature has been and continues to be poor. Libraries have long recognized the importance of library services to physically disabled individuals and this book attempts to take this service one step further by providing a guide to rehabilitation literature. It is hoped that professionals using this guide will become more aware of the literature within their own field and in related fields.

For the librarian there are several works which address the information needs of and the literature for disabled persons. These include:

>Baskin, Barbara H., and Harris, Karen H. Notes from a Different Drummer: A Guide to Juvenile Fiction Portraying the Handicapped. New York: Bowker, 1977.

>Strom, Maryalls G. Library Services to the Blind and Physically Handicapped. Metuchen, N.J.: Scarecrow Press, 1977.

>Wright, Keith C., Library and Information Services for Handicapped Individuals. Littleton, Colo.: Libraries Unlimited, 1979.

>Velleman, Ruth A. Serving Physically Disabled People: An Information Handbook for All Libraries. New York: Bowker, 1979.

However, to date, few bibliographic works exist to assist other professionals in meeting the information needs they encounter in serving physically disabled persons. There have been attempts within professional associations to compile bibliographies, but these bibliographies have been neither exhaustive nor evaluative and have had a limited distribution.

This book is offered as a guide to professionals particularly in the fields of architecture, rehabilitation counseling, health education, physical education, law, librarianship, therapeutic recreation, and health. Its objectives are to: 1) provide a listing of today's professional literature which addresses the physically disabled population, 2) evaluate the literature in terms of how it compares to related literature in that field, and 3) identify appropriate types of collections to which these materials should be added. Within each chapter the authors discuss which professionals are addressed, characteristics of the literature, and the current status of the field as reflected in the literature. Quotations which appear in the annotations are taken from the introductory material of the book cited unless otherwise stated.

This literature guide does not include all publications written in the field of physical disability. Instead, the authors have attempted to select materials on the basis of availability, quality, uniqueness, usefulness, audience, and significance to the field. Much of the literature is considered to be useful to the physically disabled individuals themselves, as well as to the professionals serving them. Librarians should find this book useful for purposes of collection development and information services.

The first three chapters cover materials written about the specific physical disabilities of mobility, visual, and hearing impairment, providing a background of information which should be useful to any professional seeking information on a specific disability. The next

PREFACE

eight chapters address the social, psychological, medical, legal, communication, and independent living aspects of the physically disabled community. Among these, Chapter 6 is a highly technical chapter dealing with the hearing impaired community and will be of interest primarily to those professionals in the fields of speech, hearing, and audiology. Another chapter has been devoted to the disabled child, Chapter 12. The author believed the needs and experiences of the developing child possessing a physical disability deserved special attention. Parents, as well as professionals, will find this to be an exceptionally useful chapter. The last three chapters are based on types of materials, i.e., federal government publications, journals, and audiovisuals.

All sources cited have been examined and evaluated by the contributing authors who, for the most part, are librarians in academic and medical libraries. This publication is an outgrowth of an LSCA (Library Services and Construction Act) Grant to establish a collection of materials for professionals serving the physically disabled. This collection, now housed at the University of Illinois, is available to anyone through interlibrary loan by contacting or visiting the:

> Library of the Health Sciences
> University of Illinois
> 506 South Mathews
> Urbana, Illinois 61801

I would like to thank Helen Baker, the principal typist for this project, for her concerned effort. I would also like to acknowledge the assistance of Julie Hamilton, Diane Kastiel, Beth Kawski, Margaret Notheisen, Ruth Peters, Jerilynn Troxell, staff of the Library of the Health Sciences, Urbana-Champaign, and the University of Illinois Library, without whose help in ordering and processing the collection and typing this manuscript, this publication would not have been possible.

Phyllis C. Self

CONTRIBUTORS

Francesca Allegri
Assistant Professor
Assistant Health Sciences Librarian
University of Illinois
Urbana, Illinois

Betsy K. Baker
Reference Librarian
Bibliographic Instruction Services Librarian
Northwestern University Library
Evanston, Illinois

Susan E. Bekiares
Assistant Professor
Documents Librarian
University of Illinois Library
Urbana, Illinois

Richard E. Bopp
Assistant Professor
Documents Librarian
University of Illinois Library
Urbana, Illinois

Nancy P. Johnson
Associate Professor
Reference Librarian
Georgia State University
Law Library
Atlanta, Georgia

Carol A. Klink
Assistant Head of Acquisitions
Library of the Health Sciences
University of Illinois at the Medical Center
Chicago, Illinois

Robert E. Kretschmer
Coordinator of the Program in Hearing Impairment
Associate Professor of Special Education
Teachers College
Columbia University
New York, New York

Dianne C. Olson
Catalog/Acquisitions Librarian
Loyola University Medical Center
Maywood, Illinois

Carol Bates Penka
Assistant Reference Librarian
Assistant Professor of Library Administration
University of Illinois Library
Urbana, Illinois

Phyllis C. Self
Associate Professor
Health Sciences Librarian
Library of the Health Sciences
University of Illinois
Urbana, Illinois

1 MOBILITY IMPAIRMENT AND BARRIER FREE DESIGN

RICHARD E. BOPP/Documents Librarian, University of Illinois
Library, Urbana, Illinois

INTRODUCTION

   Persons with impaired mobility due to injury or disease constitute a large and diverse group among the physically disabled population. Current estimates are that more than twelve million people suffer from some degree of mobility impairment.(1) Among the causes of mobility impairment are congenital conditions such as spina bifida and cerebral palsy, injuries such as spinal cord injury and amputation, and numerous diseases, including multiple sclerosis, poliomyelitis and arthritis. Various degrees of limitation in mobility also may result from stroke or any of a number of neurological or orthopedic diseases and disorders.
   Regardless of the etiology of their condition, mobility impaired individuals face similar problems and challenges in their rehabilitation and re-entry into society. One persistent problem is how to maneuver in a physical environment cluttered with architectural barriers such as steps, curbs, narrow doorways, and other structures and facilities built for the mythical "normal" individual. An even greater challenge, however, is presented by the attitudinal barriers in our society. Taught from an early age that disability connotes evil, freakishness or helplessness, disabled individuals must struggle to accept their impaired bodies

and the physical limitations imposed by disability. Psychological adjustment to disability is complicated by both the physical and attitudinal barriers disabled persons encounter in society. These physical and attitudinal barriers are prominent concerns in the literature on rehabilitation of mobility impaired persons.

This chapter reviews several categories of books on mobility impairment. It gives the greatest attention to literature on psychological and social adjustment to mobility impairment and on barrier free design for the elimination of architectural barriers (Readers are encouraged to consult Chapters IV and X for further literature relevant to psychological adjustment). General works on mobility impairments are also reviewed in this chapter, as well as works which overlap or lie outside the subject areas of other chapters. Some of these works provide introductions or beginning points for persons with little prior knowledge of disability. Examples are Bauer's Manual on Multiple Sclerosis and Cruickshank's Cerebral Palsy: A Developmental Disability. They provide the general background which is a prerequisite to intensive study of particular aspects of the rehabilitation process. Most such works, however, are directed at medical professionals, and these are reviewed in Chapter VII.

Monographic literature on psychological adjustment to specific forms of mobility impairment is rather limited. In Spinal Cord Injuries: Psychological, Social, and Vocational Adjustment, Trieschmann reviews the literature on adjustment to spinal cord injury and offers valuable suggestions both for clinical practice and for further research. A study of her bibliography reveals the large body of periodical literature on adjustment to disability. The only book-length treatment of the emotional consequences of amputation is Friedmann's The Psychological Rehabilitation of the Amputee. There are three general works on the psychological aspects of stroke, but none provides a comprehensive up-to-date treatment of the subject. Benton's Behavioral Changes in Cerebrovascular Disease is uneven in quality and overly technical, while Ullman's Behavioral Changes in Patients Following Strokes is more balanced, but is based on research now twenty-five years old. Brown's Physiological and Psychological Considerations in the Management of Stroke is practical and current, but superficial. A comprehensive treatment of the psychological aspects of stroke rehabilitation would be welcomed. The same can be said for multiple sclerosis and arthritis. Speaking generally, there are books for patients on psychological adjustment to their disabilities, and books for health care professionals on medical concerns, but few up-to-date, scholarly and comprehensive works for other professionals.

There are several compilations of essays on psychological adjustment to disability which contain chapters on specific mobility impairments. The Psychological and Social Impact of Physical Disability, edited by Marinelli and Dell Orto, contains two essays on psychological and social adjustment to paraplegia. Cobb's Medical and Psychological Aspects of Disability includes chapters on hemiplegia, cerebral palsy and amputation. Social and Psychological Aspects of Disability, edited by Stubbins, considers several aspects of adjustment to spinal cord injury. Psychological Practice With the Physically Disabled, edited by Garrett and Levine, discusses arthritis, cerebral palsy, and hemiplegia, and includes a lengthy chapter on amputation. These are all good sources for persons seeking an introduction to the psychological consequences of mobility impairments.(2)

For beginning professionals in rehabilitation fields, autobiographical accounts by disabled persons offer insights based on experience rather than on research. These works provide a valuable introduction to the problems of psychological adjustment by people who themselves have faced these problems. A large number of such autobiographies exist, and each is as unique as its author. Brickner's My Second Twenty Years: An Unexpected Life, offers observations by a forty-year-old quadriplegic on his life since his spinal cord injury at the age of twenty. The son of two psychiatrists, his analysis of his growth during his "second life" is detailed and informative. Dahlberg and Jaffe, in Stroke: A Doctor's Story of His Recovery, provide both the patient's and the physician's perspectives on the experience of stroke rehabilitation, as well as a lucid scientific discussion of the problem of asphasia following a stroke. Works such as these are as instructive in their own way as the research studies which generally receive more attention in professional literature. A selection of recent autobiographies is included in this chapter.

The literature on barrier free design is voluminous. The wealth of information on all aspects of design, for environments ranging from professional meeting rooms to outdoor recreational facilities, is in response to federal legislation such as the Architectural Barriers Act of 1968 (P.L. 90-480) and the Rehabilitation Act of 1973 (P.L. 93-112). These laws require public facilities constructed or modified with federal funds to be accessible to physically disabled individuals. Following the lead of the federal government, several states have published their own standards for accessibility to disabled persons. These tend to be very comprehensive and detailed, and they are useful to architects and planners nationwide. The best state government guidelines are Access for All: An Illustrated Handbook of Barrier Free Design for Ohio and the State of Illinois' publication, Accessibility Standards Illustrated. Selim's book on the Michigan Construction Code, and the work on Washington State barrier free design regulations by Small & Allen, are also very well conceived and written. The authoritative standards on which many state laws and regulations are based are the American National Standards Specifications for Making Buildings and Facilities Accessible to and Usable by Physically Handicapped People, published by the American National Standards Institute, Inc. These standards were first published in 1961, and have recently (1980) been revised and expanded.

MOBILITY IMPAIRMENT 5

    Monographic works on barrier free design vary greatly in format, in content, and in the audience for whom they are intended. Several organizations have published pamphlets which serve as introductions to the general topic or to barrier free design principles in particular settings. The National Center for a Barrier Free Environment's booklet, <u>Opening Doors: A Handbook on Making Facilities Accessible to Handicapped People</u>, provides an overview of physical considerations as well as information resources and funding options. For specific domestic design suggestions, the Paralyzed Veterans of America has published <u>Home in a Wheelchair: House Design Ideas for Easier Wheelchair Living</u>, written by Joseph Chasin. <u>The Planner's Guide to Barrier Free Meetings</u>, published jointly by Barrier Free Environments, Inc. and Harold Russell Associates, is an excellent guide for organizations wishing to assure that workshops, meetings and conventions are fully accessible to disabled persons.

    Among longer, more comprehensive treatments of barrier free design, several outstanding works deserve mention. <u>Design for Independent Living</u>, by Lifschez and Winslow, is unique in discussing the broader implications of barrier free design for the social, leisure and working lives of individuals with mobility impairments. This work is based on a study of the interaction between disabled people and their physical environment in Berkeley, California. This same interactional theme is at the center of Cary's <u>How to Create Interiors for the Disabled</u>. In addition to providing detailed suggestions for all aspects of interior barrier free design, Cary discusses how accessible homes improve the lives of disabled individuals and their families. Finally, Mueller takes the same broad approach in his work, <u>Designing for Functional Limitations</u>, which assists employers in planning work environments suited to the unique needs of individuals with any of a variety of mobility impairments.

    These are but a few of the many valuable works on barrier free design. In addition to these, there are several works on adapting schools and college campuses to the needs of mobility impaired students. Leisure environments such as recreation areas and shopping centers have also been addressed in the literature on barrier free design. Most of these works are very recent, and undoubtedly refect the attempt by all segments of the community to conform to the accessibility requirements of Section 504 of the Rehabilitation Act of 1973. As a result, the literature on barrier free design is about as complete and satisfactory as one could wish.

One day we will have the abundance of information on psychological adjustment that we now enjoy in the area of barrier free design. However, that is not the case as yet. It is much easier to solve the problem of architectural barriers than to understand the complexity of human reactions to disability. In similar fashion, it is easier to concentrate on physical restoration and rehabilitation than to deal with the intense emotional reactions which are inevitable consequences of disabling illness or injury. There is reason to believe, however, that the literature on psychological and social adjustment will expand in the near future. Trieschmann's review of the literature on adjustment to spinal cord injury is an important step in this development. Recent works by Roessler and Bolton, Vash, and Power and Dell Orto all demonstrate the realization that the key to rehabilitation is successful adjustment by the disabled individual and his or her family members.(3) Techniques for facilitating that adjustment will be well represented in rehabilitation literature in years to come.

NOTES

1. Goldenson, Robert M., editor-in-chief. Disability and Rehabilitation Handbook (New York, McGraw-Hill, 1978), pp. 766.
2. Annotations for these works are provided in Chapter IV.
3. See the introductory section of Chapter IV for a discussion of these works.

MOBILITY IMPAIRMENT 7

ANNOTATED BIBLIOGRAPHY

Albrecht, Gary L. <u>Reducing Public Barriers of the Severely Handicapped</u>. Chicago: Rehabilitation Institute of Chicago, 1976. 31 pp.

   A research report based on a study designed to test public response to a person in a wheelchair in need of assistance. A paraplegic was seated in a wheelchair by a curb on a Chicago street and the helping or non-helping behaviors of passersby were measured by hidden cameras and post-interaction personal interviews. The results are given in numerous statistical tables. The significant conclusion was that the behavior of the disabled person was more important than the attitude toward disability of the helper. Thus, the disabled can influence others' reactions to them. This research documents what disabled people know by experience, that able-bodied people are usually willing and eager to assist them when they require help. One valuable aspect of the study was that it occurred in a completely natural environment using ordinary, non-selected subjects. An interesting outcome of this research is that while most people have positive attitudes toward persons with disabilities and want to help them, their knowledge of disability and the capacities of disabled people is minimal. Recommended for research collections in social science and rehabilitation fields.

American Institute of Architects. Potomac Valley Chapter. <u>Barrier Free Rapid Transit</u>. Silver Spring, Md.: Potomac Valley Architects, 1969. Unpaged.

   Report prepared by Potomac Valley chapter of the American Institute of Architects on techniques and designs for making the Washington, D.C. Metro system accessible to disabled persons. Describes and illustrates options for access to the underground stations and for the design of subway cars. Certain designs and options are recommended as most suitable. Material presented here would be useful to urban planners in cities considering construction of a rapid transit system.

American National Standards Institute. <u>American National Standard Specifications for Making Buildings and Facilities Accessible to and Usable by Physically Handicapped People</u>. New York: The Institute, 1980. 68 pp.

   Revised and expanded edition of the ANSI A117.1 standards first published in 1961. Design features for all disabilities are addressed, and include exterior and interior considerations for both private and public buildings. These standards are generally regarded as the most detailed and comprehensive available, and are often used in the drafting of state and local laws and building codes. Specifications are detailed and well-illustrated by drawings. They provide <u>minimum</u> acceptable accessibility; in many cases, more is suggested and expected. This is a basic reference work which should be in all government and special libraries serving engineers, architects, urban planners or legislative personnel.

Barrier Free Environments. *Accessible Housing: A Manual on North Carolina's Building Code Requirements for Accessible Housing.* Raleigh, N.C.: The Special Office for the Handicapped, Insurance Commissioner's Office, North Carolina, Dept. of Insurance, 1980. 68 pp.

Detailed explanation and illustration of accessibility features for residential housing units required by North Carolina State Building Code. Applies to apartment buildings, condominiums, hotels, motels, residential schools, and institutions. Primary emphasis is on layout and special features in bathrooms and kitchens to facilitate maximum accessibility to persons in wheelchairs. Text differentiates between minimum requirements of the code and suggestions for voluntary maximum level of accessibility. Many drawings and model floor plans with physical specifications. Recommended for special libraries serving architects, planners, engineers, and professionals in related fields.

Bathroom Facilities Accomodating the Physically Disabled and the Aged. Ann Arbor: The School of Art, University of Michigan, 1977. 41 pp.

Results of a study undertaken by industrial design students to identify concepts and designs which maximize accessibility and convenient use of public and residential bathroom facilities by persons who are disabled or elderly. Their recommendations embody the principle that all facilities should be designed for use by all persons, with no special provisions. Various disabilities are addressed, but problems of persons in wheelchairs receive major emphasis. Illustrations and drawings depict possible layouts and various design concepts for fixtures such as tubs, stools, and vanities. Bibliography included. Useful for architects, interior design students and engineers serving these groups or professionals in related fields.

Bauer, Helmut J. *A Manual on Multiple Sclerosis.* Vienna, Austria: International Federation of Multiple Sclerosis Societies, 1977. 84 pp.

A brief manual for rehabilitation professionals on various aspects of the management of multiple sclerosis. Topics covered range from the diagnosis and medical treatment of the disease to advice on matters such as diet, sex and travel. The language is technical, but the emphasis is on practical approaches to common complications of the disease. The author has mastered the medical literature while still retaining the ability to see the patient's point of view. A valuable introduction to the subject for health professionals and others who work with patients having multiple sclerosis. Recommended for medical libraries.

Bednar, Michael J., ed. Barrier-Free Environments. Stroudsburg, Pa.: Dowden, Hutchinson and Ross, 1977. 278 pp.

A group of essays on various physical and social barriers facing physically disabled persons. Several of the essays deal, as well, with the mentally handicapped and the barriers they encounter. The emphasis is on the philosophical basis for the goal of total integration of the disabled into the mainstream of society. This philosophical basis suggests policy and planning decisions to achieve that goal. Case studies provided in the book give examples of how this is to be done. They include a project in Moline, Illinois, and several European models. The primary audience for this book is professionals and civic leaders in a position to plan and design community living environments which are barrier free. As such, it is recommended for municipal libraries and special and academic library collections in architecture, engineering, and urban planning.

Benton, Arthur L., ed. Behavioral Change in Cerebrovascular Disease. New York: Harper and Row, 1970. 257 pp.

Composed of talks given at a workshop; authors are primarily physicians, but some are clinical phychologists. Papers discuss language and psychomotor disorders following stroke, as well as rehabilitation principles for dealing with these disorders. Twenty-one papers are included. None of the papers is titled, and no introduction is provided, so reader has no clue as to focus of individual papers. There is no index, and references from all twenty-one papers are combined in one bibliography. Papers are well-informed, based on research and familiarity with literature on the topic. Not oriented toward clinical practitioners; could be useful reading for researchers, but information is rather dated.

Brickner, Richard P. My Second Twenty Years: An Unexpected Life. New York: Basic Books, 1976. 198 pp.

Brickner suffered a spinal cord injury at the age of twenty, which left him a quadriparetic (weak, but not paralyzed, in all four limbs). This autobiography, authored twenty years later, describes his new life. Written at a time when he had finally come to terms with the conditions of his "second life," it is a witty, incisive and literate account of his adjustment to disability. Throughout, he describes his feelings in the style of a novelist and analyzes them with the mind of a psychiatrist (both of his parents were, in fact, trained in psychiatry). My Second Twenty Years is full of subtle insights and delightful anecdotes. As a study in adjustment to disability, or just as a story, it is well worth reading. Recommended for public and academic libraries.

Brown, Arnold. Physiological and Psychological Considerations in the Management of Stroke. St Louis: W. H. Green, 1976. 83 pp.

Basic introduction to causes and consequences of stroke, with major emphasis on the importance of understanding psychological and emotional factors in the rehabilitation of stroke patients. Author is a physical therapist who believes strongly in the "team approach" to rehabilitation. The team, he believes, must include the patient and family members. A psychologist or social worker, to help patient and family adjust, must also be part of the team. Author is well versed in the literature of psychological adjustment to disability. Emphasis on psychological adjustment is much needed, but discussion is too brief and superficial. Adds no new knowledge to field, but useful for medical students to read because of its commitment to "the patient as a person." Recommended for libraries serving students in medical and allied health fields.

Brown, Christy. The Childhood Story of Christy Brown. London: Pan Books, 1972. 158 pp.

This is the paperback edition of Christy Brown's autobiography, originally published in 1954 under the title of My Left Foot. Brown, who was born with cerebral palsy and writes and types only with his left foot, has published two novels, one the highly acclaimed Down All the Days, an account of Irish slum life. His autobiography is written in a simple, straight-forward yet very graceful style. It relates his adjustment to life as a disabled person and the emergence, in adolescence and adulthood, of his artistic and literary interests and talents. This story provides numerous insights into both the problems encountered by a person who is congenitally disabled and the techniques of overcoming such a handicap. Recommended for general audiences as well as for professionals who work with disabled children.

Bunin, Nina; Jasperse, David; and Cooper, Susan. A Guide to Designing Accessible Outdoor Recreation Facilities. Ann Arbor, Mich.: Lake Central Regional Office of Heritage Conservation and Recreation Service, U.S. Dept. of Interior, 1980. 58 pp.

Contains practical ideas for creating accessible recreation areas. Heavily illustrated with drawings which show how accessibility can be achieved. Detailed specifications occasionally given. Types of recreational areas covered include picnic and camping areas, paths and trails, fishing and boat docks and historic sites. Emphasis on universal design (creating recreational facilities to be enjoyed by all persons) rather than on special facilities for disabled people.

Cary, Jane Randolph. How to Create Interiors for the Disabled: A Guidebook for Family and Friends. New York: Pantheon Books, 1978. 127 pp.

Most comprehensive and useful book available to disabled persons and their families on the subject of adapting one's home environment to one's physical limitations. Author is not disabled, but has visited the homes of many disabled people and gathered their ideas and techniques. She discusses all aspects of interior design, and includes chapters on exterior ramps and doorways as well. She not only discusses rooms and spaces, but also important functional considerations such as windows and lighting systems. She discusses the advantages and disadvantages of different types of furniture and equipment for those with various disabilities. More than one option is offered in most cases, to allow for individual needs or preferences. Profusely illustrated with excellent drawings. Addresses provided for manufacturers of materials and equipment. Highly recommended for public libraries and for libraries serving rehabilitation professionals, students, or practitioners in fields of architecture or interior design.

Chasin, Joseph. <u>Home in a Wheelchair: House Design Ideas for Easier Wheelchair Living</u>. Washington, D.C.: Paralyzed Veterans of America, 1978. 32 pp.

Discussion of all aspects of choosing, building, or adapting a home to meet the needs of an individual who uses a wheelchair. Author has used a wheelchair for thirty years. Primary audience is disabled individuals. More comprehensive and detailed than Garee's work. A list of longer works on individual aspects of wheelchair living is appended. Virtually every room and function is discussed with illustrations and drawings, even including lifts and elevators for two-story homes. Recommended for public libraries and for special libraries which serve engineers, architects or rehabilitation professionals.

Chasin, Joseph and Saltman, Jules. <u>The Wheelchair in the Kitchen</u>. Washington, D.C.: Paralyzed Veterans of America, 1978. 32 pp.

Outlines ways in which kitchen furniture and appliances, as well as aids for cooking, serving and eating, can be arranged, remodeled or adapted to meet the needs of a homemaker who uses a wheelchair. Illustrations and drawings are well designed to depict the suggestions given in the text. A list of safety tips to avoid injury or accidents is also included. Comprehensive, practical, clearly written, and inexpensive. Useful to occupational therapists, rehabilitation counselors, and disabled laypersons. Recommended for medical and large public libraries.

Coons, Maggie and Milner, Margaret, eds. <u>Creating an Accessible Campus</u>. Washington, D.C.: Association of Physical Plant Administrators of Universities and Colleges, 1978. 143 pp.

A comprehensive guide for those who have the responsibility for adapting college campus facilities to make them accessible to disabled students as required by Section 504 of the Rehabilitation Act of 1973. All aspects of the planning, designing and construction activities necessary to accomplish this are discussed by various individuals with personal and/or professional expertise in barrier free design. Specific problems caused by various disabilities are listed, and detailed design specifications to accommodate persons with these disabling conditions are provided. The book is well planned, researched, and illustrated. It is recommended for academic libraries as well as special libraries serving architects and engineers.

Corbet, Barry. Options: Spinal Cord Injury and the Future. 2d ed. Denver: A.B. Hirschfeld Press, 1980. 152 pp.

Corbet, a paraplegic, interviewed 54 spinal cord injured persons from around the country to show that fulfilling and exciting options are available to disabled people, just as they are to others. His subjects pursue a variety of careers, from farming to medicine. Many are married, and some are active in sports and other leisure activities. The book is intended to be read by newly disabled persons who may think that such activities are no longer realistic options for them. The 54 mini-biographies consist of verbatim thoughts and feelings by the subjects and commentary and background information by Corbet. The variety of lifestyles presented here is impressive. Should be read not only by disabled people, but by rehabilitation professionals who sometimes underestimate the abilities of their clients. Recommended for academic and public libraries and rehabilitation collections.

Craig Hospital. Family Service Department. Mobility in the Wheelchair Home. Englewood, Colo.: The Craig Hospital, 1977. 23 pp.

Overview of considerations and techniques for adapting, purchasing or building a home which allows for independent living by a person using a wheelchair. Discusses and illustrates design principles for the following features: parking and entrance to home; hallways; bedroom furniture; and the layout of bathroom and kitchen appliances and facilities. Similar in scope and content to Chasin's Home in a Wheelchair, but not as comprehensive as Chasin's work. A unique contribution, however, is a short description of an accessible mobile home. Contains an annotated bibliography for further reading. Recommended for patient libraries and large public libraries.

Cruickshank, William M., ed. Cerebral Palsy: A Developmental Disability. 3rd rev. ed. Syracuse, N.Y.: Syracuse University Press, 1976. 623 pp.

A comprehensive text for professionals and students in all rehabilitation fields. Consciously designed to encourage an interdisciplinary approach to working with individuals with cerebral palsy. Contributing authors are scholars affiliated with academic or medical institutions. Chapters summarize the state of knowledge in fields from medicine to speech therapy to social work. A comprehensive bibliography is included, as well as a detailed index by name and subject. This work is the most comprehensive introduction to the subject available, and should be in all medical, academic, and special libraries serving those who work in rehabilitation fields.

Dahlberg, Charles Clay, and Jaffe, Joseph. <u>Stroke: A Doctor's Personal Story of His Recovery</u>. New York: Norton, 1977. 200 pp.

Dr. Dahlberg, a psychiatrist, had a mild stroke in 1973. Like 50% of stroke patients, he suffered afterward from aphasia (loss of language skills). He and his friend, Dr. Jaffe, wrote this book to help both stroke patients and physicians understand the nature of aphasia and the problems the patient encounters in seeking to regain language skills lost after stroke. Dahlberg describes the stroke, his emotional reaction to it and his feelings and experiences in the months of rehabilitation which followed. Jaffe in his five chapters, discusses the nature of language and how it is affected by a stroke or other brain damage. His explanation is straight-forward, informative, and as non-technical as possible. The joint authorship works well in this book, Dahlberg presenting the human and Jaffe the scientific side of stroke rehabilitation. Recommended for medical, academic, and public libraries.

Davis, Marcella Zaleski. <u>Living With Multiple Sclerosis: A Social Psychological Analysis</u>. Springfield, Ill.: Charles C. Thomas, 1973. 71 pp.

Based on thesis research for a doctoral degree in nursing, this book examines some of the psychological and social consequences of multiple sclerosis (MS). Written for social work and health care professionals. Issues discussed include the effect of MS on self-concept and on relationships with family and friends. Suggests means for facilitating continued social interaction, such as self-help groups and clubs and recreational centers. Overall, the information in this work is not new or unique, and adds little to our understanding of coping with disability or methods of helping individuals cope.

Eareckson, Joni. <u>Joni</u>. Minneapolis: World Wide Publications, 1976. 190 pp.

Personal narrative by young woman paralyzed from neck down at age of 17. Most of the book deals with her long struggle to accept her quadriplegia as a permanent condition and to find reasons for continuing to live and enjoy her life. She discovers these in painting with her mouth and in witnessing for God as a born again Christian. Both give her an outlet for her ideas, feelings and faith, and convince her that life can still be meaningful. Simply and candidly written, her story accurately reflects the depression and anger felt by the newly disabled person. Strong religious emphasis, which will please some readers and offend others. Recommended for public libraries.

Edgar, Betsy Jordan. We Live with the Wheel Chair. Parsons, W. Va. McClain Printing Co., 1970. 122 pp.

Story of a man who lost both legs in World War II. Written by his wife, it describes his adjustment to his disability and their life together since his injury. Also contains some interesting information about medical treatments available in the 1940's for the thousands of U.S. soldiers disabled in the war. The style is mediocre, and the book espouses values somewhat out of fashion among most disabled people today, e.g., that people who overcome disabilities are brave, superior individuals who are an inspiration to society. Useful for historical perspective rather than for understanding today's disabled individual. Not recommended for most collections.

Fishman, David. Shopping Centers and the Accessibility Codes. New York: International Council of Shopping Centers, 1979. 23 pp.

Author is president of an accessibility consulting service in Santa Barbara, California. His book is written for shopping center developers, to inform them how to comply with barrier free design codes and legislation. Discusses ANSI standards which have been adopted by many state and local governments as the guidelines for accessibility. Gives specifications for features such as ramps, restrooms, drinking fountains, telephones, and parking spaces for disabled shoppers. Financial information on tax deductions and costs of barrier free features are given. Ideas for publicity and staff awareness training are mentioned. Bibliography on barrier free design included. Straight-forward approach which emphasizes financial benefits of barrier free design and legal obligations to provide accessible facililites. Well conceived and written. Should be in municipal libraries and special libraries serving planners, builders, and designers.

Friedmann, Lawrence W. The Psychological Rehabilitation of the Amputee. Springfield, Ill.: Charles C. Thomas, 1978. 157 pp.

Author is a physician specializing in rehabilitation. His book is one of the few works on this topic, and it is solidly based on both experience and knowledge of the literature on psychological aspects of disability. More emphasis is placed on understanding the amputee's state of mind than on how to integrate psychological counseling into the rehabilitation program. The organization of the book could be improved; i.e., chapters could be sub-divided into more specific topical sections. However, the author does express throughout a strong commitment to understanding the necessary emotional problems which amputation causes. Chapters on phantom limb phenomena and on the history of society's attitudes toward amputees broaden the coverage of the book. It is a valuable contribution to rehabilitation literature aimed at physicians. Recommended for medical libraries.

MOBILITY IMPAIRMENT

Garee, Betty. <u>Ideas for Making Your Home Accessible</u>. Bloomington, Ill.: Accent Press, 1978. 104 pp.

This book includes ideas, specifications and commercial products which persons in wheelchairs should study before purchasing or adapting a house to fit their needs. All information is from the computerized retrieval system, Accent on Information, a commercial service of Cheever Publishing, Inc., Bloomington, Illinois. General accessibility requirements for exterior and interior spaces are discussed and illustrated in drawings and photographs. Some detailed specifications are given, but the emphasis is on identifying problems, providing practical answers, and listing agencies and commercial suppliers which offer specialized services and equipment. A good introduction to the subject for wheelchair users and their families. It provides the information they should have before they contact a builder who, most likely, will not be aware of the design needs of disabled persons. Recommended for public libraries and patient education collections.

<u>Getting There: A Guide to Accessibility for Your Facility</u>. Sacramento: California Department of Rehabilitation, 1979. 46 pp.

Authored by professional and lay people in Sacramento and Berkeley, California. Investigates the psychological and social ramifications of the physical environment. Discusses social attitudes inherent in, and encouraged by, inaccessible design and the psychosocial benefits to disabled persons of accessible environments. Seeks to educate the reader in the principles rather than the physical specifications of barrier free design. Discusses sensory as well as mobility impairments, based on personal interviews with disabled persons who have visited accessible and inaccessible buildings and places. Illustrations depict disabled persons interacting with professionals and others in a variety of settings. The effect of the environment on social interactions is stressed throughout. Works which provided the theoretical basis for this approach are listed in an appendix. A thought-provoking work of value to architects, rehabilitation professionals, sociologists and urban planners. Highly recommended for special and academic libraries serving these audiences.

Goble, R.E.A., and Nichols, P.J.R. <u>Evaluation of a Disabled Living Unit</u>. London: Butterworths, 1971. 271 pp.

This work reports on a study of 200 patients admitted to a Disabled Living Research Unit in Oxford, England, from 1964-1966. The unit was a twelve-bed facility which conducted what we would now call training in independent living activities such as mobility, self-care and preparation for employment. The patients all suffered orthopedic or neurologic impairments following disease or injury. Patients were followed after discharge from the Disabled Living Unit to assess the degree of maintenance of the skills they had learned there. The authors conclude that social factors are more important than clinical features in the long-term rehabilitation of severely disabled persons. The disabled person's family is critically important, and the rehabilitation team must treat the family and not just the patient, if adaptation and independence are to be achieved. This work contains valuable information on many aspects of rehabilitation and is highly recommended for all medical libraries which serve rehabilitation professionals.

Goldsmith, Selwyn. <u>Designing for the Disabled</u>. 3rd. ed. London: RIBA Publications, 1976. 525 pp.

The largest, most comprehensive guide to designing and adapting all manner of buildings for use by persons with physical disabilities. Provides detailed specifications for all types and aspects of residential housing; public buildings of all purposes and uses are also discussed. Signage, a consideration overlooked in many works, is discussed fully here. Various disabilities are defined and briefly discussed, and the psychological aspects of disability are treated briefly. The book is decidedly British in its emphasis, attitude, and language, and all measurements are metric (a conversion table is provided). Appendices include a bibliography and list of British disability-related organizations.

Griesse, Rosalie. <u>The Crooked Shall Be Made Straight</u>. Atlanta: John Knox Press, 1979. 240 pp.

Forty-three-year-old minister's wife tells story of her thirty-one-year experience with scoliosis, a severe spinal curvature. She has learned to live with pain, with repeated surgical operations, and with frequent confinement in a neck-to-knees plaster cast. However, she has maintained a hopeful, positive attitude toward life and has recognized scoliosis in her two daughters at an early stage when it can be more easily corrected. Treatment of scoliosis today has improved, so that experiences such as hers are no longer necessary with early diagnosis and proper care. Her story is valuable primarily as an example of endurance and perserverence, both on her part and that of her family and friends. Recommended for public libraries.

Hackler, Emily N. <u>Stroke Rehabilitation and Re-Socialization: A Handbook for the Volunteer</u>. Irvine, Calif.: California Regional Medical Programs. Area VIII, University of California, Irvine, California College of Medicine, 1971. 35 pp.

Handbook for use in a program which utilizes volunteers as members of a stroke rehabilitation team. Responsibility of volunteer is to assist patient and family in understanding and accepting disabilities resulting from stroke, and to aid patient's re-entry into society. Training manual provides information on causes and consequences of stroke, on typical emotional reactions of patient and family, and on health care and community resources available for treatment and assistance. Suggestions are provided for dealing with predictable reactions and problems in the patient or the family. Readings for further information about stroke are included. Information is presented in outline form and should be supplemented by training sessions by a health professional. Unique and useful work. Recommended for hospital and rehabilitation libraries.

Harkness, Sarah P., and Groom, James N., Jr. Building Without Barriers For the Disabled. New York: Whitney Library of Design, 1976. 79 pp.

Brief design principles and specifications for "an environment which is more easily negotiable by all people." Emphasis on exterior access to buildings and on heavily-used interior rooms such as bathrooms and kitchens. Drawings give detailed specifications for facilities and furniture, and photographs illustrate disabled persons using bathroom and kitchen appliances. Unique feature is comparison chart showing differing specifications recommended by other publications on barrier free design. As with similar works, emphasis is on needs of persons using wheelchairs. Bibliography and index provided. Not as detailed or comprehensive as most other guides in this field. Recommended only for comprehensive collections on barrier free design.

Helms, Tom. Against All Odds. New York: Thomas Y. Crowell, 1978, 277 pp.

Excellent autobiography by a real fighter. Helms twice recovered from a broken neck and temporary quadriplegia. The first time his recovery was complete; the second time he recovered only partially and now walks with the aid of a cane. That he can walk at all is tribute to his amazing stores of determination and courage. Helms also made constructive use of the anger he felt toward fate and toward himself and others. His anger kept him believing and struggling, when others gave up on him. Unable to find a job because of his disability, he turned to writing, and his autobiography is the first fruit of his new career. Guaranteed to grip the reader. Highly recommended for public libraries.

Hirsch, Ernest A. Starting Over: the Autobiographical Account of a Psychologist's Experience with Multiple Sclerosis. North Quincy, Mass.: Christopher Publishing House, 1977. 169 pp.

A psychologist discusses his life since discovering in 1956, at age 32, that he had multiple sclerosis. He writes the book for other multiple sclerosis patients, their families and health professionals. He describes the course of the disease in his case, the adjustments he has had to make in his life and his attitude toward his disability. The book is disappointing in two respects. First, there is very little chronological order and many digressions, so that the progression of the disease and how it affects his life is hard to follow. Secondly, he excessively analyzes and explains his actions and feelings. However, since there are few autobiographies by patients with multiple sclerosis, the book would be of some value to the audiences he addresses. Hence, it could be a useful addition to public and medical libraries.

Hodgins, Eric. <u>Episode: Report on the Accident in My Skull</u>. New York: Atheneum, 1964, 272 pp.

    A journalist recounts, in a literate and intelligent fashion, his recovery from a stroke. Despite his various afflictions and setbacks, he tells his story without rancor, and indeed, with a great sense of humor. His insights into the patient's point of view are profound and should be read by every health professional. His tale is a delight to read, and would provide enjoyment to non-medical professionals and a general readership as well. The book is informative and entertaining. Although not written for any one group, it would be valuable reading for health professionals, families of stroke patients, and others. Highly recommended for medical, academic, and public libraries.

Jenkins, William M. <u>Rehabilitation of the Severely Disabled</u>. Dubuque, Iowa: Kendall/Hunt Publishing Co., 1976. 245 pp.

    Compilation of papers presented at a 1974 conference in Memphis concerning the rehabilitation of spinal-cord-injured and other disabled persons. Primarily intended for vocational counselors. Chapters provide overview of many aspects of rehabilitation, including the roles and functions of allied health professionals, such as physical and occupational therapists and orthotists. Most papers, however, deal with psychological adjustment and vocational evaluation and placement. Papers are based on practical experience rather than on research, and are aimed at practitioners. Recommended for special libraries and academic collections used by rehabilitation counseling professionals or students.

Jones, Michael Anthony. <u>Accessibility Standards Illustrated</u>. Springfield, Ill.: Capital Development Board, State of Illinois, 1978. 217 pp.

    Describes standards for accessiblity of buildings passed by the Illinois legislature in 1977. The standards are preceded by a discussion of various disabilities which create problems moving about in the physical environment. The standards themselves are presented, along with illustrations of how to implement them and with the problems which made each standard necessary. A very comprehensive, well-defined book which illustrates both the problems caused by poor design and the way to design exterior and interior environments for easy accessibility for all. Includes drawings and photographs which clearly illustrate each standard. In addition to general buildings, standards for specific-use buildings such as libraries, assembly halls, recreational facilities, hotels and motels are included. A 1982 reprint, while containing well as to urban planners, but is too specific in its audience for most library collections.

Lifchez, Raymond and Winslow, Barbara. <u>Design For Independent Living: The Environment and Physically Disabled People</u>. New York: Whitney Library of Design, 1979. 208 pp.

 A book about disabled people in Berkeley, California and how various adaptations in their environment and the support of other people allow them to live full and active lives. The lives and activities of seven disabled individuals are profiled, and their physical, social, and psychological means of coping with their disability are explained. The main part of the book focuses on common daily activities, such as work, play, eating, and grooming. Both attitudes and techniques in these areas are explored, with concrete illustrations from the lives of disabled individuals. There are numerous photographs, a bibliography, and an index. This book is innovative and uniquely valuable because the emphasis is on how the lives of individual people are affected by the environment, rather than on the physical environment, <u>per se</u>. The photographs of disabled people engaging in various daily activities are excellent supplements to the text. They convey the positive message that even severely physically limited people are capable of participating in all aspects of life. The book reads extremely well because of the imaginative and empathetic approach of the authors. Highly recommended for academic and special libraries.

Mace, Ronald L. <u>Accessibility Modifications: Guidelines for Modifications to Existing Buildings for Accessibility to the Handicapped</u>. Raleigh: North Carolina Department of Insurance, Special Office For the Handicapped, 1976. 63 pp.

 Shows how to adapt building entrances and interior facilities such as restrooms to make them accessible to and usable by physically disabled persons. The primary emphasis is on modifications such as ramps, doorways, and bathroom layouts which provide mobility for persons using wheelchairs. An attractive, well-organized book which provides many good ideas for physical accessibility to persons in wheelchairs. The drawings are exceptionally well done. Some modifications not discussed include lowered public telephones for persons in wheelchairs and braille markings in elevators to aid blind persons. A good introduction to the topic, but not as detailed or exhaustive as some other publications on barrier free design.

Marquit, Syvil. <u>Psychological Factors in the Management of Parkinson's Disease</u>. Miami, Fla.: National Parkinson Foundation Inc., n.d. 28 pp.

 Brief overview of psychological aspects of adapting to Parkinson's Disease. Author is a staff psychologist at the National Parkinson Institute in Miami. He discusses healthy and unhealthy some revisions, is generally of inferior quality. Recommended for all libraries.

Kamenetz, Herman L. The Wheelchair Book: Mobility for the Disabled. Springfield, Ill.: Charles C. Thomas, 1969. 267 pp.

Comprehensive guide to wheelchairs, their use, and the principles of prescribing them. Opens with an interesting and lengthy history of wheelchairs, followed by equally lengthy, detailed chapters on types of wheelchairs and wheelchair accessories. Finally, the author, a physiatrist, discusses prescription of wheelchairs and their operation and care by wheelchair users and/or helpers. In addition to a bibliography, index, and medical glossary, a dozen appendices provide information on travel, specialized clothing, and other matters important to wheelchair users. Recommended for all medical libraries, although an updated version is needed.

Kunder, Linda H. Barrier Free School Facilities for Handicapped Students. Arlington, Va.: Educational Research Service, 1977. 89 pp.

Designed as a planning document to help school administrators identify and correct barriers to disabled students. The publisher specializes in preparing informational documents of interest to educational researchers and administrators. In addition to providing a model building survey to facilitate accessibility, this book offers detailed specifications for designing ramps, classrooms, bathrooms and other school facilities so as to make them accessible to disabled students. Primary emphasis is given to the requirements of those in wheelchairs, but the needs of other groups such as the blind and deaf are also considered. The information in this work is specific enough that school personnel would not need to acquire any of the general works on barrier free design. However, a bibliography of such publications is included. Recommended for special education collections.

Labanowich, Stanley. Transportation Counseling for Handicapped Individuals: A Manual For Rehabilitation Professionals. Washington, D.C.: Rehabilitation Research and Training Center, George Washington University and the Transportation Alliance, 1979. 104 pp.

Written to aid rehabilitation counselors in assisting disabled individuals to assess their transportation needs and t about options for meeting those needs. Factors which should considered are discussed, and a flowchart illustrates a "coing process model." Forms for assessing clients' needs and surveying local transportation providers are included. An dix lists sources of federal funding for agencies or commu seeking to provide transportation for disabled citizens. manual would be valuable to vocational and other counselo

MOBILITY IMPAIRMENT 21

modes of adjusting to the knowledge that one has Parkinson's disease, and the psychological consequences of the physical symptoms of the disease, such as fear of falling. He then provides helpful suggestions about attitudes to cultivate and activities to pursue in order to achieve the best possible physical and psychological adjustment to the disease. This booklet is simply written yet informative. It would be useful both to laypersons and to professionals who work with persons having Parkinson's disease.

Mathews, Bryan. Multiple Sclerosis: The Facts. Oxford: Oxford University Press, 1978, 103 pp.

Brief, introductory discussion written for the general public by an Oxford Professor of Clinical Neurology. Describes current theories about causes of multiple sclerosis, symptoms and variable course of the disease, and methods of treatment from physical therapy to drugs and special diets. Sensible and non-dogmatic. Good summary for non-medical personnel. British in tone and emphasis. Easier to understand than Bauer's Manual on Multiple Sclerosis, but not as comprehensive. Recommended for public or patient libraries.

Milner, Margaret. Adapting Historic Campus Structures for Accessibility. Washington, D.C.: Association of Physical Plant Administrators of Universities and Colleges, n.d. 90 pp.

Detailed guide to principles and practices involved in adapting historic college and university campus buildings to make them usable by persons with mobility impairments. Many illustrations show how numerous institutions have made older buildings accessible to wheelchair users, while still preserving the historic structure and appearance of these buildings. Part I discusses various problems of accessibility and shows through drawings and photographs how these problems were solved on different campuses. Part II contains six detailed studies, each describing the adaptation of one historic building. Appendices include a bibliography, relevant 504 regulations, and lists of state historic preservation officers and campuses who reported accessibility projects in older buildings. This is an excellent, comprehensive work, which would be of great value to architects and campus administrators. The information it provides would also be applicable to older buildings in non-university settings. Highly recommended for academic libraries and special libraries serving architects and city planners.

Mueller, James. Designing For Functional Limitations. Washington, D.C.: Job Development Laboratory, George Washington University Rehabilitation Research and Training Center, 1979. 79 pp.

Designed to assist employers, vocational counselors, and others in "planning functional environments most sensitive to the abilities and limitations of disabled persons." Unique in its organization and emphasis upon the functional limitations which follow particular disabilities. These limitations, such as poor balance, weak upper extremities, sensory deficits, and others, are each considered in turn, with suggestions for each regarding design of a work environment which minimizes the effects of each limitation. The emphasis is upon accommodating individual disabled people, rather than on a general barrier free approach which usually considers only the requirements of wheelchair accessibility. Suggestions are given primarily in illustrations, with minimal explanation. The book shows the reader how to accommodate persons with various disabilities, but does not educate them about the disabilities themselves. Valuable for its unique approach and emphasis on work environments. Recommended for special libraries serving vocational counselors, or industrial design professionals.

National Center for a Barrier Free Environment. Accessibility Assistance: A Directory of Consultants on Environments for Handicapped People. Washington, D.C.: The Center, 1978. 202 pp.

Directory of firms and individuals who offer consulting services on barrier free design. Most listings are of architectural and engineering consultants; some interior designers, landscape architects and urban planners are also included. Directory includes: references; services which consultants provide; and previous consulting projects, all supplied by the consultants themselves. Separate listings by state and by profession; also, a name index at end of book. Very valuable for municipalities, educational institutions, businesses, and others seeking to expand accessibility of their facilities to disabled persons. Most comprehensive directory available in this area. Recommended for academic and public libraries and architectural collections.

National Center for a Barrier Free Environment. Opening Doors: A Handbook on Making Facilities Accessible to Handicapped People. Washington, D.C.: The Center, 1978. 31 pp.

A small booklet designed as an introduction to the subject of barrier free design. Short chapters summarize accessibility needs of persons with various disabilitites, strategies for action and sources of funds, federal legislation, and resources for more detailed information. Some detailed specifications and drawings, but not the detail required by planners or builders. This would be a good place to begin for anyone with no knowledge of the subject who needs a guide into the field.

New Jersey. Department of the Treasury, Division of Building and Construction. Barrier-Free Design for Providing Facilities for the Physically Handicapped in Public Buildings. Trenton, N.J.: The Division, 1977. 45 pp.

Almost entirely composed of definitions and specifications for making public buildings accessible to various groups of disabled persons. Comprehensive and specific with regard to various facilities, both interior and exterior. No illustrations and very little amplification of the regulations. The lack of illustrations limits the value of this publication. It has little educational value beyond making available to New Jersey residents the regulations for accessibility which apply in their state. Useful primarily for designers, architects, and engineers. Recommended primarily for special libraries in New Jersey. For those in other states, better works are available.

Ohio. Governor's Committee on Employment of the Handicapped. <u>Access for All: An Illustrated Handbook of Barrier Free Design for Ohio</u>. 2d. ed. Columbus: The Committee, 1978. 192 pp.

Detailed guidelines for designing new buildings and modifying older ones to make them accessible to disabled people. Includes information about categories of disability and estimates percentage of the population which has each disability. Covers all aspects of interior and exterior design, including such things as signage and lighting, which some other books omit. Also has guidelines for specific public buildings such as libraries and banks. Probably the most comprehensive and detailed of the books on accessibility published by state agencies. Provides guidelines for accommodating persons with various disabilities such as mobility, visual, and hearing impairments. Photographs as well as detailed drawings are given, illustrating techniques of providing accessibility. Highly recommended for libraries serving architects, engineers, planners, and professionals in similar fields.

Peoples Housing, Inc. <u>Housing Adaptability Guidelines</u>. Topanga, Calif.: Peoples Center for Housing Change, 1980. 39 pp.

Brief introduction, with drawings and specifications, to concept of building apartment complexes that are "adaptable" rather than "accessible." Recommends construction of units which meet minimum accessibility standards (e.g., no steps), but which are designed for able-bodied persons and adaptable for the disabled. Basically, this involves creating features in bathroom and kitchens, particularly, which can be easily and cheaply adapted for persons in wheelchairs, should such individuals desire to rent these units. Techniques for marketing this approach are discussed. This guide is brief, but outlines a unique idea for a cost-conscious society. Recommended for large public libraries and for special libraries serving professionals in planning and construction fields.

Peterson, Yen. <u>Marital Adjustment in Couples of Which One Spouse is Physically Handicapped</u>. Palo Alto, Calif.: R & E. Research Associates, 1979, 116 pp.

Study of marital adjustment of couples where one spouse is mobility-impaired to the extent of using a wheelchair. Study group is the disabled spouse, so major emphasis is on the feelings and behavior of that member of the couple. In addition to general problems of adjustment, such as role definition, intimacy, conflict resolution, and others, the study also attempted to discover if differences in adjustment can be related to the disabled spouse's sex, or to whether the disabled spouse's medical condition is static or progressive. The study concluded that some couples in the study group had developed a "disabled marriage lifestyle" different from other identifiable marriage styles in American culture. Other conclusions and suggestions for further research are given, along with numerous tables and statistical analyses. This study represents a valuable addition to an area in which few published research studies exist.

The Planner's Guide to Barrier Free Meetings. Raleigh, N.C.: and Waltham, Mass.: Barrier Free Environments, Inc., and Harold Russell Associates, 1980. 73 pp.

Detailed and comprehensive guide for organizations to use in ensuring that their meetings and conventions are optimally accessible to disabled individuals. Provides introductory information about disabilities and about laws and regulations governing accessibility. Defines special needs of persons with mobility and visual impairments. Main body of work provides excellent text and illustrations for all aspects of program accessibility, from parking and building entrances to bathroom and meeting room designs and specifications. Practical and informative; based on thorough knowledge of needs of disabled persons. Final section provides lists of organizations of disabled persons, of sources of equipment, and of sources of interpreters. Outstanding guide which should be read by meeting planners, hotel managers and architects.

Redden, Martha Ross, ed. Assuring Access for the Handicapped. San Francisco, Calif.: Jossey-Bass, 1979. 121 pp.

This work discusses some of the concerns other than architectural barriers which must be addressed in order to maximize accessibility of colleges to physically disabled students. Chapters focus on the responsibilities and challenges facing each of the groups involved: disabled students; architects; administrators; faculty members; and persons involved in various services to students. Attitudes and general approaches predominate rather than detailed plans, but the requirements of Section 504 of the Rehabilitation Act of 1973 are the basis for the discussion, and one chapter deals specifically with "legal" technicalities. The work should be available in all academic libraries where faculty, academic staff, and administrators will benefit from it. It is effective background reading for the works which deal more specifically with physical accessibility, and it provides the social and philosophical framework in which physical accessibility should be considered.

Redden, Martha Ross; Fortunato-Schwandt, Wayne; and Brown, Janet Welsh. Barrier-Free Meetings: A Guide for Professional Associations. Washington D.C.: American Association for the Advancement of Science, 1976. 73 pp.

This guide is the result of a special effort by the American Association for the Advancement of Science to make their 1976 Annual Meeting accessible to scientists with hearing, visual or mobility impairments. Preparation for both that meeting and this guide included consultation with disabled individuals and rehabilitation experts. Organization is chronological by stages of planning, and emphasizes the advance work that must be done months before the "accessible meeting" is to take place. Areas covered include: choosing and surveying the meeting site for accessibility; assessment of transportation options for disabled attendees; publicity; and interior accessibility. The provision of interpreters for deaf attendees is also discussed. Throughout, the authors demonstrate their commitment to total integration of disabled persons into professional activities. Appendices include specifications (e.g., for bathroom) and lists of organizations and publications relative to disability. Valuable and informative, but not as comprehensive as the Planner's Guide to Barrier Free Meetings.

Schweikert, Harry A., Jr. Wheelchair Bathrooms. Washington, D.C.: Paralyzed Veterans of America, 1967. 20 pp.

A small work devoted entirely to the subject of building or adapting bathrooms for the wheelchair user. The emphasis is on one's private home, rather than on public facilities. Unfortunately the bulk of the pamphlet involves a discussion of types of toilets, sinks, and bathtubs rather than on the design of the bathroom or on the many available accessories (other than grabbars, no accessories are discussed). Many of the recommendations provided in the text are obvious, and the detailed discussions of types of appliances is not the kind of information disabled people usually require. While a work on "wheelchair bathrooms" could be a useful contributioin to the literature, this pamphlet does not live up to expectations.

Selim, Georges. Barrier Free Design, A Design Manual Based on the Michigan Construction Code. Ann Arbor: The Office of Disabled Student Services, University of Michigan, 1977. 152 pp.

Author is a civil engineer at the University of Michigan. Based on the Michigan Construction Code governing exterior access and interior design of public and private buildings. Very comprehensive, including some problem areas not covered in other state accessibility guides, such as checkout lanes and doors in series. For each design feature discussed, author quotes applicable part of the Michigan Construction Code. He then elaborates upon the Code with his own recommended principles. He also makes recommendations for some buildings, such as libraries, not covered in the <u>Code</u>. Drawings illustrate his recommendations. Appendices summarize or reproduce in full a number of relevant U.S. and Michigan laws. This work compares favorably with the Illinois and Ohio guidebooks, and would be useful to architects, engineers, builders, and planners in Michigan, and in other states as well.

Sister Kenny Institute, Minneapolis. <u>Wheelchair Selection: More Than Choosing a Chair with Wheels</u>. Rev. ed. Minneapolis: The Institute, 1977. 56 pp.

Basic introduction to wheelchairs, their selection, and their accessories. Primary emphasis is on how to fit the proper type of chair to individual patients. Book is written by staff of a rehabilitation center. All aspects of selection and use of wheelchairs are considered, but the discussions are brief and rather superficial. While this book would be valuable for students and beginning health professionals, it is doubtful that it would add much to the knowledge of experienced therapists. (For an exhaustive approach, Kamenetz's volume should be consulted.) This work, because of its brevity, is recommended for collections serving students in physical and occupational therapy, nursing, or physical medicine.

Small, Robert E., and Allan, Barbara. <u>An Illustrated Handbook for Barrier Free Design: Washington State Rules and Regulations</u>. Olympia: Washington State Office of Community Development(?), 1978 (?). 72 pp.

Illustrated and annotated version of "Rules and Regulations Setting Barrier-Free Design Standards," adopted by the State of Washington in 1976. Regulations are printed in green, while the text, which amplifies the regulations and provides suggestions for implementations, is printed in black. Illustrated by photographs and by drawings which provide detailed specifications for accessibility. Discusses all aspects of exterior design and access, as well as interior facilities such as lavatories, telephones, and water fountains. Both public and residential buildings are included. Unique feature is a discussion of recommended building products, such as glass doors, elevator controls, and floor surfaces. Short list of references appended. Well organized and comprehensive. Recommended for libraries serving planners, builders, architects, engineers, and designers.

Sorenson, Robert James. <u>Design for Accessibility</u>. New York: McGraw-Hill, 1979. 264 pp.

Provides specifications for designing exterior and interior spaces, furniture and equipment to be usable by those with various disabilities. Virtually all identifiable aspects of public and private building use are considered, even including such facilities as laundry rooms, swimming pools, and garages. Each section has numerous hand drawings with specific measurements and instructions. A brief text introduces each section. Appendices include relevant sections of federal laws and a table summarizing state barrier free design legislation. Author is an architect and has written this book for fellow architects, designers, or drafts-persons. The drawings and text are separated, and both are rather technical. The bulk of the book is drawings; the text is small and refers to design considerations only. Thus, the book is valuable for those involved in exterior or interior design, but has little information for the general population or for administrators. Because of its comprehensive nature, it would be a useful addition to some special collections, but for general works on barrier free design, look elsewhere.

Trieschmann, Roberta B. Spinal Cord Injuries: Psychological, Social, and Vocational Adjustment. New York: Pergamon Press, 1980. 234 pp.

This book is the result of research into the state of the art regarding psychological, social and vocational adjustment to spinal cord injury. The author has exhaustively studied the literature on this topic and presents what we do know and what we do not know about the process of adjustment. She also discusses research problems (such as how to measure "adjustment") and points to areas where more research is needed. Her approach to rehabilitation is that it is an on-going process of learning to live with one's disability in a normal environment. As a psychologist in a rehabilitation center, she has had extensive contact with disabled persons and has been involved in the rehabilitation process. This book is extremely valuable as a summary of the current state of knowledge in rehabilitation and as a statement of a philosophy of rehabilitation in line with today's emphasis on the disabled person as a partner in the rehabilitation process. Highly recommended for medical libraries and for academic libraries which serve graduate programs in psychology and counseling.

Ullman, Montague. Behavioral Changes in Patients Following Strokes. Springfield, Ill.: Charles C. Thomas, 1962. 103 pp.

This book reports on the psychological and behavioral responses to stroke, based on a study of approximately 300 patients over a three-year period (1957-1960). A number of issues are discussed, such as sexuality after stroke, depression, and subjective reactions of patients to stroke and its resulting disabilities. Numerous case histories are used to illustrate typical patient reactions. The author, a psychiatrist, concludes that the personality of the patient, including his attitude, motivation, and previous life experiences greatly influences his psychological responses to stroke. He also suggests that a psychiatrist can play an important role in the rehabilitation of stroke patients. This work represents a beginning, but it barely scratches the surface on the subject of how rehabilitation professionals can contribute to positive attitudes and stimulate the patient's motivation. Furthermore, it is based on data collected twenty years ago. A more current and exhaustive study would be very useful.

Wittmeyer, Marilyn and Barrett, Jim. <u>Wheelchair Accessibility: Opening the Door to Housing</u>. Seattle: Health Sciences Learning Resources Center, University of Washington, 1977. 23 pp.

A brief manual outlining some basic concerns involved in making residential buildings accessible to and usable by persons in wheelchairs. All recommendations are based on physical characteristics of wheelchairs and physical limitations of the person using the wheelchair. Exterior facilities such as parking spaces, curb cuts and ramps are discussed, with desirable specifications given for each. Interior concerns include elevators, doors, telephones, light switches, and closets. Special bathroom and kitchen facilities are also described. Illustrations include photographs and drawings. This is a good basic introduction to accessible housing, particularly for disabled persons themselves or for apartment building owners and developers. Engineers and architects would need more detailed specifications. Recommended for public libraries.

2 BLINDNESS AND VISUAL IMPAIRMENT

RICHARD E. BOPP/Documents Librarian, University of Illinois Library, Urbana, Illinois

INTRODUCTION

Visual impairment occurs in many forms and degrees, from the numerous individuals whose vision is correctible to 20/20 by the use of eyeglasses, to the few individuals who see nothing at all. In between these extremes are approximately 11 million persons with varying but definitely permanent visual impairment and 1.5 million individuals whose impairment is severe enough that they cannot read ordinary print even with the aid of eyeglasses.(1) The causes of visual impairment are not well known to most people. Macular degeneration and retinitis pigmentosa are two of those little known causes. Others include diabetes, tumors, strokes, and more common conditions such as cataracts and glaucoma.(2) Many of these conditions are associated in some way with the aging process. Consequently, a large percentage of visually impaired people are elderly. As normal life expectancy increases, as the elderly constitute a proportionately larger segment of the population, the number of persons with a significant visual impairment will also increase.(3)

Visual loss affects many areas of everyday life, and the rehabilitation of visually impaired people is more complex than teaching braille reading or locomotion with a cane or guide dog.

The blinded individual must learn new ways of relating to his or her environment. Other senses, such as hearing and touch, as well as the memory, must be trained to compensate for the absence of visual cues. Along with new skills must come a new self-concept that accepts blindness while retaining confidence and optimism. New ways of communicating must be learned, as the visual aids to successful social intercourse are no longer available. Numerous techniques have been developed to assist blind persons in navigating effectively in their physical environment. This chapter surveys the literature which describes rehabilitation techniques for visually impaired and blind individuals. Also reviewed here are monographs describing the special needs of two unique groups in this population, the aging blind and the deaf-blind. The education of blind children, as an aspect of the special education field, is not, however, included, nor is the related subject of the teaching of braille reading.

A major gap in the literature on visual impairment is the lack of a comprehensive, up-to-date introductory text on the nature and consequences of blindness and the rehabilitation of visually impaired persons. Yeadon's Living with Impaired Vision briefly describes the causes and impact of blindness, but gives very little attention to rehabilitation techniques. A more complete picture may be found in Carrolls's Blindness, which is particularly valuable for its detailed discussion of the myriad ways in which loss of vision affects one's life. The rehabilitation section of this work is also well done, but it cannot inform the reader regarding the technological advances of the past twenty years. Many recently developed aids and devices are discussed in Ophthalmological Considerations in the Rehabilitation of the Blind, edited by Hoehne, Cull and Hardy. Their work, however, suffers from the lack of unity typical of many multiply-authored works. Students new to the field of blindness will want to supplement one or more of these works with some of the more detailed but narrowly defined monographs on particular aspects of the rehabilitation of the blind.

One area well covered in the literature is attitudes toward blindness and blind persons. The prevalence of negative attitudes has been explored from several angles. The Changing Status of the Blind, by Lowenfeld, is a study in the social history of blindness from antiquity to the present. It emphasizes the gradual improvement in the treatment accorded blind persons by social and political institutions. Kirtley discusses historical attitudes toward blindness as reflected in art and literature. His Psychology of Blindness also summarizes recent empirical research on these attitudes. Monbeck's Meaning of Blindness concentrates on research into the origins of our attitudes toward blindness, such as fear of blindness which affects the behavior of sighted persons toward blind individuals. Of the three, Monbeck's work is the most practical, as it points the way toward changing the negative attitudes which all authors on this topic have ably documented.

On the subject of counseling newly blinded individuals, several new approaches are reflected in the literature. Roessler and others at the University of Arkansas have developed a behaviorally based program called Personal Achievement Skills Training, which can be used with persons having physical or visual impairments.(4) Personal Achievement Skills Training for the Visually Handicapped, by Roessler and Means, applies this program to the needs of recently blinded persons. A more cognitive approach is taken by Roberts in Psychosocial Rehabilitation of the Blind. He describes the use of the principles and constructs of transactional analysis in facilitating psychological adjustment of blind adults. A more concrete contribution is offered by Scholl and Schnur, in Measures of Psychological, Vocational, and Educational Functioning in the Blind and Visually Handicapped. Their work discusses the principles of psychological evaluation of blind persons and provides brief descriptions of numerous commercially available tests of personality, intellect and vocational interests and abilities. At the other end of the spectrum, Lukoff and Whiteman discuss the many social contexts in which adjustment takes place. The Social Sources of Adjustment to Blindness summarizes research on the roles played by peers, family members, professionals and others in the blind person's psychological and social adjustment. Their work provides invaluable background information for anyone who counsels blind individuals or groups.

One group which has received considerable attention in the past five years is the senior citizen population, which includes aging persons who have been blind for years as well as many persons with aging-related visual impairments. Most writers on this subject have viewed the delivery of social services to the elderly blind and the inclusion of elderly blind persons in community programs as the key areas where ideas and information are needed. Two works provide an introduction to this topic, while two others desribe how to create successful community programs and services. The essays in Rehabilitation of the Older Blind Person, edited by Perlman, provide general information on the relationship between aging and blindness, the special needs of aging blind persons, and the role played by various professionals in meeting those needs. A publication which discusses the teaching of daily living skills and the provision of appropriate aids and devices for elderly blind persons is the American Foundation for the Blind's Introduction to Working with the Aging Person who is Visually Handicapped. The American Foundation for the Blind has also described several successful community programs for the elderly blind in How to Integrate Aging Persons Who are Visually Handicapped Into Community Senior Programs. Finally, Dickman's Outreach to the Aging Blind offers detailed information on planning and funding strategies for local agencies or government bodies seeking to generate community involvement in the provision of services and programs for the elderly visually impaired population.

Another group with unique needs are those individuals who have both severely impaired vision and severely impaired hearing.

The rubella epidemic of 1963-1965 resulted in the birth of many deaf-blind infants whose mothers had contracted rubella during pregnancy. Much of the literature has focused on the habilitation of children with this dual sensory disability. Freeman's <u>Understanding the Deaf/Blind Child</u> provides an excellent introduction to the many ways of assisting the development of these children in their pre-school years. The essays in <u>Deaf Blind Children</u>, edited by Curtis, Donlon and Wagner, stress the need for multi-disciplinary evaluation of deaf-blind children, so that their needs will be fully understood and comprehensive habilitation and education programs can be developed to meet those needs. An excellent guide for those who teach independent living skills to deaf-blind adults is Kinney's <u>Independent Living Without Sight and Hearing</u>. Kinney, an educator who is deaf and blind himself, offers personally tested techniques for the independent accomplishment of personal and social activities of everyday life. Finally, Yoken's <u>Living with Deaf-Blindness</u> profiles nine adults who are deaf and blind. Her work is an informative and very readable introduction to the subject of deaf-blindness.

Several other sources of a biographical or historical nature provide good introductory reading for students, professionals or lay persons who wish to understand the lives of the blind. Koestler's <u>The Unseen Minority</u> traces the growth of agencies and services for the blind during the past fifty years and illustrates the advances that have been made and the problems that remain in the field of rehabilitation of persons with visual impairments. The most prominent deaf-blind American, Helen Keller, has been the subject of a massive biography by Lash. <u>Helen and Teacher</u> provides a detailed yet readable study of the successes of Helen Keller, which were due in large part to her relationship with her teacher, Anne Sullivan. One of the better autobiographies by a blind person is Hartman's <u>White Coat, White Cane</u>, which relates the author's life from childhood to his completion of medical school and a residency in psychiatry. It and similar works reveal both the negative attitudes faced by blind persons and the courage and determination possessed by those individuals who succeed in spite of these social and psychological barriers.

One of the most immediate obstacles faced by the blind, however, is not attitudinal but physical. The blind person must learn how to navigate in both familiar and unfamiliar environments without visual cues. This problem is the focus of a relatively new profession, mobility training. The most comprehensive guide to this new field is <u>Foundations of Orientation and Mobility</u>, edited by Welsh and Blasch. They provide state-of-the-art reviews of various techniques of mobility, from the use of guide dogs to newly developed electronic aids. They also discuss the origins of mobility training as a profession and current research in the field of orientation and mobility. Tactual mapping is another new technique for providing orientation and mobility for blind persons. The best introduction to this subject is provided by Kidwell and Greer in <u>Sites Perception and the Nonvisual Experience</u>. This work offers extensive treatment of both the theoretical and practical aspects of tactual mapping. A more thorough discussion of various production techniques is available in <u>Tactual Mapping</u> by Wiedel and Groves. The literature on orientation and mobility techniques seems certain to expand, along with research into new aids and devices which provide greater independence to visually impaired individuals.

Research into the rehabilitation of blind and visually impaired persons is very old. Louis Braille published his code for raised dots representing letters of the alphabet in 1834. Since 1921, the American Foundation for the Blind (A.F.B.) has been funding research in areas from the development of new and improved sensory aids to the creation of more positive attitudes toward blind persons. Many of the works reviewed here were published by the A.F.B. However, advances continue to be made, both in reading devices and in orientation and mobility aids. Future works on rehabilitation of the blind should reflect the application of electronic and other technological discoveries to the task of compensating for the sensory deficits caused by visual impairments.

NOTES

1. Anne Yeadon and Dava Grayson. Living With Impaired Vision: An Introduction. (New York: American Foundation for the Blind, 1979), pp. 13.
2. Robert M. Goldenson, Editor-in-Chief. Disability and Rehabilitation Handbook. (New York: McGraw-Hill, 1978), pp. 252-253.
3. For a brief description see Richard T. Roessler and Bob L. Means. Personal Achievement Skills: An Introduction. Personal Achievement Skills Training: Discussion paper AARTC No. 932 (Fayetteville, Ark.: Arkansas Rehabilitation Research and Training Center, 1976).

ANNOTATED BIBLIOGRAPHY

American Foundation for the Blind. Directory of Agencies Serving the Visually Handicapped in the U.S. 21st edition, New York: The Foundation, 1981. 426 pp.

Comprehensive directory of agencies, medical facilities, schools, and other non-profit organizations offering education or rehabilitative services to persons with visual impairments. Listings are by state, sub-divided into three sections: Educational Services, Library Services, and Rehabilitation Services. Information provided about agencies includes: address and telephone number; funding; eligibility requirements; groups served; and type of service and aids offered. Supplementary sections list low vision clinics, dog guide schools, federal agencies, and other organizations and associations in the field of visual impairment. Essential reference tool for librarians, medical and rehabilitation personnel, social service professionals and special education teachers. Highly recommended for public libraries and medical, rehabilitation or special education collections.

American Foundation for the Blind. How to Integrate Aging Persons Who Are Visually Handicapped Into Community Senior Programs. New York: The Foundation, 1978. 35 pp.

Report of a pilot project in five New York cities to increase involvement in senior citizen programs by aged persons with severe visual impairments. Seed money was provided by the American Foundation for the Blind, but most funding and all planning and decision-making were done locally. The five participating cities were Rochester, New York, Buffalo, Syracuse, and Long Beach (a small town on Long Island). In this volume the program and results in each city are presented, along with the lessons learned during the project. A conclusion summarizes successful techniques and strategies for achieving greater integration of the aging blind into community programs. Excellent brief discussion for local social services personnel who work with the aging or the visually impaired. Recommended for public and agency libraries.

American Foundation for the Blind. An Introduction to Working with the Aging Person Who is Visually Handicapped. 2d ed. New York: The Foundation, 1977. 55 pp.

Brief outline of the needs of aging blind persons and the services and agencies available to assist them in meeting those needs. Largest section describes methods of teaching daily living skills. These skills are divided into discrete steps or procedures. Unfortunately, there are too few illustrations in this section. Federal, state and private agencies providing services or information are listed, and print sources, such as the Encyclopedia of Associations are recommended as sources of current information. A list of recommended readings is included. Aids and devices are described and ways of obtaining these are given. More useful as a guide to available information than as a guide to working with the aging blind. Recommended for social workers and counselors who work with elderly people, and for libraries in agencies which serve this population.

Asenjo, J. Albert. Rehabilitation Teaching for the Blind and Visually Disabled: The State of the Art, 1975. New York: American Foundation for the Blind, 1975. 79 pp.

Final report of a "National Workshop on Rehabilitation Teachers" held in St. Louis in 1975. Reviews the history of the profession of rehabilitation teaching, noting its growth and increased responsibility for teaching daily living skills to blind persons. Discusses issues in the professional preparation and continuing education of rehabilitation teachers. Summarizes current concepts in rehabilitating blind persons, including home training and the use of community resources and rehabilitation centers. Provides agenda of workshop and bibliography of suggested readings. Useful to students who are considering rehabilitation teaching as a profession and to professionals and para-professionals who work with the blind. Recommended for academic and rehabilitation libraries.

Barraga, Natalie C. Visual Handicaps and Learning: A Developmental Approach. Belmont, Calif.: Wadsworth Publishing Company, 1976. 113 pp.

A study of learning processes in children who have lost their vision. Author is a teacher, educator of teachers, and mother of a visually impaired child. Her text is based on research, practice and personal experience. She discusses how visual impairment affects both cognitive and affective development in children. Most of the text concerns school-age children, but importance of pre-school is emphasized. Provides theoretical framework regarding learning processes, and suggests techniques for facilitating and evaluating various learning activities. Index and bibliography included. Written primarily for students and professionals in field of special education. Recommended for academic libraries.

Bauman, Mary K. _Blindness, Visual Impairment, Deaf-Blindness: Annotated Listing of the Literature, 1953-1975_. Philadelphia: Temple University Press, 1976. 537 pp.

A monumental compilation of 3757 citations to professional books and journal articles. Divided into 35 chapters, each of which covers one aspect of the subject. Most entries have short annotations. Also appended are a list of organizations serving blind people, and 2 indexes to the bibliography, an author index and a detailed subject index. Medical literature is not included, since this is well indexed in _Index Medicus_ (this rationale overlooks the fact that _Index Medicus_ does not include monographs). Supplements are planned. This bibliography would be useful to librarians as well as to practitioners and researchers in many fields. It should be in all academic libraries.

Blea, William A. _Literature on the Deaf-Blind: An Annotated Bibliography_. Sacramento: California State Department of Education, 1976. 45 pp.

Lists and annotates books, articles and conference proceedings on the subject of education and training of deaf-blind persons. The period covered by these publications is roughly the past 100 to 130 years. The annotations are descriptive rather than evaluative, and range in length from 20 to 100 words. Many of the publications are historical rather than clinical or practical, including numerous items on famous deaf-blind individuals such as Helen Keller and Laura Bridgman. Stuckey's _Deaf-Blind Bibliography_ is more useful for identifying current research and practice in the field of deaf-blindness. This work is primarily valuable for historical purposes. Recommended for academic collections.

Carroll, Thomas J. _Blindness: What It Is, What It Does, and How to Live with It_. Boston: Little, Brown, 1961. 382 pp.

Comprehensive introduction to the problems caused by blindness and the principles and techniques of rehabilitative work with blind persons and their families. Focus is on adults who have lost their sight, rather than on children who were blinded early in life. Based on author's experience working with blind persons, rather than on research. Written in nontechnical language. Good, if slightly dated, text for beginning professionals and students in social service fields or for friends and relatives of blind individuals. Contains detailed index but no bibliography. Recommended for public and special libraries.

Curtis, Scott; Donlon, Edward T.; and Wagner, Elizabeth, ed. Deaf-Blind Children: Evaluating Their Multiple Handicaps. New York: American Foundation for the Blind, 1970. 172 pp.

Ten chapters, by various authors, discuss various aspects of evaluating deaf-blind children to understand their condition, needs and abilities, so that proper referrals and educational programs can be effected. The evaluation program described has been developed by the authors and other professionals associated with the Syracuse University Center for the Development of Blind Children. This program involves examination and evaluation by a team consisting of several medical specialists, speech, hearing and language specialists, and social work and educational professionals. Individual chapters explain the need for such evaluation, the goals of the evaluation process, and the techniques used. Provides highly useful information for professionals who work with hearing and visually impaired children. Recommended for medical, academic and rehabilitation libraries.

Dickman, Irving R. Outreach to the Aging Blind: Some Strategies for Community Action. New York: American Foundation for the Blind, 1977. 168 pp.

A guide for promoting cooperation among local agencies in identifying and serving the special needs of older persons with visual impairments. Concludes that this population, which in the past has been underserved, is now growing because of our increased longevity and consequent susceptibility to age-related visual loss. Argues for greater consumer involvement in planning services to the aging blind. Primarily an analysis of strategies employed by various communities around the country. Suggestions provided for conference planning, for publicity and for obtaining funding. A list of publications available from the American Foundation for the Blind is appended, along with sample survey forms, news releases and workshop programs. Useful primarily to local planners and social service agency personnel. Recommended for large public libraries.

Freeman, Peggy. Understanding the Deaf/Blind Child. London: Heinemann Health Books, 1975. 126 pp.

Written by a British mother of a deaf/blind child for other such parents, to teach them methods of training their children in various areas to prepare them for school and academic learning activities. Topics covered include the following: communication with deaf/blind children; social and emotional development; motor and mobility training; and learning through play activities. Author has worked with exceptional children for four years in educational settings. Her text is well-informed and written in a readable style. An appendix lists British sources of health, social, educational and economic assistance and voluntary organizations devoted to the welfare of exceptional children. A list of books for further reading is also provided. This work would be valuable reading for special educators as well as for "exceptional parents." Recommended for public and academic libraries serving special education programs.

Gloor, Balder, and Bruckner, Roland, ed. Rehabilitation of the Visually Disabled and the Blind at Different Ages. Baltimore: University Park Press, 1980. 164 pp.

Contains papers presented at an international symposium held in Basel in 1978. Speakers were ophthalmologists and physical and occupational therapists from Western European countries and the U.S.A. Twelve chapters focus on such topics as early treatment and training of congenital visual impairments; communication techniques with deaf-blind children; current research in visual disorders; and recent electronic aids for the blind and visually impaired. Published for practicing medical personnel and for those involved in basic or applied research. Chapter references and index provided. Several chapters contain illustrations. Recommended for medical and rehabilitation libraries.

Goldberg, Maxwell H. Blindness Research: The Expanding Frontiers. University Park, Pa.: The Pennsylvania State University Press, 1969. 544 pp.

Presents the proceedings of a conference held in 1967 in University Park, Pa. to discuss the problems of blind persons and to identify areas needing more research. Focus is on disciplines in the humanities and behavioral sciences and contributions which scholars in those fields can make to improving services to blind persons. Topics discussed include: effect of blindness on the family; problems of special groups, such as the aging blind and the blind adolescent; social and psychological adjustment and counseling; and occupational placement of blind persons. Some essays are now dated; others, such as those on adjustment to blindness are still useful to students and researchers. Recommended for comprehensive academic collections only.

Goldstein, Hyman. The Demography of Blindness Throughout the World. New York: American Foundation for the Blind, 1980. 324 pp.

A study of the incidence and prevalence of blindness and of the causes and costs of blindness worldwide. Also prominent is a discussion of the difficulties involved in collecting and comparing statistics on blindness because of varying definitions of "blindness" and problems in identifying blind persons, particularly in underdeveloped countries. Based on exhaustive review of available statistical studies. Contains many statistical tables, accompanied by discussion of methods used in compiling the statistics, problems with the data, etc. Unique and important both for reference and for research purposes. Recommended for academic libraries.

Hardy, Richard E., and Cull, John G., ed. <u>Social and Rehabilitation Services for the Blind</u>. Springfield, Ill.: Charles C. Thomas, 1972. 403 pp.

Twenty-five chapters by twenty-two contributors on the psychological, social and vocational rehabilitation of blind individuals. Authors are professionals in academic and clinical settings. Provides an introduction to a variety of concerns of counselors who work with the blind, such as: mobility training; vocational placement; community resources; psychological evaluation of blind persons; and physiological aspects of vision and blindness. As an introductory work, it provides a comprehensive overview for students and neophyte professionals. Contains some chapter bibliographies and a name and subject index. Recommended for academic and rehabilitation libraries.

Hartman, David, and Asbell, Bernard. <u>White Coat, White Cane</u>. Chicago: Playboy Press, 1978. 182 pp.

Autobiographical account by a psychiatrist blinded at the age of 8 as a result of a double retinal detachment. The main theme of the story is Dr. Hartman's struggle to convince teachers and medical school admissions committees that a blind man can succeed in medical school. The story is told in a concise chronological fashion, with the author's opinions about the "blind establishment," the nature and meaning of his "handicap," and the medical profession blended into the narrative. The author's style is simple and engaging. This book would appeal to a general audience, as well as to those who work with blind persons. It would also be informative reading for those on the faculties of medical schools. Recommended for public, medical and rehabilitation libraries.

Hoehne, Charles W.; Cull, John G.; and Hardy, Richard E. ed. <u>Ophthalmological Considerations in the Rehabilitation of the Blind</u>. Springfield, Ill.: Charles C. Thomas, 1980. 313 pp.

A much broader discussion of rehabilitation of visual impairments than is indicated by the title. Contains 28 chapters by authors from fields of medicine, rehabilitation counseling, and public and private service organizations. Some essays report results of research; others offer advice based on practice. Topics covered vary widely, from medical assessment to electronic aids and devices to psychological and vocational counseling. Similar in scope to, but more current than, the 1972 compilation of essays edited by Hardy and Cull. Probably the most comprehensive introduction to the subject of rehabilitation of the blind for students in non-medical rehabilitation fields. Includes subject bibliographies and name and subject indexes. Recommended for academic libraries.

Jastrzembska, Zofja S., ed. The Effects of Blindness and Other Impairments on Early Development. New York: American Foundation for the Blind, 1976. 210 pp.

Proceedings of a conference of behavioral scientists and special educators held in Ann Arbor, Michigan, in 1972. Six papers were presented on the topic of the effects of blindness on the physical and mental development of very young children. Papers are reproduced in full, with accompanying figures and tables. Also summarized are the discussions which followed each paper. Content is highly specialized; useful primarily to medical and psychological professionals who assess or treat exceptional children. Recommended for academic and research collections in early childhood development or visual impairment.

Jurgens, Mary Rose. Confrontation Between the Young Deaf-Blind Child and the Outer World: How to Make the World Surveyable by Organized Structure. Amsterdam: Swets & Zeitlinger, 1977. 57 pp.

Offers practical suggestions for teaching the deaf-blind child to organize his or her experiences in order to understand the environment. Based on known principles of learning as they apply to the special needs of children with less than normal sensory input. Text preceded by introduction explaining the principles upon which author's methods are based--principles developed at the Institute Voor Doven in Sint Michielgestel, Holland. Contains numerous illustrations. Useful information for professionals who work with deaf-blind children. Recommended for special education collections.

Kay, Leslie. Toward Objective Mobility Evaluation: Some Thoughts on a Theory. New York: American Foundation for the Blind, 1974. 55 pp.

An attempt to provide a simple theory of mobility which can be used by orientation and mobility instructors in mobility training with blind persons. Based on observations of blind and sighted persons performing various walking exercises. Defines mobility in terms of various aspects of motor coordination and the development of body control skills and skills in recognizing and understanding the physical environment. Lists nine basic skills which blind persons must learn for effective, independent mobility. Would be of use to physical therapists as well as to mobility instructors. Recommended for rehabilitation libraries.

Kidwell, Ann Middleton, and Greer, Peter Swartz. Sites Perception and the Nonvisual Experience: Designing and Manufacturing Mobility Maps. New York: American Foundation for the Blind, 1973. 192 pp.

Detailed discussion of design, construction and evaluation of tactual mobility maps for blind persons. Authors are graduate architecture students at Massachusetts Institute of Technology, who recently produced a tactual map of the MIT campus. They describe their background research on orientation methods used by the blind and on previous techniques of tactual mapping. Their work provides an excellent introduction to both topics. It is profusely illustrated and includes numerous interviews with blind persons regarding their methods of perceiving their environments and orienting themselves for independent mobility. Bibliography provided. Recommended for academic libraries and for special libraries used by professionals who work with blind individuals.

Kinney, Richard. <u>Independent Living Without Sight and Hearing</u>. Arlington Heights, Ill.: The Gray Dove, 1972. 102 pp.

Originally written as a guide for deaf-blind persons, this work is published in inkprint for the edification of professionals and lay persons who may have contact with individuals lacking useful sight and hearing. Author, himself deaf and blind, is an educator and administrator at the Hadley School for the Blind. Each chapter contains exercises through which the deaf-blind individual practices the principles and techniques presented. Kinney offers practical methods for accomplishing tasks of everyday living, from communication with others to travel and homemaking chores. The underlying theme throughout is that deaf-blind persons, lacking knowledge about their environment which others acquire through sight and hearing, must develop good mental habits, using intuition, inference and creative problem-solving to master their world. Maximizing their use of the senses of smell and touch is also essential. A work which is both positive in outlook and constructive in its concrete suggestions. Valuable awareness-raising reading for the general public as well as for social-service professionals and those in special education.

Kirtley, Donald D. <u>The Psychology of Blindness</u>. Chicago: Nelson-Hall, 1975. 312 pp.

Author is a psychologist who has been blind for twenty years. He has written a critical introduction to the theories and research on the topics of attitudes toward blindness and the effects blindness has on the behavior of blind persons. His approach to the first topic (attitudes) is more technical and more comprehensive than Monbeck's, employing Freudian and Jungian theories and an analysis of the depiction of blind persons in literature, myth and folklore. His analysis of the effects of blindness on the blind individual includes research in the areas of cognition, emotion, and social behavior. A separate chapter discusses the value of dreams in evaluating the personality of a blind individual. A scholarly work written for students and professionals in the social and behavioral sciences. Chapter bibliographies and indexes provided. Highly recommended for academic libraries.

Klemz, Astrid. Blindness and Partial Sight. Cambridge, Mass.: Woodhead-Faulkner, 1977. 150 pp.

Overview of causes and consequences of visual impairment and the techniques and principles of rehabilitation used in Britain with blind and partially sighted individuals. Comprehensive coverage of special topics such as aids and adaptations, mobility training, and special needs of blind persons who are also deaf. Provides lists of British agencies which serve blind persons and of organizations which offer educational information. Includes index and suggestions for further reading. Some sections unique to British situation, but overall a good basic introduction to the field. Provides both general guidelines and specific techniques. Language is nontechnical. Recommended for academic and public libraries.

Koestler, Frances A. The Unseen Minority: A Social History of Blindness in the United States. New York: David McKay Co., 1976. 559 pp.

A history of blind persons in American society from the early 1920s to the early 1970s. Commissioned in 1970 by the American Foundation for the Blind (A.F.B.) as it approached its fiftieth anniversary (1921-1971). Thus the A.F.B. figures prominently in the pages of this history of the growth of services for the blind. Illustrates the changing attitudes toward blindness among both blind and sighted Americans. Valuable chiefly as a history of the contributions of individuals to the various organizations devoted to providing social and educational services to blind persons. Technological and political developments given less attention. Good source for professionals wishing extensive background on goals and philosophies underlying services to the blind. Recommended for large academic libraries.

Lash, Joseph P. Helen and Teacher: The Story of Helen Keller and Anne Sullivan Macy. New York: Delacorte Press/Seymour Lawrence, 1980. 809 pp.

Monumental work by noted biographer. Covers century from Anne Sullivan's birth in 1866 to Helen Keller's death in 1968. Based on several Helen Keller archival collections and the papers of Anne Sullivan Macy. Many of these papers have never before been consulted by an independent, scholarly biographer. Story is predominantly of Helen Keller, although Anne Sullivan's influence is so profound that her life and Helen's are intimately intertwined. A scholarly, complete, and extremely readable work. Includes chronological outline, detailed index, bibliography, and an appendix on "Helen's Religion." Valuable as a biography, or for background on history of education and habilitation of deaf-blind persons. Recommended for public and academic libraries.

Lowenfeld, Berthold. The Changing Status of the Blind: from Separation to Integration. Springfield, Ill.: Charles C. Thomas, 1975. 336 pp.

A history of the social status of blind persons from antiquity to the mid 1970s. Unifying theme is the extent to which the blind have been accepted as participants in society. Author believes that social integration of the blind has gradually replaced their isolation. This process began in the nineteenth century and is still not complete because of some remaining negative attitudes, adverse socio-economic conditions, and some private and public programs which still segregate blind persons. Well written, based on primary sources. Contains an extensive bibliography and a name and subject index. Provides an excellent history of attitudes toward and services for the blind. Useful for students in rehabilitation, social work and allied fields. Recommended for academic libraries.

Lukoff, Irving F.; Cohen, Oscar; and others. Attitudes Toward Blind Persons. New York: American Foundation for the Blind, 1972. 74 pp.

Contains presentations from the National Invitational Symposium on Attitudes Toward Blindness, sponsored by the American Foundation for the Blind in 1971. The symposium was designed to stimulate local and regional action to combat negative attitudes toward blindness and discrimination against blind individuals. Presentations on attitudes and prejudice in society at large, among rehabilitation agencies and professionals, and among families of blind persons. Based on review of literature and on practical experience. Contains analysis and recommendations for strategies to foster more positive attitudes. Useful reading for professionals in psychology, social science or rehabilitation. Recommended for academic and rehabilitation libraries.

Lukoff, Irving F., and Whiteman, Martin. The Social Sources of Adjustment to Blindness. New York: American Foundation for the Blind, 1970. 291 pp.

An investigation of how various social forces affect the adjustment patterns of blind persons. Social forces studied include family members, organizations of and for the blind, rehabilitation agencies, and the attitudes and behaviors of the blind toward other blind persons. Particular attention is paid to how these forces affect the self-image and degree of dependence or independence exhibited by blind individuals. Previous sociological and psychological studies of blindness are reviewed. This study includes many statistical tables. Footnotes but no bibliography or index provided. Valuable as a research model for sociology students. Essential reading for professionals who work with blind persons. Highly recommended for academic and rehabilitation libraries.

Meighan, Thomas. An Investigation of the Self Concept of Blind and Visually Handicapped Adolescents. New York: American Foundation for the Blind, 1971. 43 pp.

Study by a special education professor of the various ways in which blindness affects the self concept of adolescents. Intended to increase awareness of psychological response to blindness and of the unique needs of blind persons, including the need for understanding and acceptance by society. Based on distribution of the Tennessee Self Concept Scale to a sample of 203 visually impaired adolescents. Results showed that the visually impaired students scored significantly lower than the norm on this exam. Important reading for counselors who work with blind youth. Valuable also for students and researchers in psychology. Recommended for academic and special education collections.

Monbeck, Michael. The Meaning of Blindness: Attitudes Toward Blindness and Blind People. Bloomington: Indiana University Press, 1973. 214 pp.

Author has served as editor of several publications in area of visual impairment, including Talking Book Topics and New Outlook for the Blind. His interest in the subject of attitudes toward blindness arose out of contact with blind people and with sighted people who know of his interest in the rehabilitation of blind persons. His book is an investigation of the origins of our attitudes toward blindness and blind individuals. Based on a thorough review of current and past research. Focus is on both the real and symbolic attributes of sight and blindness, and the fear sighted people have both of blindness and blind people. Extensive bibliography provided. The work is very well written and should be read by students of psychology and anyone who works with blind persons. Recommended for academic and special libraries.

National Federation of the Blind. Blindness and Disorders of the Eye. Baltimore: The Federation, 1976. 24 pp.

Brief, clearly written description of normal eye function, of leading causes of visual impairment and of services offered to blind individuals by the National Federation of the Blind. Consultant for this work is an ophthalmologist. Written for lay persons with no medical background. Glossary and list of further readings are provided. Useful as an introduction of the topic or as a reference source on disorders of vision. Recommended for public libraries.

Perlman, Leonard G., ed. The Rehabilitation of the Older Blind Person: A Shared Responsibility. Washington: National Rehabilitation Association, 1977. 130 pp.

Reproduces papers and summarizes discussions from the Second Mary E. Switzer Memorial Seminar, held in New York, January

17-19, 1977. Participants were rehabilitation personnel who work directly with blind persons through public or private agencies. First chapter provides background on aging and blindness, and final four chapters focus on issues in the effective delivery of services to older visually impaired persons. Each chapter includes a "Summary of Implications for Action", based on discussions which followed the presentation of the paper. Provides practical information and raises important issues for those who work with the elderly or the blind. Useful for rehabilitation personnel, social workers and staff of various public and private social agencies. Recommended for public and rehabilitation libraries.

Pfaffenberger, Clarence J.; Scott, John P.; Fuller, John L.; Ginsburg, Benson E.; and Bielfelt, Sherman W. Guide Dogs for the Blind: Their Selection, Development, and Training. Amsterdam: Elsevier Scientific Publishing Co., 1976. 225 pp.

Monograph by several authors reporting the results of research in the mid-1960s on the subject of selecting and training guide dogs for the blind. Research was conducted at Guide Dogs for the Blind, Inc., in San Rafael, California. Chapters summarize various aspects of guide dog training, including selective breeding, testing, and the relationship between the guide dog and the blind individual. The final chapter highlights the most important findings of the research project. The majority of persons who work with the blind have no need for the information in this book. However, anyone involved in breeding or training dogs to guide the blind would find it extremely valuable. Recommended only for libraries with comprehensive collections on services for the blind.

Potok, Andrew. Ordinary Daylight: Portrait of an Artist Going Blind. New York: Holt, Rinehart and Winston, 1980. 290 pp.

Contains valuable insights into the reaction of author to his loss of vision due to retinitis pigmentosa; but the title is somewhat of a misnomer. Most of the book concerns author's pilgrimage to England to see a woman who claims to cure diseases by having her patients stung by bees. An illustration of how intelligent people can submit to ridiculous quackery to preserve their health and normal functioning. His style is literate and easy to read; the bees cure assumes perhaps too large a place in the story. At end of his stay in England, author rejects bees and begins to accept his blindness and forge a new life. Important for its insights into adjustment to disability. Recommended for public, academic and rehabilitation libraries.

Roberts, Alvin. Psychosocial Rehabilitation of the Blind. Springfield, Ill.: Charles C. Thomas, 1973. 83 pp.

Application of principles of transactional analysis to the task of understanding and facilitating adjustment to blindness.

First three chapters explain how transactional analysis is used to understand an individual's behavior. Final three chapters discuss how this knowledge can be applied to work with blind persons. Emphasis is on adventitiously blinded persons (those who lose their vision after age five). Author describes techniques for promoting psychological adjustment of blind persons and for training psychological counselors who work with the blind. Special chapter on aging and blindness. Index but no bibliography. Useful because of its concrete, practical approach. Written for educators, social workers and rehabilitation counselors. Recommended for rehabilitation libraries.

Robinson, Robert Lee, ed. *Blinded Veterans of the Vietnam Era.* New York: American Foundation for the Blind, 1973. 33 pp.

Highlights of proceedings of a conference sponsored by the American Federation of the Blind in 1972 to investigate the problems of the 1000 or so blinded Vietnam veterans. Participants were physicians, social workers and other professionals who work with the blind in Veterans Administration hospitals or in state and private agencies. Their papers and remarks are not reproduced in full, but summarized. Most of the discussion centered around medical, prosthetic and rehabilitation services provided by the V.A. Names and addresses of participants are provided. May be useful to some rehabilitation personnel or researchers as the only monograph available on this topic. Not recommended for most libraries.

Roessler, Richard T. and Means, Bob L. *Personal Achievement Skills Training for the Visually Handicapped.* Fayetteville, Ark.: Arkansas Rehabilitation Research and Training Center, 1977. 107 pp.

Instructor's manual for applying principles of "Personal Achievement Skills Training" (PAS) package in group counseling with visually impaired persons. PAS training, developed by Roessler and others, involves training in interpersonal skills, in goal-setting and in self-understanding. PAS training with the visually handicapped differs little from its use with other disabled groups. The manual provides an introduction to the philosophy and goals of the training, followed by a description of the long series of group and individual activities which comprise the training. Short list of references appended. Valuable reading for rehabilitation personnel. Recommended for rehabilitation libraries.

Routh, Thomas. *Rehabilitation Counseling of the Blind.* Springfield, Ill.: Charles C. Thomas, 1970. 85 pp.

Brief discussion of the principles and techniques of vocational counseling of newly blinded individuals. Topics covered include interviewing, evaluating and guiding blind clients in the selection of an appropriate career. Group and individual counseling in psychological adjustment to blindness also discussed. Useful for its application of general principles of rehabilitation of the disabled to specific handicap of blindness. Somewhat dated in its emphasis on employment as the primary goal of rehabilitation. Very up-to-date, however, in its insistence that counselors are only helpers; the blind person must make his own career choice. Valuable as an introductory text for workers new to the field. No bibliography or references. Recommended for rehabilitation libraries.

Salmon, F. Cuthbert. The Preparation of Orientation and Mobility Maps for the Visually and Physically Handicapped. Stillwater, Okla.: Oklahoma State University School of Architecture, 1977. 24 pp.

Brief introduction to techniques of producing tactual or mobility maps for persons with visual or mobility impairments. Describes preparation of tactual map of Oklahoma State University campus and of a booklet in print and braille which explains the map and introduces the university to new students and staff. Useful for raising the awareness of campus administrators to the need for such maps and to the fact that costs for such projects are minimal. For guidance in producing such a map, the work by Kidwell and Greer is more comprehensive and detailed. Recommended for academic libraries.

Scholl, Geraldine, and Schnur, Ronald. Measures of Psychological, Vocational, and Educational Functioning in the Blind and Visually Handicapped. New York: American Foundation for the Blind, 1976. 95 pp.

Lists and briefly describes personality and aptitude tests for the evaluation of the intellectual, vocational, educational and psychological functioning of visually impaired persons. Also provides numerous references for more detailed descriptions of the tests, studies of their validity, guides to their use, etc. Intended for psychologists, guidance counselors and educators who are not specifically trained in evaluating blind persons. Brief introduction offers general information on blindness and guidelines for assessing behavior and abilities of clients. Valuable reference work for school psychologists and rehabilitation counselors. Recommended for special and academic libraries.

Scott, Robert A. The Making of Blind Men: A Study of Adult Socialization. New Brunswick, N.J.: Russell Sage Foundation, 1969. 145 pp.

Sociological analysis of the ways in which professionals and others affect the personalities of their blind clients. Argues that "the disability of blindness is a learned social role" inculcated by the agencies which rehabilitate the blind and by sighted society generally. Based on research studies, records and reports of agencies, and nearly 200 personal interviews of blind individuals and agency personnel. Includes an extensive bibliography. Essential reading for rehabilitation personnel, psychologists, social workers and sociologists. Highly recommended for academic and rehabilitation libraries.

Sensory Aids Foundation, comp. Sensory Aids for Employment of Blind and Visually Impaired Persons: a Resource Guide. New York: American Foundation for the Blind, 1978. 210 pp.

A catalog of commercially available sensory aids for visually impaired persons. Produced by the Sensory Aids Foundation, a non-profit corporation which funds and directs research into techniques and aids which facilitate independence by visually impaired persons. This catalog is the result of one such research project, directed at the development of new employment options for persons with visual impairment. Aids which assist such persons in employment settings are listed alphabetically by generic name. Each entry provides a non-evaluative description of the aid, discusses its potential uses in employment programs, gives addresses of distributors, and discusses availability and cost. Illustrations included for some items. There are indexes by manufacturer or vendor, by device, and by the occupational codes used in the Dictionary of Occupational Titles. Essential reference tool for counselors in vocational rehabilitation programs. Recommended for rehabilitation libraries.

Sloan, Louise L. Reading Aids for the Partially Sighted: A Systematic Classification and Procedure for Prescribing. Baltimore: Williams and Wilkins, 1977. 150 pp.

Introduction to principles and procedures for selecting appropriate reading aids for persons with impaired vision. Discusses the various magnifying lenses and equipment which are available, and considers lighting and other factors which promote use of residual vision for purposes of everyday reading. Chapters also on ophthalmological examination and on unique needs of children in the area of reading aids. Contains many illustrations and charts. Appendices provide case histories and discuss reasons for success or failure in the use of reading aids. Chapter references, but no bibliography included. Contains much useful information for medical and rehabilitation personnel. Recommended for medical and rehabilitation libraries.

Stocker, Claudel S. Listening for the Visually Impaired (A Teaching Manual). Springfield, Ill.: Charles C. Thomas, 1973. 167 pp.

Written in the belief that increased efficiency of other senses in blind persons is not automatic but learned, and therefore can be taught. Program described is the outcome of a project to develop methods of improved listening ability conducted at the Kansas Rehabilitation Center for the Blind. Emphasis is on teaching the blind person to discriminate between different sounds, to focus on the important sounds, and to understand how one's emotions affect one's interpretation of what is heard. The manual also seeks to enhance the listener's ability to create mental images based on what is heard, and to improve his or her recall and retention of important information conveyed through speech. Provides instructions for the teachers and describes the exercises which promote these skills. No index or bibliography provided. An excellent work for those involved in the rehabilitation of recently blinded persons. Recommended for rehabilitation and special education libraries.

Stuckey, Kenneth A., comp. Deaf-Blind Bibliography. Rev. ed. Watertown, Mass.: The Perkins School for the Blind and New England Regional Center for Services to Deaf-Blind Children, 1977. 186 pp.

Comprehensive compilation of sources of information in many formats on the subject of the dual handicap of deafness and blindness. Lists books and journal articles; some listings are annotated. Divided into numerous chapters, according to topics such as medical concerns, motor and language development, psychological and social aspects, and education and training. Contains annotated list of audiovisual productions. Unique lists such as conference proceedings, professional newsletters and organizational sources of information are also provided. Excellent source for educational and rehabilitation personnel or researchers. Recommended for academic, rehabilitation, and special education collections.

Sullivan, Tom and Gill, Derek. If You Could See What I Hear. New York: New American Library, 1975. 183 pp.

Autobiography by musician, composer and television personality blinded in infancy by an overdose of oxygen in his incubator. Story of a disabled person determined that his visual impairment would not stop him from living a full, exciting life. Perhaps overly dramatic in recounting his adventures and daring escapades; consequently less educational about subject of blindness than it could be. Makes for good recreational reading. Recommended for public libraries.

Welsh, Richard L., and Blasch, Bruce B., ed. Foundations of Orientation and Mobility. New York: American Foundation for the Blind, 1980. 672 pp.

The most comprehensive text on the current theory and practice of mobility training for visually impaired persons. Editors have worked as mobility instructors, have taught mobility training specialists and have written extensively on the subject. Text includes 20 chapters by 22 authors who work in the practice, research and teaching of mobility training. Topics discussed include kinesiology, the use of auditory and tactual senses in spatial orientation, mobility aids and devices which aid mobility,

mobility training with multiply handicapped blind persons, and the use of dog guides. This text will help students, professionals and others understand the complexity of mobility training. It is not designed as a manual, but as a summary of current knowledge in the many aspects of non-visual orientation and mobility. Includes chapter bibliographies and a general index. Highly recommended for large medical libraries, for academic libraries and for special libraries serving rehabilitation personnel.

Welsh, Richard L., and Wiener, William. Travel in Adverse Weather Conditions. New York: American Foundation for the Blind, 1976. 20 pp.

Monograph based on first conference devoted solely to the problem of orientation and mobility in adverse weather (e.g., snow, ice) without vision. This 1975 conference was attended by mobility instructors, academic professionals and visually impaired lay persons. Presentations and discussions were followed by field testing of the suggested techniques and procedures. This work summarizes the various problems and solutions discussed and experienced during the conference. Contains many practical ideas presented in clear language. Useful for mobility instructors, rehabilitation counselors or family and friends of blind persons. Recommended for rehabilitation and public libraries.

Widerberg, Lloyd, and Kaarlela, Ruth. Basic Components of Orientation and Movement Techniques. Kalamazoo, Mich.: College of Health and Human Services, Western Michigan University, 1977. 19 pp.

Provides a brief outline of orientation and mobility techniques useful to a blind individual. Intended as a reference manual for rehabilitation teachers already familiar with general principles of teaching blind persons. Divided into two sections, one of which describes procedures for mobility with a sighted guide, and the other techniques of independent orientation and mobility. Provides a detailed outline of procedures, but no background information. Would be useful for rehabilitation professionals already familiar with needs of blind clients, or for families of blind persons. Recommended for libraries serving professionals who counsel the blind.

Wiedel, Joseph W., and Groves, Paul A. Tactual Mapping: Design, Reproduction, Reading and Interpretation. College Park, Md.: University of Maryland, 1972. 116 pp.

Report of a research project whose goal was the production of "well designed, easily reproducible, large-scale mobility and orientation maps for use by the visually handicapped." Authors are cartographers at the University of Maryland. They are concerned with the problems involved in creating maps of neighborhoods, shopping malls, or large buildings, such as the Library of Congress. More practical in focus, with less theory than is found in the work by Kidwell and Greer. Discusses different production methods, various symbols used and the scope of information which is required by blind map readers. Provides a good technical background for anyone wishing to create a tactual map. Recommended for academic and rehabilitation libraries.

Yeadon, Anne, and Grayson, Dava. Living With Impaired Vision: An Introduction. New York: American Foundation for the Blind, 1979. 75 pp.

An excellent introduction to all aspects of visual impairment. Subjects briefly discussed include: causes of visual impairment, attitudes toward blind people, educational and self-help techniques and devices, and the problems of blind persons who suffer other impairments in addition to blindness. A list of recommended further reading as well as a chapter on agencies and organizations who work with blind people are also provided. This book should be in all public and academic libraries, and in appropriate special libraries.

Yoken, Carol. Living with Deaf-Blindness: Nine Profiles. Washington, D.C.: National Academy of Gallaudet College, 1979. 175 pp.

This book is the culmination of a project at Gallaudet College to provide first-hand information about the lives of deaf-blind individuals to students who might be considering careers working with this population. The deaf-blind population (estimated at 21,000 in the U.S.A.) is unique in that communicating with deaf-blind persons requires special knowledge and skills. Ms. Yoken possesses these, and spent many hours interviewing 9 deaf-blind individuals and their relatives and friends to compile these intimate accounts of their daily lives. Each chapter contains about equal amounts of first- and third-person descriptions, the third person parts provided by friends or by the observations of the author. An interesting and unique contribution which should be in many academic and large public library collections as well as all collections concerned with deaf and/or blind persons.

3 DEAFNESS AND HEARING IMPAIRMENT

RICHARD E. BOPP/Documents Librarian, University of Illinois Library, Urbana, Illinois

INTRODUCTION

This volume has just one chapter which addresses a specific problem of a single disabled group, namely that on communication difficulties in deaf persons (Chapter VI). The history of the rehabilitation of deaf individuals reveals that, until recently, that was the salient issue in the literature of the field. A "holy war"(1) has raged for decades between proponents of the two schools of thought on solving the communication problems of the deaf. These opposing schools are the oralists, who emphasize the use of residual hearing and speechreading skills, and the proponents of manual communication, who advocate the use of sign language. This "holy war" plays a prominent role as well in the present chapter, which reviews the literature on the psychological and social consequences of deafness and hearing impairment as well as the many general works on deafness. Fortunately, the fanaticism that fueled this battle is dying out, and other important and long neglected issues in the rehabilitation of hearing impaired persons are beginning to receive the attention they deserve.

The psychological and social consequences of deafness or hearing impairment vary both with the degree of impairment the individual experiences and with the age at which the impairment occurs.(2) Individuals with a mild hearing loss, or with even a severe hearing loss acquired in adolescence or later, will have mastered the English (or other) language, and will suffer only the psychological consequences of impaired oral-aural communication. However, an individual born deaf, or one suffering profound hearing loss in infancy, will have great difficulty not only with communication, but with mastering the language on which any form of communication depends.

Language and communication difficulties have wide ranging social and psychological consequences for hearing-impaired individuals. Historically, prelingually deafened persons have had great difficulty learning to speak or read the speech of others, and have formed their own sub-culture with its own social network based on manual communication. Their inability to communicate in the hearing world has had economic effects as well, since their educational and occupational advancement in all areas is hindered by their poor language skills. Even those individuals who have mastered the English language, and can speak it well and read the speech of others, often encounter social difficulties because of their deafness. And trying to pass for hearing in a hearing world has psychological consequences, as Schowe has observed in <u>Identity Crisis in Deafness</u>. It is because of the growing awareness of the many psychological ramifications of language and communication problems that the method of total communication, employing any mode and combinations of modes that will work, has met with such broad acceptance in recent years.(3)

An understanding of the psychological and social consequences of the communication difficulties faced by hearing impaired individuals must be based on a thorough knowledge of the nature of hearing impairment, the principles of treating and habilitating hearing-impaired individuals, the history of deafness and educational theories regarding deaf children, and the personal experience of deafness as recorded by deaf authors. For this reason, general works on deafness and/or hearing impairment will be discussed first in this chapter, followed by an overview of the many studies on the psychological and social aspects of deafness. An assessment of the current status of research and writing on deafness, emphasizing new and broader approaches to rehabilitation of deaf individuals, concludes this introductory essay.

There are several useful texts and compilations of essays designed to introduce new students to the study of hearing impairment. The most comprehensive of these is Hearing and Hearing Impairment, edited by Bradford and Hardy. In fifty essays by fifty-seven authors, it covers all aspects of the field, from physiological to psychological, sociological, educational and historical. Many texts focus more heavily on one or two subject areas, and would thus be useful primarily to students preparing for professional careers in those areas. Moores' Educating the Deaf: Psychology, Principles and Practices is the best of these. While written for future teachers, it contains extensive information on psychological and social concerns which are intimately related to educational success. Other works are more clinical in nature and would be useful to students of audiology, auditory and speech training, or hearing aid research. Two good clinical texts are Ballantyne's Deafness and Hearing and Deafness, edited by Davis and Silverman. Ballantyne's work provides a British point of view, whereas the authors of Hearing and Deafness reflect the approach taken at the Central Institute for the Deaf in St. Louis. A similar work, which also gives cursory treatment to psychological and educational concerns, is Jaffe's Hearing Loss in Children. For the most part, these works are intended for an academic or medical audience and would be most useful as texts in structured courses.

There are a number of briefer works which also serve an introductory purpose and would be useful in a broader range of settings. Less technical and detailed, they could educate lay persons, paraprofessionals or professionals interested in broadening their knowledge or updating their skills. The most comprehensive of these is Lawrence's compilation, Focus on Deafness, which reprints a wide selection of articles from professional journals on many aspects of deafness. A briefer work, which is designed primarily to raise the awareness of lay and professional readers regarding the experience of deafness, is Watson's Readings on Deafness. Many of the essays compiled by Watson were written by persons who are themselves deaf. Gallaudet College has published a similar work for a more specialized audience, An Orientation to Deafness for Social Workers. For those who prefer an integrated narrative by a single author, Benderly's Dancing Without Music is a very readable introduction to deafness and is particularly strong on the "holy war" between oralists and advocates of manual communication. She writes as one who understands both the objective results of research and the subjective experiences of deaf individuals.

  The experiences of deaf persons are also available first hand, although fewer deaf than mobility-impaired persons have written personal narratives. Wright's Deafness is literate and informative, but the author's life--he attended Oxford University and has since distinguished himself as a poet and translator--is not typical. It does demonstrate the importance of the age at which one loses hearing: he lost his at age 7, after he had developed good language skills. More representative of the lives of deaf Americans are Hazards of Deafness by Holcomb and A Deaf Adult Speaks Out by Jacobs. Both works are designed to sensitize hearing people to the needs and desires of deaf persons. Jacobs writes seriously about the evils of oralism and the need for total communication, while Holcomb describes hundreds of unique experiences, some funny and some tragic, which deaf individuals encounter daily because of their hearing impairment. Finally, for those with literary interests, The Deaf Experience, edited by Batson and Bergman, offers selections from fictional and biographical works, past and present, by or about deaf persons. These works offer extremely important imformation, because most individuals in our society have had less exposure to deafness (and the lives of deaf individuals) than to any other disability.

Works for professionals on the psychological and social aspects and consequences of deafness vary greatly in emphasis and format. Authors and intended audiences range from the fields of psychiatry, social work and psychology, to education and counseling. There has been a noticeable and important shift in focus from the problems of deaf individuals to the interaction between deaf persons and their environment. Psychological adjustment to deafness is seen as involving a deaf person's family and educational environment, and also his/her relationships with both the hearing world and the deaf sub-culture. This trend is part of the general movement toward recognizing that the psychological effects of any disability can be lessened by a hospitable environment or worsened by an inhospitable one.(4)

For introductory purposes, two old but still useful texts on the psychology of deafness are Levine's Psychology of Deafness (1960) and Myklebust's Psychology of Deafness (2nd ed. 1964). These two basic works are very different in content and usefulness. Myklebust's work is broader in scope and designed for clinicians or for students or researchers in an academic setting. It is based on numerous research studies and contains many references for further reading. Levine's work, on the other hand, contains more practical information on evaluation and counseling techniques. It would be more useful for those engaged in working with deaf individuals in a rehabilitation or educational setting, or for students of social work, psychology or education. However, such individuals would get a more current perspective by reading her later work, The Ecology of Early Deafness (described below).

There are several valuable monographs written specifically for those who counsel deaf individuals. Psychology of Deafness for Rehabilitation Counselors, edited by Bolton, reviews the literature on the intellectual, social, vocational and psychological development of deaf individuals. Its authors are primarily academicians and researchers. Counseling with Deaf People, edited by Sussman and Stewart, concentrates on the practical aspects of counseling and on the education and training of individuals to work with deaf persons. While also based on recent research studies, it is less academic in style and focuses more on the counseling process than on the characteristics of the deaf population. For religious counselors and ministers who work with the deaf, the best of several recent works is Yount's Be Opened! An Introduction to Ministry with the Deaf.

The cutting edge of research on deafness in recent years has centered on the study of the deaf child and the effects of environmental influences upon the development of deaf children. It is this research, particularly as it relates to the family environment, which has partially defused the oralist-manualist war and has provided a more constructive framework for the study of the habilitation of deaf children. An early example of this trend is Mindel and Vernon's They Grow in Silence: The Deaf Child and His Family, an outgrowth of research at Michael Reese Hospital in Chicago. Mindel and Vernon seek to understand deafness from the point of view of the deaf person and his or her family, rather than of the hearing society and the deaf education establishment. In similar fashion, the study by Schlesinger and Meadow, Sound and Sign: Childhood Deafness and Mental Health, stresses the social environment of deaf children as an important contributor to their developmental problems. Finally, two very recent works add to the emphasis upon the environmental forces which shape deaf children. Meadow's Deafness and Child Development assesses the importance of numerous family, social and educational factors on the cognitive, psychological and social behavior patterns of deaf children. The very title of Levine's recent work, The Ecology of Early Deafness, amply illustrates the change in focus of research and practice in the field of deafness. This text is in some ways an update of her 1960 text mentioned above, but the focus and tone have changed entirely. While still providing information on techniques and tests for evaluating deaf clients, the author now precedes this material with a long discussion on "early environmental influences" on the development of the deaf child.

This healthy trend in the literature on deafness is likely to continue and to broaden, as researchers allow the perspectives and experiences of the deaf community to contribute to their understanding of deafness. Already, a study of the adult deaf community from the inside has appeared. Higgins' Outsiders in a Hearing World: A Sociology of Deafness is based on intensive interviews with seventy-five deaf adults in the Chicago area. The author was accepted into this community as one of their own because he is the son of deaf parents. His study focuses both on the traditional problem in deafness research--communication--and on the attitudes among both deaf and hearing people which cause the deaf person to view the hearing world as a hostile environment.

Further literature on deafness, then, seems destined to escape from the confines of the war over modes of communication. No doubt this controversy will still generate heat, because of the psychological and social implications and consequences of the choice between oral and manual communication. As Schowe has described it, in Identity Crisis in Deafness, the war has its real basis, not in the mode of communication, but in the decision to identify with other deaf people (and communicate manually) or to try to succeed in the hearing world through speech and speechreading. But because of the work of Meadow, Schlesinger, Levine, Higgins, and others, the problems caused by deafness can no longer be viewed simply in terms of communication and language deficiencies. The growing awareness of the importance of the environments of deaf individuals has broadened our approach to the rehabilitation of the deaf and their families. Future research and practice promise more understanding and less heat.

NOTES

1. Beryl Lieff, Dancing Without Music: Deafness in America (Garden City, N.Y.: Anchor Press/Doubleday, 1980), VII.
2. For a brief summary, see Robert E. Kretschmer, "Living with a Hearing Impairment," Illinois Libraries 63, no. 7 (September 1981): pp. 515-520.
3. For a further discussion of the issues raised in this paragraph, see also the chapter "Communication for the Deaf and Hearing Impaired" (Chapter VI).
4. For a further discussion of this trend, see "The Social and Psychological Contexts of Physical Disability" Chapter IV.

ANNOTATED BIBLIOGRAPHY

Ballantyne, John. Deafness. 3rd ed. Edinburgh: Churchill Livingstone, 1977. 250 pp.

   Basic text emphasizing physical and physiological aspects of hearing and hearing loss. Author is a British otologist. Most of his text deals with causes of deafness, with diagnostic and audiological tests and with hearing aids. Short chapters included on psychological and rehabilitation considerations. Lengthy chapter on causes of deafness in childhood and on educational methods with deaf children. Appendices include a directory of British organizations for the deaf, an index and a bibliography. Useful and reasonably non-technical introduction to physical aspects of hearing and deafness. Recommended for academic and medical libraries.

Batson, Trenton W., and Bergman, Eugene, eds. The Deaf Experience: An Anthology of Literature by and about the Deaf. 2d ed. South Waterford, Me.: Merriam-Eddy Company, 1976. 400 pp.

   Selections from a variety of autobiographical and fictional accounts of deafness from the past 150 years. Illustrates attitudes toward the deaf as seen in literature and insights into their own experiences by deaf writers. All selections are introduced and discussed by the editors. Nineteenth-century authors include Dickens and Turgenev, while the twentieth century is represented by Eudora Welty and Bernard Malamud, among others. The autobiographical accounts by deaf writers are from both the nineteenth and twentieth centuries. This work could be a valuable sourcebook for introductory courses on deafness, and is recommended for academic libraries.

Becker, Gaylene. <u>Growing Old in Silence</u>. Berkeley: University of California Press, 1980. 148 pp.

    Study of life experiences and social organization of elderly deaf persons in San Francisco Bay Area. Based on author's doctoral thesis in anthropology. Emphasis on effects of early life experiences on individuals' ability to adapt to the aging process. Concludes that elderly deaf persons who learned to cope with their disability early in life developed skills and resources for dealing with the problems that accompany old age. The support of their peers in the deaf community also prepares deaf persons for the necessary interdependence of old age. Excellent study of individual adaptation to disability and the important role of social relationships with other deaf persons in successful adaptation. Based on personal research and a review of the literature. Written in a clear and concise style. Valuable for students, professionals and others interested in aging and/or deafness. Highly recommended for academic and large public libraries.

Bender, Ruth E. <u>The Conquest of Deafness; a History of the Long Struggle to Make Possible Normal Living to Those Handicapped by Lack of Normal Hearing</u>. Rev. ed. Cleveland: The Press of Case Western Reserve University, 1970. 243 pp.

    Comprehensive history of man's understanding and treatment of hearing loss from earliest recorded history to the present day (1970). Based on primary and secondary sources. Many quotations from writings of various periods. Author's style and method of presentation are direct and straightforward, but rather dull. Mostly narrative with minimal interpretation or commentary. Contains useful factual information, such as biographical accounts of prominent historical figures in education of the deaf. Extensive bibliography and index included. Recommended for comprehensive academic collections.

Benderly, Beryl Lieff. <u>Dancing Without Music: Deafness in America</u>. Garden City, N.J.: Anchor Press/Doubleday, 1980. 302 pp.

    Lively, informed discussion of what it means to be deaf today in America, and of the controversies over modes of communication used by deaf and hearing-impaired individuals. Author says oralists and proponents of manual communication are engaged in a holy war. One must choose sides in a fight where there is conflicting evidence, and where prejudice rather than reason determines one's choice. She discusses the social and psychological aspects of growing up deaf, including the core problem of how language is learned. The advantages and disadvantages of both oral and manual communication for the deaf persons and their family are given in a readable and fairly objective manner (a bias against oralism does appear). She brings a combination of reason and conviction to her discussion of the goals and problems of mainstreaming deaf children in regular schools. Her well-written narrative fluently blends the historical background with the current status of each topic and controversy she discusses. An excellent, readable introduction to the psychological, social and educational consequences of deafness. Highly recommended for public and academic libraries.

Bolton, Brian, ed. Psychology of Deafness for Rehabilitation Counselors. Baltimore: University Park Press, 1976. 156 pp.

Discussion of psychological aspects of deafness for counselors who will be working with deaf young adults. Authors are academicians who have had experience in both research and practice with deaf persons. Topics discussed include language acquisition, intellectual and academic functioning, personality and social development, and vocational development of deaf persons. Essays are based on a review of recent literature in each area. The general consensus is that deaf persons are relatively immature, in all of these areas, and that better methods of early intervention are needed. Recommended for academic and rehabilitation collections.

Bradford, Larry J., and Hardy, William G., eds. Hearing and Hearing Impairment. New York: Grune & Stratton, 1979. 653 pp.

Monumental compilation of 50 essays by 57 authors, each of which addresses a different aspect of hearing impairment, from diagnosis and assessment to learning aids and educational and vocational programs and services. Authors are prominent researchers and practitioners in many fields, such as law, social work, many branches of medicine, psychology, and education. No one philosophy of rehabilitation or education predominates - the essays are designed to reflect a variety of views and approaches. The form of the essays ranges from reports of research to overviews of a specific topic or activity. Useful text for an introduction to hearing impairment in all of its contexts: medical, psychological, social, educational and vocational. Recommended for academic libraries.

Davis, Hallowell, and Silverman, S. Richard, eds. Hearing and Deafness. 4th ed. New York: Holt, Rinehart & Winston, 1978. 552 pp.

Basic introduction to hearing, hearing loss, evaluation of hearing loss (audiology) and rehabilitative techniques used with persons with hearing impairments. Editors and most contributors are at Central Institute for the Deaf in St. Louis. Emphasis is on oral approach (auditory training, hearing aids and speech reading), although one short chapter discusses manual communication. Chapters on psychology of deafness and on education of hearing-impaired children, but more emphasis on physical and medical causes, diagnosis and treatments. Good beginning text for students of audiology, because it combines technical aspects of hearing and hearing loss with consideration of psychological and educational consequences of hearing impairment. Recommended for academic libraries and special library collections on deafness.

The Deaf Man and the World: Work, Love, Worship, Play. New Orleans: Council of Organizations Serving the Deaf, 1969. 96 pp.

Proceedings of a national forum in February 1969, sponsored by the Council of Organizations Serving the Deaf. Rather than focusing on the usual topics, such as educational programs or communications, the sponsors chose to concentrate on the real life experiences of deaf individuals in the crucial areas of work, play, love, and worship. In each area, speakers offered presentations which were followed by discussion; only summaries of the discussions are published here. Authors are practitioners in their respective fields and discuss practical rather than research topics, presenting techniques based on their experiences and pointing out areas where more work is needed. The largest part of the book, dealing with the world of love, discusses family problems and counseling techniques as well as methods for fostering personal independence in, and community integration of, deaf persons. Unique in its desire to focus on general aspects of the interaction between deaf persons and their environment which are lost in the common emphasis on modes of communication. Valuable reading for those who work with deaf persons. Recommended for rehabilitation collections.

Fellendorf, George W. Bibliography on Deafness: the Volta Review 1899-1976; American Annals of the Deaf 1847-1976. Rev. ed. Washington, D.C.: Alexander Graham Bell Association for the Deaf, 1977. 272 pp.

Consists of two indexes, subject and author, to substantive articles which appeared in "The Volta Review" or "American Annals of the Deaf" through 1976. The subject index is organized under approximately thirty headings, from aphasia to technological devices. Entries for each journal are separated, and are listed chronologically, rather than alphabetically by author, to show the historical progression of literature on each topic. Although this bibliography contains only a part of the literature on deafness, it is valuable because of the importance and longevity of the two journals it indexes. It would be particularly useful for historical background in any area relating to deafness. Recommended for academic collections in special education or speech and hearing sciences.

Frisna, Robert, ed. A Bicentennial Monograph on Hearing Impairment: Trends in the U.S.A. Washington, D.C.: Alexander Graham Bell Association for the Deaf, Inc., 1976. 148 pp.

Series of essays on various aspects of deafness by prominent professionals in their fields. Stated purpose is to provide an overview of recent progress and an assessment of the current status of each area included. Topics covered range from medical and psychological assessment to devices such as hearing aids and telecommunication devices for the deaf (TDD's). Chapters on manual and total communication systems make this a comprehensive and balanced work. Not as detailed or complete as the more recent Hearing and Hearing Impairment, edited by Bradford and Hardy. Does provide a useful overview of the field for students and practitioners. Recommended for comprehensive academic or special library collections on deafness.

Furth, Hans G. Thinking Without Language: Psychological Implications of Deafness. New York: Free Press, 1966. 236 pp.

Analysis of the relationship between thinking and language, with specific reference to language-deficient deaf children. Concludes that thinking does not depend on language, that oralism is thus not the only effective educational system for deaf children, and that verbal thinking may be overemphasized generally in American educational theories and practices. Based on scientific research, but written in nontechnical language. Provocative work of interest to students and researchers in education and many social science fields. Contains bibliography and index. Highly recommended for academic libraries.

Gannon, Jack R. Deaf Heritage: A Narrative History of Deaf America. Silver Spring, Md.: National Association of the Deaf, 1981. 483 pp.

History of all aspects of the lives of deaf Americans from the early nineteenth century to 1980. Extensive coverage of developments in education for the deaf, in services to the deaf, and in associations, activities and organizations of the deaf. Emphasis on individuals who were influential in education, technology, communications, and advocacy. Separate chapters on sports, on publications of deaf persons, and on American Sign Language. Notes, extensive bibliography and detailed index are appended. Excellent introductory work for students, professionals and the general public. Some bias against oral-aural approach to communication methods and in favor of manual communication. Recommended for public and academic libraries.

Gregory, Susan. The Deaf Child and His Family. New York: John Wiley and Sons, 1976. 256 pp.

Designed to "paint a picture" of the everyday life of the young (1-6 years old) deaf child and his or her family. Based on interviews with 122 British mothers of deaf children. Compares and contrasts the life of deaf children with that of hearing children as depicted in similar studies based on interviews with mothers of hearing children. Offers intimate view of deaf children in their natural environments, provided by those who best understand them, their families. Prominent topics which the mothers discuss are: their feelings about having a deaf child, the attitudes of others, the effect on family life, communication problems, and common child-rearing concerns such as discipline, play activities and relationships between children. Author intersperses mothers' reports with her own comments and conclusions. Picture that emerges is that each deaf child is unique and individual but that deaf children are handicapped in many ways, socially and intellectually, because of the difficulty they experience in understanding and communicating. Appendices discuss survey and interview techniques. Unique in its emphasis on presenting the point of view of a large number of parents of deaf children. Recommended for public and academic libraries.

A Guide to College/Career Programs for Deaf Students. Washington, D.C.: Gallaudet College Press, 1978. 99 pp.

Lists, by state, 60 colleges, universities and technical institutes which offer programs or services for deaf students. For each institution, provides information on accreditation, enrollment, admission requirements, annual tuition and room and board, areas of study and degrees offered, and special services (e.g., interpreters) provided. Index by major areas of study allows reader to find all schools offering programs in a specific subject area. Invaluable reference work for public and school libraries and for guidance and vocational counselors who work with deaf students.

Hardy, Richard E., and Cull, John G., eds. Educational and Psychosocial Aspects of Deafness. Springfield, Ill.: Charles C. Thomas, 1974. 197 pp.

A collection of essays by recognized authorities in the field of counseling with the deaf. Designed as a practical guide for counselors, social workers, psychologists and other professionals. The work has no central focus. Topics discussed range from the history of the National Association of the Deaf to psychological consequences of deafness to work adjustment for deaf persons. Two chapters provide useful lists, such as postsecondary schools for deaf students and schools offering degrees in rehabilitation of the deaf. Approach varies from review of research to presentation of use studies. Individual chapters might be useful supplementary reading for students of hearing impairment or special education. Most professionals will want more detailed and current information. Recommended for comprehensive academic library collections.

Higgins, Paul C. Outsiders in a Hearing World: A Sociology of Deafness. Beverly Hills, Calif.: Sage Publications, 1980. 205 pp.

A sociological study of the deaf community and its individual members by a sociologist who was accepted into that community because his parents are deaf. Based on intensive interviews with seventy-five deaf adults of varying age, sex, and educational background. Author concluded that the deaf community is divided into distinguishable groups and cliques, but members share common interests, experiences, activities, and points of view. Their sense of identity is enhanced and reinforced by participation in the deaf community. Even though they are beginning to shed their ambivalence about their deafness, and take more pride in it, as other minority groups are doing, their integration into the hearing world is hindered by the communication barriers their deafness creates. Thus, they are "outsiders" not only in terms of attitudes (stigma of their disability), but in ways that are more difficult to overcome. A valuable, informed view of the lives of deaf individuals, this work is recommended for all academic libraries.

Holcomb, Roy K. Hazards of Deafness. Northridge, Calif.: Joyce Media, 1977. 109 pp.

Collection of 662 humorous and/or tragic everyday experiences which befall deaf persons because of their hearing disability. Each situation is described in a short paragraph; they vary from home and transportation problems to experiences in social situations and employment. Author is a deaf man involved in educating deaf children and is a pioneer of the practice of total communication. Good and easy way to understand some of the problems faced by deaf people every day in activities which hearing people take for granted. Also shows how insensitive some hearing people can be. Valuable tool for consciousness-raising. Recommended for public and academic libraries.

Jacobs, Leo M. A Deaf Adult Speaks Out. Washington, D.C.: Gallaudet College Press, 1974. 145 pp.

A teacher of the deaf who is himself deaf writes about deafness and castigates traditional (oralist) methods of teaching deaf children. He talks about the wide implications of hearing loss for personality development, and illustrates his points with personal experiences and scientific literature. He aims to sensitize hearing persons to the world of deafness and stresses that total communication--employing any and all means of communicating with the deaf--is what deaf people want and need. The author was born deaf of deaf parents and is now married to a deaf woman; they have a deaf and a hearing daughter. Thus, he has wide experience of his subject both as a person and as a teacher. The book is written for a general audience with little knowledge of deafness. It contains a glossary and a bibliography. A second edition containing a new chapter on mainstreaming and a panel discussion involving seven deaf adults, has recently been published. Recommended for public libraries and undergraduate college libraries.

Jaffe, Burton F., ed. Hearing Loss in Children: A Comprehensive Text. Baltimore: University Park Press, 1977. 784 pp.

    Designed as an authoritative volume on the causes, types and effects of hearing impairment in children. Fifty-seven chapters by numerous authors. Primary emphasis on physiological and audiological aspects. Shorter sections on developmental consequences of hearing loss and on educational and habilititative principles. Most useful for broadening the knowledge of medical specialists, but could be used by other professionals who want to deepen their understanding of medical aspects of hearing impairments. Recommended for medical and academic libraries.

Lawrence, Edgar D., comp. Focus on Deafness: Selected Readings on Deafness for Paraprofessionals. Washington, D.C.: University Press of America. 1978. 278 pp.

    Compilation of previously published articles on various aspects of deafness. They are "selected readings," but why they are "for paraprofessionals" is not clear: most originally appeared in professional journals. The information is current: most original publication dates are mid-1970's. Topics addressed include: communication; psychology of deafness; employment; and social and family relationships. Authors are well-known in their fields. Provides a good introduction to the subject of deafness. Would be useful reading in special education or various social science courses. Recommended for academic libraries.

Lawrence, Edgar D. Ministering to the Silent Majority. Springfield, Mo.: Gospel Publishing House, 1978. 92 pp.

    Written by an ordained minister in the Assemblies of God Church, this small paperback seeks to introduce ministers, students, and others to the considerations and knowledge required to work with deaf people in group settings such as church and Sunday School. The author has experience working with deaf people and is familiar with the facts and literature about deafness. He translates his knowledge and experience into practical advice for ministers who are beginning a church program for the deaf. He covers areas such as administrative issues and communication modes and methods. The book is well-informed, thoughtfully written, and would be a good addition to religious education collections.

Levine, Edna Simon. The Ecology of Early Deafness: Guide to Fashioning Environments and Psychological Assessments. New York: Columbia University Press, 1981. 422 pp.

    Focus of this work is on the influence various environments exert on the psychological development of prelingually deafened children. Within this framework, author describes techniques for the psychological evaluation of deaf clients, interspersing technical aspects with case histories and anecdotes supplied by deaf individuals and parents of deaf children. Thesis throughout is that "the psychological examination is ... an assessment of a deaf individual's shaping environment as much as of the individual per se." Author has produced a monograph that breaks new ground in its theoretical approach, while at the same time providing the information on psychological tests and measures found in a reference work. Appendices provide details on several psychological tests and techniques, a list of test publishers and distributors, as well as a short list of published bibliographical sources. Highly recommended for academic and special library collections on deafness and/or psychology.

Levine, Edna Simon. The Psychology of Deafness: Techniques of Appraisal for Rehabilitation. New York: Columbia University Press, 1960. 383 pp.

One of the first comprehensive analyses of the psychological implications of deafness and of the psychological evaluation of hearing impaired individuals by rehabilitation counselors. The book is divided into four parts: Part I discusses the importance of hearing in early development and the psycholinguistic and psychosocial consequences of deafness in the child; Part II outlines some of the general psychological principles involved in working with a disabled person; Part III, the major part of this book, applies these principles to the psychological evaluation of deaf children and adults and discusses available and appropriate tests to use; Part IV points out areas where future research is needed. Author also provides a glossary, an extensive bibliography, and several appendices. One of the pioneering works in its field, it has now largely been superceded by the same author's Ecology of Early Deafness (1981). While still a valuable part of a comprehensive collection, it is not recommended for those seeking a current introduction to the field of deafness.

Liben, Lynn S., ed. Deaf Children: Developmental Perspectives. New York: Academic Press, 1978. 246 pp.

Compilation of essays written expressly for this work by prominent psychologists and educators specializing in deafness (e.g., Meadow, Moores, Schlesinger). All were members of a study group of the Society for Research in Child Development formed to consider "theoretical and practical implications of research on the development of deaf children." The dozen chapters address primarily the issues of how deafness affects psychological development and how deaf children acquire language and cognitive skills. Within these broad areas, individual authors focus on topics such as parent-child relations, the relationship between sign language and proficiency in reading and writing skills, and the value of Ericksonian and Piagetian perspectives in understanding the development of deaf children. The editor, in an introductory chapter, ably and succinctly summarizes in clear and non-technical language recent research on the prominent developmental issues of family life, modes of communication, and educational programs. An excellent overview for students or researchers in the areas of psychology and education of deaf children. Recommended for academic libraries.

Mathis, Steve L., ed. International Directory of Services for the Deaf. Washington, D.C.: International Center on Deafness, Gallaudet College, 1980. 231 pp.

Lists primarily schools for deaf persons, by country, for all nations except the U.S.A. Provides addresses and information on number of pupils and age group served. Separate listings for organizations, social service agencies, vocational rehabilitation agencies, and athletic organizations. Updated every 4-6 years. Valuable for reference purposes, but would not be used extensively except in specialized settings.

Meadow, Kathryn P. Deafness and Child Development. Berkeley: University of California Press, 1980. 236 pp.

Overview of current state of knowledge concerning various developmental problems faced by deaf children. Designed to provide educators of deaf children with framework necessary for understanding the behavior and capabilities of their deaf or hearing impaired students. Author reports research results in areas of cognitive, language, social, and psychological development of deaf children, as well as describing studies concerning the prevalence of various behavioral problems among deaf children. Lengthy chapter on how deaf child's environment--family, school, community--affects his or her psychological and educational functioning. Final chapter provides author's interpretation of research findings and her recommendations for improving the education of deaf children (e.g., she favors total communication). Lengthy, comprehensive bibliography and an index are appended. This work is essential reading for students, researchers and practitioners in the field of deaf education and allied social service fields. Highly recommended for special education collections.

Mindel, Eugene D., and Vernon, McCay. They Grow in Silence: The Deaf Child and His Family. Silver Spring, Md.: National Association of the Deaf, 1971. 118 pp.

Critical discussion of causes and consequences of deafness in children and of current educational theories and techniques. Authors are a child psychiatrist and a psychologist who were part of a team which studied the psychosocial problems of deaf persons at the Michael Reese Hospital in Chicago in the late 1960s. They attack the traditional oral approach to educating the deaf child on the grounds that it is both wrong and illusory to try to make the deaf child conform to a world of spoken communication. Oralism, they maintain, is a failure. They cite many studies which show that total communication is a more effective method of language acquisition and education. They also discuss causes of deafness and methods of audiological assessment, as well as family responses to a deaf child, and the social and intellectual development of the deaf child. This work is a well-researched introduction to the social and educational consequences of deafness. Its bias is that of the deaf person and his family, rather than that of the traditional deaf education establishment. It is a statement which should be read by all students preparing for careers in the field of deafness, as well as by those already working with deaf children and their families. Recommended for academic and large public libraries.

Montgomery, George, ed. Of Sound and Mind: Papers on Deafness, Personality and Mental Health. Edinburgh: Scottish Workshop Publications, 1978. 165 pp.

Compilation of papers presented at a series of one-day conferences sponsored by the Scottish Workshop with the Deaf, a non-profit association of deaf and hearing professionals in various fields of social work and mental health work with deaf persons. Several of the authors are deaf, and most authors are involved in both research and practice with the deaf community. Papers vary from theoretical discussions to reports of research to statements based on personal experience. The common theme is the psychological consequences of deafness, and techniques for assessing and treating mental health problems encountered by deaf persons. Recommended for large academic collections.

Moores, Donald F. Educating the Deaf: Psychology, Principles, and Practices. Boston: Houghton Mifflin, 1978. 347 pp.

A broader work than the title implies. A basic overview of "the educational and psychological implications of deafness." Provides basic information on many aspects of deafness, such as causes, modes of communication, intellectual functioning and various teaching methods. There are also chapters on broader topics such as psychological and social adjustment and the impact of a deaf child on the family. Two chapters discuss the history of educational theories and methods with deaf children. Extensive bibliography, including a separate section of references on sign language acquisition. Excellent beginning text for students or professionals in fields other than deaf education. Recommended for academic libraries.

Myklebust, Helmer R. The Psychology of Deafness: Sensory Deprivation. 3rd ed. New York: Grune and Stratton, 1964. 423 pp.

Standard text on deafness and its psychological implications. Focuses heavily on the effect of deafness on the acquisition of language in both its spoken and written forms. Also describes research into the cognitive, emotional and social development of deaf individuals. Describes causes and incidence of deafness and other disorders or disabilities which sometimes accompany deafness. A useful introduction to the subject of deafness, but badly in need of updating to incorporate recent research findings. Recommended for comprehensive academic collections only. Levine's Ecology of Early Deafness is preferred for students and practitioners.

National Conference on Program Development for and With Deaf People. Proceedings. Washington, D.C.: Office of Public Service Programs, Gallaudet College and the Cooperative Extension Service, University of Maryland, 1973. 131 pp.

Proceedings of a conference designed to provide information to state extension services and vocational rehabilitation personnel on principles and techniques for including deaf persons in extension programs. Based on pilot program for deaf homemakers jointly conducted by the University of Maryland cooperative Extension Service and the Office of Public Service Programs of Gallaudet College. Numerous speakers discussed the needs and problems of deaf adults and children, the importance of sign language in relating to deaf persons, community resources for program planning and various techniques of reaching out to deaf persons and their families. Presentations reproduced here are brief, practical, and based on personal experience. Eight appendices supplement the text and provide more detailed information in several areas. Useful guide for university extension or social service agency personnel. Recommended for large academic and rehabilitation libraries.

An Orientation to Deafness for Social Workers: Papers from the Workshop, March 18-20, 1975. Washington, D.C.: Gallaudet College, 1975. 88 pp.

A selection of papers presented at a special workshop on deafness for social workers, sponsored in 1975 by the Public Service and Social Work departments of Gallaudet College. Authors are professionals who work with deaf persons, as well as deaf persons themselves and family members of deaf persons. All have intimate experience with deafness, and are well-qualified to heighten the awareness and broaden the understanding of readers of this volume. Topics covered include, in addition to social work with deaf clients, psychological and social consequences of deafness, the needs of special groups such as elderly deaf persons, and communication and educational techniques with deaf persons. While not detailed or comprehensive, this work would be useful for students or professionals seeking a brief introduction to the topic of deafness. Recommended for academic and social service agency libraries.

Ovellette, Sue E., and Lloyd, Glenn T., eds. Independent Living Skills for the Severely Handicapped Deaf Person Preparing to Enter Gainful Employment. Silver Spring, Md.: American Deafness and Rehabilitation Association, 1979. 103 pp.

For an evaluation of this work, see Chapter 5.

Pentz, Croft M. Ministry to the Deaf. Elizabeth, N.J.: Croft M. Pentz, 1978. 91 pp.

Author is a minister in the Assemblies of God Church and has extensive experience working with deaf people in religious and educational settings. The book consists of practical advice for ministers and other religious workers in conducting church services or Sunday School and in counseling with the deaf. This book shows more religious zeal and less familiarity with professional literature than Lawrence's "Ministering to the Silent Majority." The Rev. Pentz has strong fundamentalist views which intrude upon his subject continually. Not recommended for professional collections.

Petal, Marla. Independent Living and Deafness: Incorporating Deaf Clients into the Independent Living Network. Houston: The Institute for Rehabilitation and Research, 1980. 30 pp.

For an evaluation of this work, see Chapter 5.

Regional Directory of Services for Deaf Persons. Washington, D.C.: Office of Information and Resources for the Handicapped, U.S. Office of Education, 1980. 10 volumes.

Consists of ten pamphlet sized volumes, one for each of the ten Health, Education and Welfare Regions in the U.S. Each volume has the same introductory sections on national organizations and agencies, and on the certification system for interpreters for the deaf. Regional services are listed by state. They include certified interpreters in that state and the names and addresses of agencies which provide educational, vocational or social services to deaf individuals. Officers of associations of the deaf in each state are listed as well. Also included is a summary of state laws relating to the rights of deaf persons to an interpreter in legal and other situations. These volumes would be valuable reference works for public libraries and for rehabilitation agency collections.

Russo, Anthony. The God of the Deaf Adolescent: An Inside View. New York: Paulist Press, 1975. 278 pp.

Reports design and results of a study of Roman Catholic deaf adolescents with regard to their idea of God. Using a control group of hearing adolescents, the study shows how deafness affects thinking, in this case abstract thinking about God. Recommendations for effectively teaching deaf persons about God are given at the conclusion. Written by a priest for religious teachers who work with deaf persons. A theological background is required to appreciate the significance of this study. The study was limited to deaf adolescents reared in a Christian culture (although some professed atheism). An important, scholarly study, but of value primarily to theologians and clergymen. Recommended for theology and deafness collections.

Schein, Jerome D., and Delk, Marcus T., Jr. <u>The Deaf Population of the United States</u>. Silver Spring, Md.: National Association of the Deaf, 1974. 336 pp.

Based on the National Census of the Deaf Population (NCDP) conducted in 1971-1972 by the National Association of the Deaf and the Deafness Research and Training Center at New York University under a grant from the Rehabilitation Services Administsration. Target population was those individuals who lost (or never had) ability to hear and understand speech before age 19, i.e., prevocationally deaf persons. Goal was to provide accurate data for planning for educational and vocational rehabilitation and placement of these deaf individuals. Characteristics studied in the NCDP include education, mode of communication, economic status, family composition and occupational status. The final chapter and 5 appendices contain information on technical aspects of the design and execution of the NCDP. This work is unique and informative and is essential for academic and special library collections on deafness.

Schein, Jerome D., ed. <u>Education and Rehabilitation of Deaf Persons with Other Disabilities</u>. New York: Deafness Research and Training Center, School of Education, New York University, 1974. 85 pp.

Ten essays address the special needs of deaf individuals who also have a physical, mental, emotional or learning disability. Emphasis is on the development of programs and the delivery of services to this group, estimated at 20-40 percent of the deaf population. Essays are brief and serve as introductions to their topics, which range from audiological assessment to educational programs for multiply handicapped deaf children. Includes comprehensive bibliography on deaf persons with other disabilities. Useful primarily for students new to the field of deafness. Recommended for academic libraries.

Schlesinger, Hilde S., and Meadow, Kathryn P. <u>Sound and Sign: Childhood Deafness and Mental Health</u>. Berkeley: University of California Press, 1972. 265 pp.

Collaborative effort by a psychiatrist (Schlesinger) and a sociologist (Meadow) who work with deaf individuals in a psychiatric institute and in a residential school for the deaf, respectively. Their work is a synthesis of developmental theory and sociological research. Schlesinger adapts developmental theories, primarily Eriksonian, to the situation of deaf children and adolescents, while Meadow reports on developmental problems experienced by deaf children in home and school settings. Both authors stress the social environment -- family, teachers, peers -- in which the child's psychological and cognitive development occurs, and identify it as the source of developmental problems and the focus of intervention. They also discuss training needs for professionals if an effective community mental health program for deaf persons is to be established. Numerous statistical tables, as well as an extensive bibliography are appended. Essential reading for mental health and social service professionals. Recommended for academic collections in special education, mental health, psychology and deafness.

Schowe, Ben M. Identity Crisis in Deafness: A Humanistic Perspective. Tempe, Ariz.: Scholars Press. 1979. 152 pp.

Author is a deaf man, 85 years old, who has long been involved in the movement for deaf equality. His thesis is that, because deafness carries a stigma, the deaf person faces a crisis in his identity: should he strive to be as "normal" as possible (denying his disability) or should he identify with the deaf community (a separate and unequal minority). Author's approach is "humanistic" in the sense that it is based upon experience, intuition and wide reading rather than on scientific studies. He proposes that deaf individuals must learn "the art of being deaf" and that this is best learned by associating with the deaf community, not in vain attempts (although some may succeed at that) to deny one's deafness and pass for hearing in the hearing world. Schowe's style is informal, allusive, and epigrammatic, making his book interesting to read, but not always easy to follow. His work is a valuable addition to the literature on the social psychology of deafness, and should be read by all deaf individuals and by the professionals who work with them. Recommended for academic, public library and rehabilitation collections.

Silver, Rawley A. Shout in Silence: Visual Arts and the Deaf. New York: Metropolitan Museum of Art, 1976. 41 pp.

Reproduces drawings and paintings by deaf individuals of all ages, with commentary by Rawley Silver, an art therapist and painter. He discusses the role of artistic creations as non-verbal forms of understanding and expression for deaf persons. In essence, he sees art as an alternative form of thought and communication for persons deficient in language skills. Their art can also be useful to psychologists in assessing their cognitive abilities, interests, and needs. Author also reports results of several research studies he conducted on the subject of the artistic aptitude of deaf children. Recommended for academic and special education collections.

Sussman, Allen E., and Stewart, Larry G., eds. Counseling with Deaf People. New York: New York University School of Education, Deafness Research and Training Center, 1971. 158 pp.

A series of essays attempting to evaluate the current status of professional counseling of deaf persons in the context of general psychological counseling. The authors are about evenly divided between counseling educators and professional counselors of the deaf. The first 2 chapters present the social and psychological problems common to deaf people because of their deafness and the curent status of professional counseling with deaf clients. The remaining 3 chapters discuss the training of counselors and the practice of counseling, both in general and as they apply to deaf persons. This text is designed for counseling students and psychologists, as an introduction to the principles of counseling as they apply to counseling the deaf. It should be in all academic collections which support degree programs in counseling or special education.

Watson, Douglas, ed. Readings on Deafness. New York: New York University School of Education. Deafness Research and Training Center, 1973. 138 pp.

Reprints of previously published papers chosen for their ability to introduce both lay and professional readers to the experience of deafness, and to motivate them to learn more about deaf people and the programs which seek to educate or otherwise assist deaf people. The authors of the various essays are professionals in the field of rehabilitation of the deaf; several are themselves deaf, and thus eminently qualified to communicate and interpret their experiences and to evaluate the programs and services designed to serve them. This collection of essays is valuable chiefly as an introduction to deafness for lay people, students or rehabilitation professionals with little previous contact with deaf people. Recommended for academic and large public library collections.

Wright, David. Deafness. New York: Stein and Day, 1969. 212 p.

Author is a poet and scholar born and reared in South Africa and educated at Oriel College, Oxford. The first half of the book is an autobiography which concentrates primarily on educational and cultural factors in his development. The second half of the book is a history of the education of deaf people and attitudes toward deafness. Author was deafened at age 7 due to scarlet fever. Since he had already acquired language skills, the effects of deafness on his development are not as great as they would have been had he been born deaf. He writes more about cultural conditions in South Africa and England than about deafness, which has not been a dominant force in his life. Thus, the book is more objective but less informative about deafness than some other autobiographies by disabled people. One of the few autobiographies by a deaf person. Well-written book by a well-educated and cultured person who happens to be deaf. Recommended for academic and large public libraries.

Yount, William R. Be Opened! An Introduction to Minstry with the Deaf. Nashville: Broadman Press, 1976. 225 pp.

Excellent introduction to the subject of deafness for anyone who is planning to work with deaf persons. Designed for seminary students and lay religious workers, but would also be useful to social services personnel. Primary objective is to explain types of hearing impairment, and psychological, social, and educational aspects of deafness. Author has taught a course on ministry with the deaf, and this work was written as a text for that course. Based on literature by professionals in the field of deafness and by deaf persons themselves. Many suggestions for further reading and an excellent bibliography. Up-to-date in its emphasis and its understanding of deaf individuals as people who are like anyone else except that they cannot hear. Best work available for religious workers with the deaf.

4 SOCIAL AND PSYCHOLOGICAL CONTEXTS OF PHYSICAL DISABILITY

RICHARD E. BOPP/Documents Librarian, University of Illinois Library, Urbana, Illinois

INTRODUCTION

The works which this chapter reviews provide an introduction to the rehabilitation process and to the psychological and social aspects of physical disability--areas which have come to be recognized as essential components of rehabilitation programs. Not so long ago, rehabilitation was defined solely in terms of the physical restoration of disabled persons for a return to gainful employment. In the past decade, however, a broader view of the needs of disabled individuals and the goals of rehabilitation has emerged. The independent living movement (see Chapter 5) and the current American emphasis upon personal fulfillment have contributed to the recognition of psychological and social adjustment to disability as a prime concern of rehabilitation professionals.(1) In addition, greater appreciation of attitudinal barriers faced by disabled persons has stimulated interest in the effects of disability on social relationships, including the family, peer groups, and society at large. Increasingly, the definition of rehabilitation has expanded to include not only physical restoration but also a psychological transformation of the individual, allowing him to accept his disability, and a social transformation of the environment, so that disabled persons will be accepted as full and equal members of society.(2)

Within this theoretical framework, the works discussed here fall naturally into several broad areas. Some have been written for the general public or for a general professional audience. These seek to raise the awareness of readers regarding the daily lives of disabled people and the ways in which professionals can assist them. Other works focus on the individual's adjustment to disability and are written for a broad range of professionals who counsel disabled persons. A third group discusses interventions in the hospital setting which can aid the disabled patient in coping with his changed body. A fourth deals with the social context, in the home and in the community. Many of these works in groups three and four are written for professionals or advanced students in the social sciences or allied health fields. A fifth group, however, is intended for students or professionals in any field related to rehabilitation. These texts provide a broad introduction to the history and principles of rehabilitation. Finally, there have been a number of studies in recent years of rehabilitation practices in European countries, particularly Britain, which offer an opportunity to compare American and European goals and methods in the rehabilitation of physically disabled persons.

Among introductory works, the best text for students in rehabilitation-related fields is Goldenson's, Disability and Rehabilitation Handbook. It provides a readable, well-organized and comprehensive introduction to physical disability and to rehabilitation in all of its aspects. The most detailed guide to the current practice and theory of rehabilitation is Wright's Total Rehabilitation. Because of its encyclopedic nature, it is most effectively used with advanced students or as a reference source for practicing professionals, particularly those in rehabilitation counseling. A briefer text, useful for beginning students, is Bitter's Introduction to Rehabilitation, which provides a good overview of the history and principles of vocational rehabilitation. It is more traditional, however, than the works of Wright and Goldenson, and does not discuss in depth newer concepts of rehabilitation, such as independent living. All three of these works give a basic outline of the rehabilitation process and of the roles played by various professional personnel, by health and social service organizations, and by state and federal government agencies.

Rather than describing the rehabilitation process, many works for the general public introduce the lives of physically disabled persons. Their goal is to "rehabilitate" society by dispelling the myths that for so long have been associated with disabling conditions. The best book in this genre is Kleinfield's The Hidden Minority. Each chapter of this fascinating work describes the life of an individual with a particular disability, illuminating in the process the various obstacles disabled people face and their methods of dealing with these problems. A briefer work, which gives more emphasis to disabled children and their families, is Cohen's Special People. Organized by subject, it both illustrates the lives of disabled persons and advocates more enlightened attitudes and services. A more sophisticated and influential approach to advocacy is provided by Bowe's Handicapping America and Rehabilitating America, which describe the problems faced by disabled Americans and offer a comprehensive social program for solving them. Bowe's basic thesis is that monetary investments in rehabilitation and in the removal of barriers to disabled persons are recovered with interest by the contributions which these individuals can make to society if both they and it are "rehabilitated". Bowe has also authored the recent Comeback, which profiles six individuals who pursue successful careers in spite of disabilities such as blindness, deafness and paralysis.

Successful adaptation to severe disabilty-- how it is achieved and what obstacles must be overcome to achieve it-- has been the subject of an increasing number of monographs over the

past twenty years or so. The classic work which has provided the
framework for this discussion since its publication in 1960 is
Wright's Physical Disability-- A Psychological Approach. Wright
identifies the common psychological consequences of disability
and outlines a number of coping stategies. In the past few years,
however, new ground has been broken by several authors who offer
more current and detailed analyses of the process of psychological adjustment. In Psychosocial Adjustment to Disability,
Roessler and Bolton offer a program called "Personal Achievement
Skills Training" for use with recently disabled individuals.
Based on a thorough review of behavioral research, it stresses
the importance of group counseling and the achievement of concrete goals for building self-esteem and confidence. Also behavioral in approach is the work of DeLoach and Greer, Adjustment to
Severe Physical Disability: A Metamorphosis. Both authors are academic professionals who base their work on the results of research as well as on their own experience as disabled individuals. Their strategy for adjustment places greater emphasis upon
the stigma which attaches to disability and the techniques by
which the disabled person can incorporate his disability into a
successful self-image in the face of this stigma. Finally, Vash's
Psychology of Disability also combines personal experience with
research in an up-to-date discussion of the issues and problems
involved in successful adaptation to disability. Like DeLoach and
Grier, Vash lays great stress on the environment as the overrid-
ing problem for a recently disabled individual. Her work is more
practical and less theoretical in its approach, suggesting a
greater variety of professional interventions and placing the subject of adjustment in the broader context of other life experiences such as employment, recreation, and family life. Both of
these works, however, share the view of disabled individuals and
their professional advocates that psychological adjustment does
not depend solely on the disabled individual but also upon a
greater adaptation of the environment which constantly affects

the disabled person's self-concept through physical and social interactions.

Such a broad view of the process of adjustment is not held by most authors of works on this subject for health professionals. An exception is Shontz, whose The Psychological Aspects of Physical Illness and Disability rejects the medical model and argues for a more holistic view of the patient with a physical disability. He agrees with disabled consumers that the focus of rehabilitation should be on the whole person and his entire life situation, not just on the disability. An excellent and comprehensive guide to group therapy in a clinical setting is provided in Group Counseling and Physical Disability, edited by Lasky and Dell Orto. Peer group counseling and family support groups are among the techniques discussed in this work for health care providers. Up-to-date but more traditional in their approach are two recent works for health professionals, Behavioral Problems and the Disabled, edited by Bishop, and Greif and Matarazzo's work, Behavioral Approaches to Rehabilitation. These books provide practical suggestions to hospital personnel for dealing with behavioral consequences of disability such as anxiety, depression and aggression. Their focus is more on "managing a patient" than on assisting an individual in the process of reconstructing his or her identity and lifestyle.

By contrast, the works describing social aspects and consequences of physical disability share the broader view of rehabilitation found in most recent studies of psychological adjustment. The seminal work in this area is Safilios-Rothschild's The Sociology and Social Psychology of Disability and Rehabilitation. She views rehabilitation as a social (not physical) process, and she discusses the social influences exerted by professionals in their interactions with their disabled clients. Another work which views rehabilitation in a social context is Role of the Family in the Rehabilitation of the Physically Disabled, edited by Power and Dell Orto. The authors of this compilation see disability as an event which affects a family, not an individual; consequently, the entire family can and should be part of the rehabilitation process. Their work is written particularly for health care providers. An excellent work with a similar perspective for teachers and others who work with disabled children is Buscaglia's <u>The Disabled and Their Parents: A Counseling Challenge</u>.

Two compilations of previously published essays provide an overview of both the psychological and social consequences of physical disability. The more comprehensive of the two is <u>Social and Psychological Aspects of Disability</u>, edited by Stubbins. While placing the greatest emphasis on sociological topics, it covers a broad range of issues and disabilities, and is interdisciplinary both in its intended audience and in the backgrounds of its contributors. Attitudes toward disabled persons, on the other hand, is a subject given more coverage in <u>The Psychological and Social Impact of Physical Disability</u>, edited by Marinelli and Dell Orto. There is a greater emphasis in this work on psychological adjustment. Some overlapping of essays exists in these two works, but they complement each other well, and both provide useful background reading for students or professionals interested in the psychological and social adjustment necessitated by physical disability.

Works which portray the experiences of disabled persons and the ideas and techniques of rehabilitation workers in European countries also make valuable reading for American students and practitioners in rehabilitation fields. Their authors write from the same perspectives and have the same goals as the authors of the works on American rehabilitation, which heightens their value for comparative analysis. For instance, <u>Disability in Britain</u>, edited by Walker and Townsend, offers a similar social program to that of Bowe for achieving full integration of disabled persons into society. Its contributors are more militant than Bowe, but they have the same goal of raising the level of public awareness regarding the abilities and problems of disabled persons and the benefits to society from investment in rehabilitation. In similar fashion, Handicap in a Social World, edited by Brechin, Liddiard, and Swain, provides an array of essays on social and psychological aspects of life with a disability which can be compared to the works of Stubbins and Marinelli and Dell Orto. Other works, however, provide insights into the uniqueness of European conditions and programs. Blaxter's The Meaning of Disability illustrates the perceived needs of British disabled individuals and assesses the degree to which public and private agencies do or do not recognize and meet those needs. For other European countries, two valuable studies are available to American readers. Carnes' European Rehabilitation examines the social and vocational services for disabled persons in five European countries and compares these services to each other and to those offered in the United States. Personal Relationships, the Handicapped and the Community, edited by Lancaster-Gaye, focuses on psychological problems faced by disabled persons in four northern European societies, particularly marital and sexual problems exacerbated by the attitudes of those societies toward disabled persons. Indeed, a perusal of these works indicates that while some European societies have superior economic and social programs, Americans appear to be more progressive in their attitudes toward disabled individuals.

American interest in the lives of disabled persons is made evident by the proliferation in recent years of books about the physically disabled. Almost all of the works discussed above have been published in the past five years. This literary explosion is undoubtedly a consequence of the increased numbers and visibility of disabled persons and the growing involvement of the federal government in rehabilitation programs following the landmark Rehabilitation Act of 1973 (P.L.93-112). The broadening of the definition and scope of rehabilitation, noted above, is a result of the demand by disabled Americans that they be accorded full and equal participation in American society. This demand has made it necessary for rehabilitation professionals to concern themselves not only with medical and vocational restoration, but with the psychological and social consequences of disability which impede the full integration of disabled persons in various aspects of social life. It is now apparent that both the disabled individual and society's response to that individual require rehabilitating. As much recent literature shows, rehabilitation professionals have begun to accept that challenge.

NOTES

1. For a discussion of changing views on rehabilitation, see Gerben De Jong, The Movement for Independent Living: Origins, Ideology and Implications for Disability Research. (Boston: Medical Rehabilitation Institute, Tufts-New England Medical Center, 1978).
2. This is the approach taken by, among others, Carolyn Vash, in Psychology of Disability. (New York: Springer, 1981).

ANNOTATED BIBLIOGRAPHY

Albrecht, Gary L., ed. The Sociology of Physical Disability and Rehabilitation. Pittsburgh: University of Pittsburgh Press, 1976. 303 pp.

   Eleven essays written specifically for this volume by academic psychologists and sociologists. Differing greatly in theoretical approach, all deal either with the interaction between the disabled person and others or with the organization and delivery of rehabilitation services. The book has no unifying theme. Some of the issues discussed include: self-concept of the physically disabled person; labeling theory as it relates to rehabilitation; family responses to disability; and alternatives to rehabilitation services and programs as they existed in the mid-1970s. Each chapter has its own bibliography, and there are Subject and Name Indexes. Individual chapters would be valuable reading for students and researchers in psychology and sociology. For most students, however, the integrated text by Safilios-Rothschild offers a better introduction and overview of the sociological aspects of disability and rehabilitation. Recommended for academic libraries.

SOCIAL AND PSYCHOLOGICAL CONTEXTS 85

Barnes, Ellen; Berrigan, Carol; and Biklen, Douglas. <u>What's the Difference? Teaching Positive Attitudes Toward People with Disabilities</u>. Syracuse, N.Y.: Human Policy Press, 1978. 165 pp.

    This book is an introduction to teaching positive attitudes toward disabled people. It describes ninety-four activities teachers can use to help children examine their attitudes and increase their understanding of what it means to be disabled. There are also chapters providing background information about various disabilities and offering suggestions for organizing the classroom and the learning activities. Materials required for each activity are listed.

    "Resources" section lists and annotates print and nonprint materials about various disabilities. Includes lists of organizations. This section gives reference value to the book. The activities section is an excellent source for teaching attitudes, since most suggested activities require discussion and creative thinking by the students. For teachers, a good source of information, ideas, techniques, and resources available. Because more disabled children are being integrated into regular classroom, this book is very timely. Recommended for public and school libraries.

Berger, Gilda. <u>Physical Disabilities</u>. New York: Watts, 1979. 119 pp.

    Introduction to causes and consequences of a variety of disabling or chronic disorders. Discusses neuromuscular diseases such as polio, multiple sclerosis and muscular dystrophy, chronic health problems such as asthma, diabetes, and heart disease, and sensory impairments such as blindness and deafness. Introductory chapters discuss attitudes toward disability and other problems faced by disabled persons. Emphasis, however, is on what disabled persons can accomplish if given the proper physical and social environment. Written on basic level for older children or adults with low reading level. Discussion is informal and positive throughout. Recommended for school and public libraries.

Bishop, Duane S., ed. <u>Behavioral Problems and the Disabled: Assessment and Management</u>. Baltimore: Williams and Wilkins, 1980. 473 pp.

    Contains twenty essays on various behavioral problems which may surface in a person's struggle to cope with a disability. Written for health care professionals in rehabilitation settings, to assist them in identifying and treating psychological and social problems exhibited by their patients or clients. Authors are psychiatrists, psychologists, and social workers. They describe problems such as anxiety, sexual dysfunction, aggressive behavior, use of drugs, and other behavior patterns which can be treated with proper techniques and sensitivity. Most chapters contain illustrative case studies. Chapters have footnotes, but there is no bibliography. Essential reading for professionals in rehabilitation centers. Highly recommended for academic and rehabilitation-oriented special and medical libraries.

Bitter, James A. Introduction to Rehabilitation. St. Louis: C. V. Mosby, 1979. 271 pp.

   Introductory text, written primarily for students in rehabilitation counseling and for professionals in various rehabilitation-related fields. Places major emphasis upon vocational aspects of rehabilitation, but includes information on other aspects as well. Outlines history of rehabilitation programs in the U.S. and the principles of evaluation and counseling used by rehabilitation counselors. Describes nature and consequences of most common disabilities and the roles played by various professionals in the rehabilitation process. A list of readings is included in each of the ten chapters. An appendix lists colleges and universities with federally supported educational programs in rehabilitation fields. Recommended primarily for academic libraries.

Blaxter, Mildred. The Meaning of Disability: a Sociological Study of Impairment. London: Heinemann, 1976. 259 pp.

   Study of the lives of 194 disabled British adults during the year following their discharge from "a large teaching hospital." Broad range of disabling conditions is included. Aim was to ascertain what kinds of needs and problems the subjects experienced, and to learn how and to what degree social service and other societal institutions responded to these needs and problems: i.e., do needs and problems as perceived by the disabled person coincide with or differ from the perceptions of the social service professionals? Problem areas studied included personal care, employment, family and social relationships, and financial difficulties. Author concludes that services to the disabled "are in a state of considerable confusion regarding whom to help and how best to provide assistance." Though based on British conditions, offers thought-provoking information for American rehabilitation professionals. Recommended for academic libraries and for special libraries with rehabilitation clientele.

Boswell, David M., and Wingrove, Janet M., eds. The Handicapped Person in the Community: A Reader and Sourcebook. London: Tavistock, 1974. 500 pp.

   Formerly used as the reader and sourcebook for course with same title in England's Open University. Course is designed for professionals, to broaden their knowledge of interdisciplinary aspects and approaches in field of rehabilitation. Most chapters previously appeared in print elsewhere. Focus is on social and psychological aspects of disability, such as: attitudes toward the disabled; effect of disability on the family; residential care; social policies; and delivery of social services. Authors

SOCIAL AND PSYCHOLOGICAL CONTEXTS

include professionals and academics in various fields and disabled laypersons or family members. Practice rather than research oriented. Majority of chapters reflect British experiences. Still useful even though it has been replaced as a course text by Brechin, et. al., Handicap in a Social World. Recommended for academic and rehabilitation library collections.

Bowe, Frank. <u>Comeback: Six Remarkable People Who Triumphed Over Disability</u>. New York: Harper & Row, 1981. 172 pp.

Short biographies (twenty or thirty pages each) of six individuals who, in spite of a physical, mental or sensory disability, have forged successful careers in diverse areas, from psychology to biochemistry. Most were disabled in early childhood, all before reaching the age of adulthood. Individuals profiled are interesting and important not only because of their disability, but because of the contribution they have made to society. Author is deaf, and in final chapter adds his "Reflections" on their lives, providing child-rearing advice to parents of disabled children. Work is designed to illustrate the potential of disabled people, with a strong determination to succeed on their part, and a hospitable environment at home, school and work. Contains short bibliography and list of sources of information on disabilities. Good awareness-raising book for general audience or for friends and relatives of disabled children. Recommended for public libraries.

Bowe, Frank. <u>Handicapping America: Barriers to Disabled People</u>. New York: Harper & Row, 1978. 254 pp.

This work, by a prominent deaf American, points out how disabled people are kept from full participation in our society by architectural and attitudinal barriers which severely restrict their ability to find housing, employment, education and recreation. In excluding these 36 million disabled individuals, we handicap American society by depriving it of the contributions they could make and by consigning them to dependency on various welfare benefits. The book details the daily lives and problems faced by people with varying disabilities, while pointing out what they can acccomplish in a barrier-free environment. An important awareness-raising book which should be in all public and academic libraries.

Bowe Frank. <u>Rehabilitating America: Toward Independence for Disabled and Elderly People</u>. New York: Harper & Row, 1980. 203 pp.

Author is deaf, and was first Executive Director of American Coalition of Citizens with Disabilities. This work is the sequel and answer to Bowe's previous work, <u>Handicapping America</u>. In the present volume, Dr. Bowe proposes a five-point plan, costing $22 billion/year, to invest funds in changing our physical environment and rehabilitating disabled persons so that they can become contributing members of the working force, rather than drains on the economy. Not to invest this money, Bowe believes, will cost $150 billion in lost taxes, social security and other payments to dependent disabled people. Thus, the cost of "rehabilitating" America is far less than that of continuing to "handicap" America. The book is well-documented and is an important contribution to the controversy over the cost of making our society more responsive to disabled and elderly persons. Recommended for public and academic library collections.

Brechin, Ann; Liddiard, Penny; and Swain, John, eds. Handicap in a Social World. Sevenoaks, Kent, England: Hodder and Stoughton, 1981. 344 pp.

Replaces Boswell and Wingrove's work as the reader and sourcebook for the course "Handicapped Person in the Community" in Britain's Open University. Like the course itself, the forty-one chapters are directed at professionals or lay people who work with disabled persons in any capacity. Readings are taken from a variety of sources, including American works. Authors are professionals and disabled individuals. In most cases, the material presented is a short selection from a book or journal article. Topics range from self-image to social and family relationships to professional counseling. Very little overlap with previous sourcebook; most readings were originally published in the late 1970s. Very useful selection of practical experiences and theoretical approaches. Could be used in undergraduate courses in social sciences, allied health fields, or special education. Recommended for academic libraries.

Browne, J. A.; Kirlin, Betty A.; and Watt, Susan, eds. Rehabilitation Services and the Social Work Role: Challenge for Change. Baltimore: Williams and Wilkins, 1981. 371 pp.

Contains an introduction, conclusion, and thirty-six topical essays on the role and practice of social work in rehabilitation settings, and on the education of social workers for practice in rehabilitation settings. Authors are from numerous disciplines, including medicine, education, and various social sciences, in addition to social work. They include academics, practitioners, and four disabled consumers. Topics addressed include: social work principles for specific groups or settings; relationships with other professionals; methods of interdisciplinary teamwork; and theoretical bases for the role of social workers in assisting the physically disabled and their families. The multi-disciplinary nature of the rehabilitation effort is stressed throughout. Excellent text for medical or rehabilitation social workers or for students contemplating those specialties. Highly recommended for academic libraries which support social work or rehabilitation curricula.

Buscaglia, Leo F. ed. The Disabled and Their Parents: A Counseling Challenge. Thorofare, N.J.: C. B. Slack, 1975. 393 pp.

SOCIAL AND PSYCHOLOGICAL CONTEXTS 89

Humanistic challenge to social workers, psychologists, and teachers to provide more sensitive and comprehensive counseling services to disabled persons and their families. All disabilities and age groups considered, but emphasis is on physically disabled children and their parents. Takes "family therapy" approach (entire family is affected by and must cope with disability). Up-to-date in its emphasis on personal adjustment and maximum self-fulfillment for the disabled person as the primary goals of the rehabilitation process. Also emphasizes the value of listening to and learning from disabled people and their family members. Some chapters written by well-known experts (e.g., Sol Gordon on sexuality), others by disabled persons or family members. Designed primarily to heighten the awareness of counselors regarding the needs, problems, desires, and capabilities of their clients. Extensive bibliography and an annotated list of "suggested reading". Highly recommended for all who work with disabled persons.

Campling, Jo, ed. Images of Ourselves: Women with Disabilities Talking. London: Routledge and Kegan Paul, 1981. 140 pp.

Contains 25 short essays by disabled Englishwomen. Authors discuss various aspects of their lives, focusing both upon practical concerns such as clothing and employment, and on more difficult problems like social relationships and sexuality. Some issues are specific to women; others are not. These essays show clearly the affect on disabled women of societal attitudes based upon negative stereotypes. Most of the women have mobility impairments; a few have sensory or neurological disabilities. Some are congentially disabled, while others were disabled in adulthood. Provides many insights into the experience of disability, particularly as it affects women. Recommended for women's studies collections and for general academic and public library collections.

Carnes, Giles D. European Rehabilitation: Service Providers and Programs. East Lansing: University Centers for International Rehabilitation, Michigan State University, 1979. 305 pp.

Comparative study of social, economic, and vocational rehabilitation programs in five European countries: Great Britain; Sweden; the Netherlands; France; and Yugoslavia. Based on author's extensive interviews with rehabilitation workers in these countries and on internal administrative documents, not written for public consumption, which illustrate the philosophy of rehabilitation in each country. Emphasis on content of programs, on training programs for rehabilitation counselors, on attitudes of counselors toward their clients, and on the perceived goals of the rehabilitation process in each country. Among many conclusions, author finds that disabled persons in Europe receive far greater social, medical, and financial benefits than do American disabled persons. However, as a consequence, they are less motivated toward economic independence. In many areas, American rehabilitation counselors, social workers, administrators and researchers could learn from both the successes and the failures of European rehabilitation programs. This work is well-researched, and is highly recommended for academic libraries and for special libraries which serve rehabilitation professionals.

Carver, Vida, and Rodda, Michael. Disability and the Environment. New York: Schocken Books, 1978. 123 pp.

Explores the implications for disabled persons of an environment (physical and social) which for centuries has been designed to meet the needs of average, able-bodied individuals. Argues that, in addition to rehabilitating the disabled individual for a return to society, attention should be focused on changing the environment to make it suitable for a wider range of human physical, social, and mental capacities. Individual chapters explore this theme for disabled children, disabled adults, and elderly disabled individuals. Considers concepts and studies from other European countries and from the U.S.A., but based primarily on British experience. Bibliography and index included. Provides a good introduction to sociological aspects of disability. Useful reading for students and professionals in the social science and social services fields. Recommended for academic libraries.

Cobb, A. Beatrix, ed. Medical and Psychological Aspects of Disability. Springfield, Ill.: Charles C. Thomas, 1973. 365 pp.

Compilation of sixteen essays, each of which discusses the psychological and/or medical aspects of a specific disabling condition. Disabilities addressed range from heart disease and epilepsy to deafness and blindness. Essays summarize the state of knowledge and current rehabilitation principles in each field. Intended audience consists of students and practitioners in field of rehabilitation counseling. Authors include physicians in Lubbock, Texas area who participated in teaching a course in "Medical Aspects of Disability" at Texas Tech University. Other authors are authorities in rehabilitation counseling from around the nation. Valuable introduction for those new to field of rehabilitation; advanced students or experienced practitioners might broaden their knowledge of the psychological aspects of those particular disabilities to which they have had little exposure. Recommended for academic and medical libraries.

Cohen, Shirley. Special People: A Brighter Future for Everyone with Physical, Mental, and Emotional Disabilities. Englewood Cliffs, N.J.: Prentice-Hall, 1977. 177 pp.

An introduction to disability, written by a special education professor, to raise the consciousness of lay persons about the abilities of disabled people. Author discusses attitudinal barriers faced by the disabled because of traditional views of disability based on fear and ignorance. Chapters focus on what it is like to be a disabled child, the parent of a disabled child, and a disabled adult seeking productivity and equal access. Many case histories and examples from literature included. Emphasis on creating more positive, accepting attitudes toward those with physical or mental disabilities. Very readable; written with intelligence and sensitivity. Highly recommended for public libraries.

Cornelius, Debra A., ed. Barrier Awareness: Attitudes Toward People with Disabilities. Washington, D.C.: Regional Rehabilitation Research Institute on Attitudinal, Legal and Leisure Barriers, George Washington University, 1981. 72 pp.

A brief but valuable introduction to the attitudinal barriers faced by persons with physical or developmental disabilities. Described in the preface as "a synthesis" of the ten booklets in the Barrier Awareness Series (each of which is available separately, from the same publisher). Each chapter deals with a specific category of disability, e.g. mobility, vision, hearing, mental retardation. A unique feature is the chapter on attitudes toward "hidden" disabilities, such as ostomies, cancer, diabetes, and epilepsy. Each chapter presents several myths about disabled individuals, followed by an explanation of the actual abilities and life styles of the disabled. Several "Scenes" illustrate in fictional form how disabled persons are treated or thought of in inappropriate fashion in everyday social, employment, and recreational settings. Practical advice on correct behavior toward disabled persons is also provided. An excellent awareness-raising book for lay persons and those new to the field of rehabilitation services. Recommended for public and rehabilitation libraries.

Cull, John G., and Hardy, Richard E. Rehabilitation Techniques in Severe Disability: Case Studies. Springfield, Ill.: Charles C. Thomas, 1974. 238 pp.

Introductory chapter on physchological reactions to disability, followed by thirteen disability-specific chapters containing primarily case studies and questions for group discussion. Intended as companion to Severe Disabilities (also edited by Hardy and Cull). Disabilities addressed include mobility, visual and hearing impairments as well as chronic conditions such as diabetes and arthritis. Each chapter provides references for further reading. Designed for use in courses in rehabilitation counseling, social work, and other social service areas. Authors are academicians in rehabilitation counseling and practitioners in governmental or private agencies. Unique approach which would be of significant value to its intended audience. Recommended for academic libraries.

Dean, Russell J. N. New Life for Millions: Rehabilitation for America's Disabled. New York: Hastings House, 1972. 180 pp.

A social history of the growth of rehabilitation in the Twentieth Century. Focuses primarily on the leading individuals, rather than on the programs or organizations which facilitated the expansion of the rehabilitation field which we see today. Changes in attitudes, and scientific and technological developments which made rehabilitation possible, are illustrated as well. Provides many facts about people and organizations not available elsewhere. Narrative is smooth, but treatment of most topics is brief and superficial. Useful work for those wanting historical background, particularly regarding individual leaders in the field. Recommended for public and academic libraries.

DeLoach, Charlene and Greer, Bobby G. Adjustment to Severe Physical Disability: A Metamorphosis. New York: McGraw-Hill, 1981. 310 pp.

Outlines the psychological and social problems faced by disabled persons and the methods of facilitating adjustment to disability. Both authors have physical disabilities, and both are faculty at Memphis State University. They wrote this work to provide students of rehabilitation counseling with a text based on research, practice and experience. Focus is on societal stereotypes regarding disability which must be overcome by the disabled individuals as those individuals reconstruct their self-concept to incorporate the fact of permanent disability. Useful appendixes provide list of recommended books, serials and films on physical disability, and an annotated list of personal narratives by disabled persons. Highly recommended for scholars, practitioners and students. Essential for any library collection on disability.

Eisenberg, Myron G.; Griggins, Cynthia; and Duval, Richard J., eds. Disabled People as Second-Class Citizens. New York: Springer, 1982. 300 pp.

This work is Volume 2 of the Springer Series on Rehabilitation. It contains nineteen essays written especially for this volume by authors from various academic backgrounds. Most authors have worked directly with disabled persons in social, psychological and medical settings; several are themselves disabled. The essays are designed to raise the awareness of rehabilitation professionals regarding the societal barriers facing disabled persons after they are physically rehabilitated. Topics discussed include: social and institutional sources and expressions of discrimination; coping mechanisms for disabled persons to employ in settings where discrimination occurs; and consumer activism and independent living concepts as strategies for changing social attitudes and behaviors. The style and content of the essays vary greatly. A few summarize the research on a given topic, while others offer ideas based on personal experience. Thoroughly up-to-date in its emphasis on the environment as a handicapping force, this work is highly recommended for academic, large public, and rehabilitation libraries.

SOCIAL AND PSYCHOLOGICAL CONTEXTS 93

Firing, Martel. <u>The Physically Impaired Population of the United States</u>. San Francisco: Firing & Associates, 1978. 114 pp.

Provides statistics on the number of Americans who have permanent or chronic physical impairments resulting from disease, injury or congenital malformation. Data taken from various reports published by the National Center for Health Statistics. Organized by type of impairment, by age, and by state. Only permanent impairments are considered. Intended as an "information source for decision-makers in business and government." Includes bibliography of sources of statistics and an appendix discussing methodological technicalities. Useful reference source for planners, governmental agencies, researchers, advocates and librarians. Recommended for academic and special libraries.

Garrett, James F., and Levine, Edna S. eds. <u>Rehabilitation Practices with the Physically Disabled</u>. New York: Columbia University Press, 1973. 569 pp.

Sixteen chapters, most of which concern specific disabilities, comprise this compilation. Disabilities discussed include cancer, heart disease, cerebral palsy, amputation, deafness, and blindness, among others. Chapters are lengthy and provide a good introduction to medical, psychological and vocational rehabilitation principles. A long introductory chapter describes the "fundamentals" of rehabilitation in general terms and provides a framework for the chapters on specific disabilities. Offers more detailed discussions than the works edited by Cull and Hardy, but like those works is somewhat dated. Useful for beginning students; recommended for academic libraries.

Goldenson, Robert M. ed. <u>Disability and Rehabilitation Handbook</u>. New York: McGraw-Hill, 1978. 846 pp.

Comprehensive guide, by multiple authors, to the nature of disability, to methods of rehabilitation, and to community services for disabled individuals. Authors are professionals from many fields and disabled individuals. Divided into four lengthy sections. Part I describes various aspects of rehabilitation, from psychological adjustment to educational, vocational, and recreational programs. Part 2 provides brief descriptions of the origin and treatment of approximately forty disabling disorders. Part 3 describes rehabilitation professions and facilities and includes a number of illustrative case histories of rehabilitated individuals. Part 4 provides lengthy listings of sources of information such as directories, periodicals and voluntary organizations. This work provides a wealth of information on all aspects of disability and rehabilitation. An invaluable reference source for practicing professionals, it is also an excellent introduction to the field for students. Highly recommended for academic, medical and rehabilitation libraries.

Greif, Elaine, and Matarazzo, Ruth G. Behavioral Approaches to Rehabilitation: Coping with Change. New York: Springer, 1982. 158 pp.

    Third volume in the Springer Series on Rehabilitation. Written for "therapists and caretakers of patients whose functioning has been impaired by injury or disease". Emphasis on practical solutions to problems faced by patients and staff in a rehabilitation setting. Based on a behavioral approach to the study of adjustment to disability and professional interventions which facilitate adjustment by patient and family members. Separate chapters deal with specific situations such as anxious patients, elderly patients, brain-injured patients, etc. The unique needs of staff who work in rehabilitation settings are described in a chapter on stress management for professionals. A lengthy case history in the final chapter illustrates the application of many of the principles described in previous chapters. Several appendices contain lists, graphs, and charts amplifying material presented in the text. Bibliography and index provided. Useful text for students or professionals in rehabilitation field. Similar in approach to the works by Bishop and by DeLoach and Grier, but oriented more toward the medical setting. Recommended for health sciences and academic libraries.

Hardy, Richard E. and Cull, John G., eds. Severe Disabilities: Social and Rehabilitation Approaches. Springfield, Ill.: Charles C. Thomas, 1974. 317 pp.

    Compilation of fourteen essays, each of which introduces the principles involved in the rehabilitation of persons with a particular physical or mental disability or chronic health problem. Authors are academicians and practitioners in psychology, education and rehabilitation counseling. Each essay comprises a summary of current research and practice. Might be useful as optional reading for students. As a text it suffers from the absence of an introductory chapter presenting general principles applicable to all disabilities or in some way providing an overview or integrated framework. Index, but no bibliography. Newer works by Stubbins and by Marinelli and Dell Orto provide more current perspectives. Recommended only for comprehensive collections.

Hartbauer, R. E. Counseling in Communicative Disorders. Springfield, Ill.: Charles C. Thomas, 1978. 323 pp.

    Collection of essays on the topic of counseling persons with disorders of language, speech or hearing. Some focus on family counseling; all emphasize the psychological and emotional problems of clients rather than the clinical or physical causes of the disorder. Numerous communication disorders are discussed, including stuttering, aphasia, deafness, cleft palate, layngectomy, and cerebral palsy. All focus on pragmatic counseling techniques or unique problems of specific groups of clients. Chapter bibliographies and general name and subject indexes are provided.

SOCIAL AND PSYCHOLOGICAL CONTEXTS   95

Well-conceived and highly useful text for students and practitioners in speech pathology, audiology, medicine, social work, psychology, and special education. Recommended for academic and health sciences libraries.

Haskins, James. Who are the Handicapped? Garden City, N.Y.: Doubleday, 1978. 109 pp.

Written for a general audience, to increase understanding of the lives of disabled people and to counteract the prejudice that may be directed against them because they are "different". Author attempts to show that disabled people are not in fact so different, but that they are "people" first and, incidentally, disabled. Thus, they have more similarities than differences with the able-bodied majority. After a brief discussion of attitudes, the bulk of the work provides an introduction to the nature of major disabilities, such as visual, hearing, orthopedic or mental impairments. Illustrations from literature and from the lives of disabled individuals accompany the factual information provided. A glossary and a bibliography are appended. A good basic introduction to disability; recommended for public libraries.

Institute for Information Studies. Learning to Live with Disability: A Guidebook for Families. Falls Church, Va.: The Institute, 1980. 80 pp.

An introduction to psychological and social aspects of disability for family members and others significantly involved with assisting the disabled person in developing coping strategies and an independent, productive lifestyle. Would also be useful to social workers, rehabilitation counselors and other social service professionals. Topics discussed include emotional reactions to disability, common problems faced by the disabled person and family members, and techniques and resources for solving those problems. Provides information on relevant legislation, methods of using agency resources, and techniques of consumerism and advocacy. Up-to-date and practical information and advice are offered. Includes annotated lists of books and periodicals for further reading and of agencies and organizations which provide information and services. Recommended for public and rehabilitation libraries.

Katz, Irwin. Stigma: A Social Psychological Analysis. Hillsdale, N.J.: Lawrence Erlbaum Associates, 1981. 140 pp.

Based on extensive studies of the attitudes held by white, able-bodied persons toward two groups regarded as deviant and disadvantaged, namely blacks and disabled persons. Designed to test the theory that these attitudes are conflicting and ambivalent, including both hostile and compassionate elements which are exhibited in differing situations and contexts. In various experiments, the behavior of individuals toward stigmitized persons (e.g., disabled persons) tended to be either more positive or more negative than toward non-stigmatized persons under the same conditions. Ambivalence as the attitudinal determinant of this behavior was not definitively proven, however. Provides extensive discussion of research on attitudes toward stigmatized persons. Includes extensive list of references. Valuable primarily to students and researchers in the fields of psychology and sociology. Recommended for academic libraries.

Kleinfield, Sonny. The Hidden Minority: a Profile of Handicapped Americans. Boston: Little, Brown, 1979. 213 pp.

Excellent introduction to the lives of disabled people, primarily those with severe mobility impairments. Each chapter deals with a particular aspect of their lives, such as housing, education, transportation, employment, and legal rights. Author skillfuly uses interviews with various disabled persons to illustrate and illuminate the problems and issues in each area. His story is informative and easy to read. Valuable addition for public, high school or college libraries. Appendix lists organizations which provide assistance and/or information. Highly recommended for general audiences.

Lancaster-Gaye, Derek, ed. Personal Relationships, the Handicapped and the Community: Some European Thoughts and Solutions. London: Routledge & Kegan Paul for the International Cerebral Palsy Society, 1972. 150 pp.

Twelve chapters concentrate on various social consequences of physical disability and how European societies and institutions have responded to these consequences. The first four chapters discuss group living arrangements for physically disabled persons in the United Kingdom, Denmark, Sweden, and Holland. The focus in each chapter is on describing those residential settings which can serve as models for other countries to follow. The final eight chapters discuss sexual and marital problems faced by physically disabled persons and offer some solutions to their problems which have been developed in the same four European countries. These chapters discuss societal attitudes toward the sexuality of disabled persons, sexual problems and experiences of disabled persons, and therapeutic intervention principles and techniques. This compilation of European experiences and ideas is brief, but provides valuable information not available elsewhere. Recommended for academic and medical or rehabilitation collections.

Lasky, Robert G., and Dell Orto, Arthur E., eds. Group Counseling and Physical Disability: A Rehabilitation and Health Care Perspective. North Scituate, Mass: Duxbury Press, 1979. 385 pp.

Thirty-nine essays on use of group therapeutic techniques with disabled persons and/or families of disabled persons. Most programs geared to health care settings. Authors are professionals in clinical or academic settings; most essays are reprinted from scholarly journals. Unique and valuable features include suggested individual exercises and structured group experiences for raising the awareness of health professionals. Various physical disabilities discussed, as well as kidney disorders, heart disease, and visual impairment. Excellent reading for professionals and students in rehabilitation and health fields. Highly recommended for academic, medical and rehabilitation libraries.

Lees, Dennis, and Shaw, Stella, eds. Impairment, Disability and Handicap: a Multi-disciplinary View. London: Heinemann, 1974. 193 pp.

Published papers presented at a conference on "the cost of human impairment", sponsored by Britain's Social Science Research Council in March 1973. The papers discuss economic aspects of disability and legal aspects of compensation for personal injury. Authors are economists and other social scientists. Examples of topics addressed are the cost of home care for disabled persons, the cost of impairments resulting from automobile accidents, and the measurement of prevalence of and psychological cost of disability. Appendices provide statistical information on disability in Britain and a summary of benefit programs available to disabled persons. Individual papers might be of interest to sociologists, economists, and administrators of social service organizations. Recommended for comprehensive academic collections only.

Lindemann, James E. Psychological and Behavioral Aspects of Physical Disability: a Manual for Health Practitioners. New York: Plenum, 1981. 426 pp.

Contains fourteen chapters, each of which describes a physical disability or genetic disorder and discusses techniques and considerations for evaluating and treating the psychological consequences of that disability. Of ten contributors, most are psychologists and pediatricians working in the Crippled Children's Division of the Oregon Health Sciences University. The disabilities discussed are for the most part childhood conditions (e.g., hemophilia, cerebral palsy and spina bifida). Some typically adult disabilities, such as stroke and multiple sclerosis, are omitted. The strength of this work is in its consistency of format. Although chapters are by different authors and about unique conditions, each chapter follows the same basic outline, from a discussion of the prevalence, etiology and psychological problems typically encountered, to principles of assessment and intervention. References and sources of further information are appended to each chapter. Provides current information for pediatricians, psychologists and social workers who treat disabled children and adolescents. Recommended for medical libraries.

Marinelli, Robert P., and Dell Orto, Arthur E., eds. The Psychological and Social Impact of Physical Disability. New York: Springer, 1977. 414 pp.

Compilation of previously published essays by authors from various professional fields. Attitudes toward disabled people, the impact of disability on sexuality, and theories and therapies relating to psychological adjustment are some of the subjects discussed. Style and content varies from paper to paper; some present personal viewpoints, others argue conclusions based upon research or experience in the field. A few review the literature. A recurring theme is the problem of self-worth due to prevalent negative attitudes toward disability which the disabled person has internalized. Counseling techniques to deal with emotional and social problems are presented as well. Most essays relate to mobility impaired persons. Recommended for academic, medical and rehabilitation libraries.

McDaniel, James W. Physical Disability and Human Behavior. 2d. ed. New York: Pergamon Press, 1976. 165 pp.

Author is a psychologist at the University of Colorado Medical School. Summarizes current knowledge about the psychological effects and consequences of physical disability. Reviews recent research on numerous aspects of human behavior in medical and rehabilitation settings. Topics covered include: attitudes toward disabled persons; emotional reactions to illness and disability; effects of disability on social development; and the role of motivation in rehabilitation. Contains brief summaries of theoretical approaches, such as Adler's individual psychology and Parsons' social role theory, as they relate to physical disability. Chapter bibliographies and subject index provided. Useful text for advanced students in behavioral psychology, medicine or other fields related to rehabilitation. Recommended for medical and academic libraries.

McDevitt, George M., ed. The Handicapped Experience: Some Humanistic Perspectives. Baltimore: University of Baltimore, 1979. 96 pp.

Proceedings of three seminars held on successive Saturdays in October 1978 at the University of Baltimore. The three topics addressed at these seminars were: images of the disabled in literature and the media; mainstreaming; and civil rights legislation, as it relates to disabled persons. Speakers were primarily academicians and educators. Emphasis of the talks reproduced here is on understanding the attitudes in our society toward disabled persons as reflected in literature, legislation and educational practices. Most unique are the talks by Harold Krents, the blind attorney and author, and the sketch "Lily the Tumbling Tumbleweed" by Lily Tomlin. Recommended for public and academic libraries.

Neff, Walter S., ed. Rehabilitation Psychology. Washington, D.C.: American Psychological Association, 1971. 331 pp.

Contains papers presented at the National Conference on the Psychological Aspects of Disability, held in Monterey, Calif., in 1970. Authors are academic researchers in fields of psychology and other social sciences. Topics addressed include: theory and methods of work evaluation and work adjustment; attitudes toward disabled persons; special problems of poor and minority persons; and suggestions for future research. Each chapter is based on a thorough review of recent research. As a state-of-the-art compilation, it is now out-of-date, however. May still be useful supplementary reading for graduate students in the psychology of rehabilitation. Each chapter includes an extensive list of references. Recommended for comprehensive academic collections only.

Power, Paul W. and Dell Orto, Arthur E. eds. Role of the Family in the Rehabilitation of the Physically Disabled. Baltimore: University Park Press, 1980. 554 pp.

Written for all allied health professionals, this work presents current knowledge on the effects disability has on family members, and on the potential of family members as a resource in the rehabilitation process. It argues that physical disability and rehabilitation should be viewed from the perspective not solely of the disabled individual, but of the family unit as well. Combines personal statements by disabled persons and family members with previously published professional literature and essays written specifically for this book. Goal is to show health professionals how to aid family members in adjusting to disability and how to help them assist disabled individuals in their adjustment and rehabilitation. Various physical disabilities are discussed, including chronic and terminal conditions. A comprehensive, innovative and creative work. Suggestions for further reading are provided. Indispensible to health professionals, psychologists and social workers in rehabilitation and family therapy settings. Highly recommended for academic and rehabilitation libraries.

Robinault, Isabel P., and Cary, Caverlee. Community Resources for the Social Adjustment of Severely Disabled Persons: Options for Involvement. New York: I.C.D. Rehabilitation and Research Center, 1980. 128 pp.

Discusses resources and agencies for the social adjustment needed by disabled persons to become full members of society. Important aspects of social adjustment such as sexuality, leisure activities, and transporation are introduced, and sources of information or research studies are listed for the reader to seek more in-depth knowledge. The national and community agencies included range from professional and academic organizations to self-help and disabled consumer groups. The unique aspect of this publication is its integration of print and agency resources into a single volume with a good subject breakdown. It is directed at social service workers, counselors, beginning rehabilitation professionals, and active disabled lay people. Recommended for rehabilitation collections.

Roessler, Richard T., and Means, Bob L. Personal Achievement Skills: An Introduction. Fayetteville, Ark.: Arkansas Rehabilitation Research and Training Center, 1976. 18 pp.

Introduces program for teaching rehabilitation clients the personal and social skills required for success in a competitive world. These skills, which facilitate life planning and the definition and achievement of appropriate goals, are taught through group activities and lessons. This pamphlet explains both the philosophy and the methods of personal achievement skills training. Training materials are described, and training programs for instructors, offered at the Arkansas Rehabilitation Research and Training Center, are discussed. Contains short list of references. Offers a systematic program for helping disabled individuals to reconstruct their lives. Highly recommended for rehabilitation, medical, and academic libraries.

Roessler, Richard and Bolton, Brian. Psychosocial Adjustment to Disability. Baltimore: University Park Press, 1978. 184 pp.

Authors are faculty at Arkansas Rehabilitation Research and Training Center, where for six years they studied psychosocial adjustment to disability. Based on that research and the research of others, they have developed specific training techniques for maximizing adjustment to any of numerous disabilities. In the area of psychological adjustment, they have developed a strategy called "Personal Achievement Skills" training, which stresses the identification and achievement of realistic and appropriate goals in an organized, step-by-step fashion. This is done in a group counseling setting, which enhances social as well as personal skills. A chapter on spinal cord injury discusses psychological problems and use of personal achievement skills program with this population. "Physical Fitness" and "Behavioral Analysis" are other aspects of successful adjustment for which Roessler and Bolton have devised training packages. A comprehensive work which offers practical techniques for rehabilitation professionals based on research and a thorough literature review. Essential reading for allied health and counseling professionals. Highly recommended for academic and rehabilitation libraries.

Safilios-Rothschild, Constantina. The Sociology and Social Psychology of Disability and Rehabilitation. New York: Random House, 1970. 326 pp.

Hailed in the introduction by T. J. Litman as "the first major, comprehensive sociological exploration of the world of the disabled". A study of the entire rehabilitation process, including aspects of adjustment by the disabled individual, societal attitudes toward disability and rehabilitation, and the goals and attitudes of those professsionals who are involved in the rehabilitation of physically disabled persons. Rehabilitation is viewed both as a social institution and as a social movement, and the author in both cases discusses areas where more research is needed to enforce and expand the services provided to disabled persons. Interdisciplinary in approach, in the literature which is reviewed, and in the audience for whom the book is intended. Excellent introduction to concepts and practices in rehabilitation and to the process of adjustment to disability by the disabled person. Valuable text for students and professionals in social services, medical and allied health fields, psychology, sociology and other social sciences. Highly recommended for academic and health sciences libraries.

Savitz, Harriet May. Consider...Understanding Disability as a Way of Life. Minneapolis: Sister Kenny Institute, 1975. 35 pp.

This pamphlet is an introduction to the life of individuals having physical disabilities. It illustrates in a very readable style the emotional and physical barriers these individuals face and offers suggestions for overcoming them. It also discusses education and employment opportunities, disabling diseases, and organizations to aid the disabled. This publication provides only superficial coverage and should be used only for an introduction to problems and solutions for physically disabled individuals. It would be useful to a recently disabled individual or to the student new to the area of rehabilitation. Recommended for public libraries and for academic or special libraries serving undergraduate students in rehabilitation fields.

Schroedel, John G. Attitudes Toward Persons With Disabilities: A Compendium of Related Literature. Albertson, N.Y.: Human Resources Center, 1979. 171 pp.

Provides bibliographic citations and descriptive abstracts for 110 journal articles and research studies on the topic of attitudes toward disabled persons. Abstracts describe purpose, methods, results, and significance of each study. Abstracts are grouped into three subject-related chapters: "Techniques of Changing Attitudes"; "Social Interaction"; and "Employer Attitudes". Each chapter has an introductory essay, several pages in length, summarizing the literature abstracted in that chapter. Each essay also serves as a subject index to its chapter, pointing out subject subdivisions and the studies abstracted in each subdivision. This work is useful primarily as a summary of past research for those contemplating research studies in the area of the social psychology of disability. Author indexed appendix. Recommended for academic collections in the social sciences and for special libraries in rehabilitation counseling.

Seligman, Milton, ed. Group Counseling and Group Psychotherapy with Rehabilitation Clients. Springfield, Ill.: Charles C. Thomas, 1977. 335 pp.

Contains fifteen essays on the topic of group counseling techniques in rehabilitation settings. Three chapters discuss general aspects of group therapy, while twelve address the use of groups in the treatment of specific disabilities. Most populations included in this volume are not persons with physical disabilities, but prison inmates, terminally ill persons, drug or alcohol abusers, etc. Physically disabled populations discussed include stroke patients, visually impaired persons and deaf individuals. Essays are practical, oriented toward professionals in psychology, social work, and psychiatry. Recommended for academic libraries.

Shontz, Franklin C. The Psychological Aspects of Physical Illness and Disability. New York: Macmillan, 1975. 294 pp.

Provides theoretical groundwork for a holistic approach to psychological reactions to disability and appropriate techniques for aiding the individual's adjustment to the fact of illness or disability. Attacks the medical model for its mechanistic approach and its tendency to expect the patient to conform to hospital needs. Asserts individuality of each patient and necessity for understanding his or her whole life situation, not just the part of the person affected by disability. Based on behavioral research into relationships between mind and body and between person and environment. An important work for health professionals, psychologists, and social workers in medical and/or rehabilitation settings. Highly recommended for medical and academic libraries.

Spiegel, Allen D., and Podair, Simon. Rehabilitating People with Disabilities into the Mainstream of Society. Park Ridge, N.J.: Noyes Medical, 1981. 350 pp.

Compiles thirty-eight previously published journal articles on selected important issues related to the rehabilitation and integration into society of persons with physical disabilities. Most articles are from late 1970's. Authors are professionals in various fields. Content of the chapters varies from reports of research to summaries of the current situation in the field. Topics addressed include: attitudinal barriers; transportation; housing; education; employment; and recreation. Provides selective rather than comprehensive coverage in each area. Could be useful as supplementary reading for students in rehabilitation fields. Recommended for comprehensive academic collections.

Stubbins, Joseph, ed. Social and Psychological Aspects of Disability. Baltimore: University Park Press, 1977. 617 pp.

Compilation of fifty-four previously published papers. Some overlap with essays reprinted in work by Marinelli and Dell Orto. More emphasis, however, on social and sociological aspects of disability. Also several excerpts from accounts of disability and rehabilitation by disabled persons. Broader focus than other works in this area, both in terms of disabilities covered and aspects of rehabilitation which are discussed. Several essays each on problems of body image, work and leisure, and treatment environments. Wide variety in approach, but all essays directed at practicing rehabilitation professionals. Most essays based on practice or literature review rather than original research. Intended as an interdisciplinary overview of rehabilitation, which will acquaint professionals in one specialty with the ideas and experiences of other specialties. Essential reading for all professionals who work with disabled persons. Recommended for academic, rehabilitation and health-related special libraries.

Thomas, David. The Experience of Handicap. London: Methuen, 1982. 209 pp.

Uses both recent research and excerpts from personal narratives by disabled persons to portray the experience of disablement. Written for teachers, social workers and others who interact with the disabled. Four of the ten chapters deal specifically with the handicapped children and their families. Other topics addressed include psychological and social consequences of disability and the role played by society in transforming a disability into a handicap. Very current in its emphasis upon the value of learning from disabled persons. Based on wide reading of American and British literature. Extensive list of references provided. Highly recommended for academic and large public libraries.

Varela, Rita A. Self-Help Groups in Rehabilitation. Washington, D.C.: The American Coalition of Citizens With Disabilities, 1979. 72 pp.

Author was Project Coordinator of a study of the role of self-help organizations in vocational rehabilitation, conducted with a federal grant by the American Coalition of Citizens with Disabilities (ACCD). Brief discussion of the reasons and options for greater involvement by disabled persons in the rehabilitation programs which affect their lives. Outlines provisions of Rehabilitation Act of 1973 which mandate participation by disabled persons in vocational rehabilitation plans and decisions. Offers examples of successful techniques for greater professional-client cooperation on more equal terms. An appendix by Frank Bowe discusses the results of an ACCD survey of the policies and attitudes of vocational rehabilitation directors toward consumer participation in program planning. An annotated bibliography on disabled consumer self-advocacy is also included. Valuable reading for rehabilitation professionals and for disabled consumers. Recommended for rehabilitation and social sciences collections.

Vash, Carolyn. The Psychology of Disability. New York: Springer, 1981. 268 pp.

This is the first volume of the Springer Series on Rehabilitation. Dr. Vash is a psychologist who is also disabled. She brings to her work twenty years of experience as a psychologist and thirty years of experience as a post-polio disabled woman. Her approach is thus based on experience, research and reflection. While thoroughly grounded in scientific theory, it is written in clear, non-technical language. It is aimed at rehabilitation and allied health professionals. In Part I, the author offers "a phenomenological accounting" of the daily lives of disabled persons, concentrating on individuals' internal reactions to various environmental stimuli and on some of the interpersonal aspects of disability. Environmental situations include family, employment, recreation, and intimacy. Part II describes ways in which both disabled individuals and their environment can be changed to make the interactions between them more pleasant and productive. Psychotherapy, peer counseling and legal advocacy are some of the interventions discussed. An annotated bibliography and index are appended. This work is an excellent text for students and professionals in all rehabilitation fields, and for students of psychology and other social sciences as well. Highly recommended for academic and special libraries.

Walker, Alan, and Townsend, Peter, eds. Disability in Britain: A Manifesto of Rights. Oxford: Martin Robertson, 1981. 220 pp.

Conceived and authored by lay and professional members of the Disability Alliance, a British advocacy organization dissatisfied with Britain's programs for disabled persons. Aim is to inform the British people of the problems faced by disabled persons, and to document the need for improved social, financial, and employment services. Authors discuss the numbers of Britains with various disabling conditions and the response of government programs for disabled persons. They offer suggestions for achieving full social and economic participation of disabled persons in British society. Individual chapters focus on the unique problems of specific groups, such as disabled children and their families, disabled women and elderly disabled persons. Valuable critical introduction to the current status of programs for disabled persons in Britain. Useful for comparison with American social and economic programs. Recommended for academic libraries.

Wright, Beatrice A. Physical Disability - A Psychological Approach. New York: Harper and Row, 1960. 408 pp.

Classic work from which contemporary study of psychological aspects of disability begins. A study in "somatopsychology": the study of how variations in physique affect a person's thought and behavior directly or through the reactions of others. Author discusses effects of disability on an individual's social status, personal self-concept and feelings of self-esteem, and interrelationships with others. She also considers how family, friends, and rehabilitation personnel can facilitate a positive self-concept and constructive social relationships. Special chapters on unique problems of disability in childhood and in adolescence. Strong emphasis on importance of including disabled person in planning and decision-making in rehabilitation process. Presents many theories and generalizations based on exhaustive study of the literature as well as personal experiences by disabled individuals. Highly recommended for any professional collection dealing with physical disability and rehabilitation.

Wright, George Nelson. *Total Rehabilitation*. Boston: Little, Brown, 1980, 830 pp.

The most comprehensive text available for those wishing an informed discussion of current knowledge and practice in all aspects of rehabilitaiton. Based on a thorough review of the literature (5000 titles were screened) and a broad view of the meaning of rehabilitation which includes psychological and social adjustment and training for independent living, as well as the more traditional vocational services. The book is tightly organized into forty chapters, many of which contain glossaries of terms and sources of further information in their subject areas. Describes history, theory, and current principles and practices in areas from family counseling to work evaluation. Would be very valuable both to students, as an introduction, and to practitioners, as a reference work. Extensive bibliography included. Highly recommended for academic and special libraries.

Yuker, Harold E., and Block, J. Richard. *Challenging Barriers to Change: Attitudes Toward the Disabled*. Albertson, N.Y.: Human Resources Center, 1979. 66 pp.

Substance of keynote presentations at the annual meeting of the Canadian Rehabilitation Council in Toronto in 1977. Authors are psychology faculty at Hofstra University and research consultants to the Human Resources Center. In addition to a discussion of the nature and importance of attitudes as barriers to disabled people, the authors include comments on an informal study they conducted of the audience to whom they were speaking. Techniques for changing attitudes of people toward the disabled are presented as well. An appendix reproduces the "Attitudes towards Disabled Persons Scale", a test divised by Yuker and Block in 1957. Useful introductory treatment of its topic. Recommended for academic and rehabilitation libraries.

5 INDEPENDENT LIVING

PHYLLIS C. SELF/Health Sciences Librarian, Library of
the Health Sciences, University of Illinois, Urbana, Illinois

INTRODUCTION

The technological advancements made in the areas of medical research and bioengineering in the 1960s and 1970s have made possible new freedoms for individuals with physical disabilities and now permit even the most severely physically disabled individuals to have greater control of their lives. For example, mouth-oriented electronic devices are now being used by individuals to control movement, communication, and the environment. Yet, only a fraction of disabled individuals benefit from existing technology. The holistic health model, which emphasizes the total individual rather than the disability, goes beyond the traditional medical models of diagnosis and treatment and does much to encourage the concept of independent living within the medical profession.

The concept of independent living is based on the premises that disabled individuals have the right to make independent decisions and the right to services of the general community including counseling, job placement, transportation, attendant care, health maintenance, preventive services, recreational activities, and many other programs and services. These services are ensured by Title VII of Public Law 95-602, Rehabilitation Comprehensive

Services, and Developmental Disabilities Amendments of 1978. The purpose of the Act and its amendments was to remove barriers and obstacles and reduce an individual's dependency on the family and/or public support. As a result of such legislation a number of federally funded "Centers for Independent Living" have developed. These centers train newly disabled adults in the skills they will need to rejoin the community as full participants in spite of their disability.

The most famous of these centers is the Center for Independent Living located in Berkeley, California. An important aspect of the Berkeley Center is that many services are provided by peers who can be used as role models. The Berkeley Center has served as a model for others because of its innovative approaches including peer counseling.

The topic of independent living is extremely broad, ranging from activities of daily living, and personal care and assistive devices, to programs and services. Therefore, this chapter has been divided into three categories to cover the topic of independent living more effectively. The three categories are: "Activities of Daily Living," "Aids and Devices," and "Independent Living Programs and Facilities." The largest concentration of literature wihin each of these components is directed toward the orthopedically or mobility impaired. Because this group represents the largest portion of individuals with physical disabilities it seems only natural this fact be reflected in the literature. Most of the publications are intended to train or prepare the orthopedically and mobility impaired individual to live more independently and could be used by those individuals, their family, and/or therapists. Several are directed toward children but the majority are to assist the physically disabled adult. The bibliography does include books aimed at visually impaired persons, hearing impaired persons, one-handers, arthritic patients, disabled homemakers, and attendants, although there are only a few in each of these areas. The reader is encouraged to use the chapter in its entirety because there are many publications that deal with two and sometimes three of these components. Such titles were placed in the area of their primary concentration as expressed in the author's introduction. The reader should use the same approach and use related chapters such "Physical Education, Recreation, and Travel," "Health Education", and the specific physical disabilities: "Mobility Impairments and Barrier Free Design," "Blindness and Visual Impairment," and "Deafness and Hearing Impairment."

The complexity of problems posed by physical disabilities makes even the most simple task seem insurmountable. Therefore, solutions and "how-to" information to assist individuals in their daily living needs and methods to conserve energy are essential. These activities represent psychologically the most important activities for persons with physical disabilities endeavoring to gain independence. Within the category "Activities of Daily Living" much of the material cited is in the format of manuals and guides providing "how-to" information. The largest number of publications in this category is in personal management which includes hygiene, grooming, child care, and the social graces. Most of the publications are directed toward the mobility impaired but there are three very good publications available to assist the visually impaired in their personal management. In 1974 the American Foundation for the Blind published two such guides: A Step-by-Step Guide to Personal Management for Blind Persons and Anne Yeadon's Toward Independence. Although both books describe many of the same activities, the purpose of Toward Independence is to introduce the "use of instructional objectives in the teaching of severely visually impaired persons" and as such is specifically directed toward educators. Lieberman's Daily Living Skills: A Manual for Educating Visually Impaired Students, a two-volume publication, is much more comprehensive than the other two and includes sports activities, care of pets, budget concepts, and many other activities which are not described in the above mentioned publications. Although this is an excellent manual and is available through Educational Resources Information Center (ERIC), some users may find it difficult to read because it is reproduced from microfiche. All of these publications lack illustrations which is a recurring phenomenon within the visual impairment literature.

Another area which has received attention is clothing for the handicapped. Clothing is essential to an individual's well-being and sense of dignity and worth and has a tremendous effect on how people feel about themselves. The kinds of clothing which meet fashion trends and the individual's functional requirements, contribute to a physically disabled person's social and psychological adjustment. Both Bowar's Clothing for the Handicapped and Kernaleguen's Clothing Designs for the Handicapped are excellent resources for the seamstress. Illustrations and instructions are useful and physically the books are easy to use while working at the sewing machine. Kernaleguen includes many more designs for such items as knapsack bags, walker carry-alls, belt pockets, wash bags and mits. Macartney's Clothes Sense is useful because of its illustrations and use of dressing techniques and aids which are seldom described as well in other books on this subject.

Many publications have been written on such topics as adapting clothing, dressing, personal management and eating, but only a few publications have been written on the subjects of furniture and home mechanics for which there is a great need. Utrup's Home Mechanics for the Visually Impaired, developed in response to teaching a home mechanics course at the Michigan Rehabilitation Center for the Blind is an extremely useful teaching manual to instruct the visually impaired in basic home repairs and maintenance.

Although reference books and bibliogrphies have not been included in this chapter one very fine publication which should not be overlooked and covers both physical and mental disability is Rehabilitation for Independent Living: a selected bibliography,

INDEPENDENT LIVING   111

1982. It is published by the President's Committee on Employment of the Handicapped and can be obtained from the Superintendent of Documents, U.S. Government Printing Office, Washington, D.C. 20402. Although it is not an all inclusive bibliography, it does list books, pamphlets, and films which should be in any independent living collection.

The category "Aids and Devices" is extremely informative because most of us are totally unfamiliar with the aids and appliances used by the disabled. The largest concentration of literature within this category is again directed toward individuals who are mobility impaired with most of the material discussing the various assistive devices involved in lifting and transporting the individual and performing activities of daily living. Prosthetic devices have been excluded from this literature guide.

Most of the publications are devoted to assisting the adolescent or adult with only a very few intended to assist the developing child (see **Chapter 12, the Disabled Child**). Ruth B. Hofmann's How to Build Special Furniture and Equipment for Handicapped Children is an excellent resource for both the family of a disabled child and for staff in a children's rehabilitation center. It is beautifully illustrated and provides explicit instructions on how-to construct tables, chairs, and other pieces of furniture from scraps of wood. Another publication that provides how-to build information is Bergen's Selected Equipment for Pediatric Rehabilitation. This book describes equipment designed and/or modified by therapists at Blythedale Children's Hospital in Valhalla, New York. The value of this publication is its description of the problems and solutions to which the equipment and therapy is intended. Both Aids for Children and Equipment for the Disabled: Disabled Child are catalogs and lists of equipment which are commercially available.

The next largest area of literature within this category deals with the technological advances and devices for communication and education of the deaf, visually impaired, and mobility impaired. LaRocca and Turem in The Application of Technological Developments to Physically Disabled People provide an excellent overview of technology and its effects on physically disabled people. The research forming the basis for this publication was funded by the National Science Foundation and as such consumer awareness and advocacy groups will find this book extremely useful because of its authenticity and frankness.

Few publications discuss medical devices and equipment and even fewer discuss the equipment industry. Clearfield's Medical Devices and Equipment for the Disabled, examines the products used by disabled consumers through a discussion of actual case studies. It provides an excellent overview of a very lucrative medical equipment industry from a consumer protection viewpoint.

The best collection of materials in the category "Aids and Devices" is the eleven volume series entitled, "Equipment for the Disabled." Topic covered include: communication, clothing, home management, outdoor transport, wheelchairs, leisure and gardening, personal care, housing and furniture, hoists and walking aids, and the disabled child. The entire series is well-illustrated and well-organized. Unfortunately, it is limited to British manufactured products which may not be available in the United States and may be difficult to obtain.

Other topics in which literature exists within this category deal with clothing, personal care, hand controls for driving, exercise, and leisure. Although all the publications cited within this category are intended to be used by occupational and physical therapists, educators and staff members at rehabilitation centers, many items would be useful to individuals with physical disabilities as well as their family and friends.

A goal of most parents is to develop independence in their children. But to accomplish this task with disabled children is difficult. Disabled children present special needs and represent a very small potential market for the production of technological devices to overcome their educational and functional needs which

INDEPENDENT LIVING   113

invariably hinders the production of technological devices. Therefore, more publications in this area would be extremely valuable for children who are developing their independence as well as counselors and therapists working with parents who are adjusting to their child's needs for independence.

The third and final category of this chapter, "Independent Living - Programs and Facilities" is devoted to those materials describing the development and management of independent living programs and other programs or centers which would assist an individual with physical disabilities to live a more independent life. The best introductions to independent living are Cole's New Options and her New Options Training Manual. She describes the independent living program at New Options Transitional Living Project in Houston, Texas and outlines eleven training modules in the program. Both of these publications would be useful to severely disabled persons wanting placement in and to rehabilitation professionals searching for model independent living programs.

In contrast to New Options which describes a particular independent living program, Susan Pflueger's Independent Living serves as a review of independent living services. Because it contains reports of programs in California, Massachusetts, Texas, and Colorado, it is useful for the purpose of comparison for individuals establishing independent living programs and individuals desiring to be consumers of such programs. For a more global view of independent living Living Independently: Three Views of the European Experience with Implications for the United States, edited by Jean A. Cole, provides excellent descriptions of european service programs by experts in the field: Lex and Joyce Frieden and Gini Laurie.

A number of publications, such as Frieden's ILRU Source Book: A Technical Assistance Manual on Independent Living exist to assist administrators in developing and operating independent living programs for the blind and mobility impaired, but only a few publications such as Carnell's Development, Management and Evaluation of Community Speech and Hearing Centers are directed toward the hearing impaired. It is intended to assist individuality in establishing a community speech and hearing center and to encourage improvement in currently existing centers. Fishler's Development of Work Programs for the Multihandicapped, is a useful "how-to" manual on planning, organizing, and operating an industrial oriented work activities center for the severly disabled adult whereas Rehabilitation Centers for the Blind and Visually Impaired: the State of the Art was produced in response to the many developments and changes in working with the visually impaired. This report published by the American Foundation for the Blind discusses the goals, services, financing, and evaluations of rehabilitation centers for the visually impaired.

Included within this category are publications dealing with behaviors, skills, and standards necessary for disabled persons within independent living programs as well as for training rehabilitation personnel. Kathy M. Walton, et. al. in Independent Living Techniques and Concepts: Level of Use vs. Importance to Independent Living as Perceived by Professionals in Rehabilitation provides insight into the gap which exists between the levels at which these techniques and concepts are used in the field. Only when the gap is closed will professionals be better trained and respond to the needs of the physically disabled in their quest for independence.

The movement for independent living, which has grown since the passage of Public Law 95-602, has made significant contributions to the lives of physically disabled individuals as reflected by the changing nature of literature in this area. Two very important thoughts which are repeatedly emphasized are independent living is a process not a place and disabled people have the right to choose -- to make their own decisions. This process involves learning activities of daily living and using aids and devices appropriate to individual needs. These provide the framework by which physically disabled individuals can exercise their right of freedom of choice in the pursuit of their individual life styles.

ANNOTATED BIBLIOGRAPHY:
Activities of Daily Living

American Foundation for the Blind. <u>A Step-by-Step Guide to Personal Management for Blind Persons</u>. 2d ed. New York: American Foundation for the Blind, 1974. 120 pp.

Now in its second edition this guide is a result of collaborative thinking and experience of a large number of people from diverse backgrounds across the country. This workbook is designed to be useful to blind persons, their family and instructors. It covers all aspects of personal management including hygiene, grooming, clothing, homemaking and home repair, child care and the social graces. Each item discussed includes an orientation to the topic, the technique and equipment to be used, and helpful hints. The lack of illustrations limits the usefulness of this publication, but it contains an excellent list of references to guide the user to other sources. Recommended for home economics and rehabilitation collections and public libraries.

Andersen, Vincent W. <u>Exercises and Self-Care Activities for Quadriplegic People</u>. n.p.: Artistocrat Publishers, 1976. 143 pp.

This manual is written for the quadriplegic patient desiring to follow a "self-rehabilitation" program as well as for professionals working with quadriplegics. It contains descriptive as well as pictorial information of exercises, devices, and techniques for physical rehabilitation. Chapters and exercises are arranged to follow the average progression of rehabilitation. It is well-illustrated and appears to be an excellent resource. Recommended for public and medical libraries.

Anderson, Hoyt. <u>The Disabled Homemaker</u>. Springfield, Ill.: Charles C. Thomas, 1981. 343 pp.

Although this book is written for disabled individuals, it would be useful as a training aid for professionals working with individuals who are wanting to lead more independent lives. It includes an excellent Living Skills Profile for which disabled persons can analyze their own abilities to live independently. The book provides practical advice and techniques for cooking, cleaning, childcare, adapting clothing, furniture, and many other activities.

It contains many fine illustrations and recent photographs which make this a most appealing publication to todays disabled population than many of its predecessors. It concludes with

Appendices to Clothing Suppliers and Manufacturers, Distributors, and Resources useful to disabled people, an excellent list of Suggested Readings, and an Index. An excellent addition to any public library or independent living collection.

Arthritis Foundation. <u>Self-Help Manual for Patients With Arthritis</u>. 2d ed. Atlanta: Arthritis Foundation, 1980. 246 pp.

This manual would be useful for people with various types and in various stages of arthritis. It is based on the two principles of conserving energy and protecting joints and describes how to perform certain activities with or without the use of devices. It is extremely well-written, illustrated, and up-to-date. The authors have included price and source information for materials they have described and bibliographies for further reading. The manual includes a list of helpful agencies and organizations and periodicals in the field of arthritis. It is a must for anyone afflicted with arthritis. Recommended for rehabilitation collections.

Baker, Bruce L.; Brightman, Alan J.; Heifetz, Louis J.; and Murphy, Diane M. <u>Toilet Training</u>. Champaign, Ill.: Research Press 1977. 83 pp.

Another excellent manual in the "Skills Training Series for Children With Special Needs." It identifies and describes the very basic and necessary steps to toilet training and emphasizes the importance in record-keeping. The manual is well-organized, easy to use, and effectively illustrated. Would be useful to parents and trainers of parents. Recommended for public and medical libraries.

Baron, Henrietta. <u>Everybody Can Cook: Techniques for the Handicapped V. 1 Breakfast (Student Manual)</u>. <u>Everybody Can Cook Techniques for the Handicapped V. 1 Breakfast (Teacher Manual)</u>. Seattle: Special Child Publications, 1977. 190 pp.

"This course of study is a procedural, step-by-step lesson plan for teachers of home economics for the orthopedically handicapped and retarded." The author has developed a course that is more than a list of recipes but a guide to selecting and preparing nutritional meals, setting an attractive table, and cleaning a kitchen. Both the student and the teacher's manuals are well-illustrated and are excellent reference books. The teacher's manual can be easily adapted by home economists to work on a specific technique or skill by using the Index of Tools and Processes. Each recipe includes the objectives of the lesson, the teaching techniques to be employed, the tools needed, the food content, and illustrations. This work can be useful to family and friends of orthopedic disabled individuals. It is an excellent resource. Recommended for home economic and rehabilitation collections. Volumes 2 and 3 do not appear to be published at this time, according to <u>Books in Print</u>.

INDEPENDENT LIVING 117

Beasley, Mary Catherine; Burns, Dorothy; and Weiss, Janis. <u>Adapt Your Own: A Clothing Brochure for People With Special Needs</u>. Tuscaloosa: University of Alabama, 1977. 14 pp.

    This brochure suggests ways of adapting clothing for specific handicapping conditions and lists features to consider when purchasing clothing to be adapted. It is well-organized, easy to use, contains good illustrations and an excellent list of additional references on this subject. The brochure should be useful to people with handicaps, their families and those professionals who work with them. Recommended for home economic and rehabilitation collections.

Blakeslee, Mary E. <u>The Wheelchair Gourmet: A Cookbook for the Disabled</u>. New York: Beaufort Books, Inc., 1981. 219 pp.

    Written in a humorous style this cookbook gives pragmatic and useful information for the wheelchair cook. It provides helpful hints in organizing a kitchen and recipes for quick, simple, but good tasting foods. Recipes are divided by sections dealing with specific appliances: blender, microwave oven, wok, slow-cooker, electric mixer, food processor, electric skillet, and toaster oven and is subdivided by appetizers, breakfast foods, soups, salads, vegetables, main dishes and desserts. The author emphasizes the importance of finding recipes that suit the cook's needs rather than making cooking a drag. "You can always find another recipe that's just as good and far easier than the one that sentences you to six hours of hard labor over a hot wok." Recommended for public libraries and home economic and rehabilitation collections.

Bowar, Miriam T. <u>Clothing for the Handicapped: Fashion Adaptations for Adults and Children</u>. Minneapolis: Sister Kenny Institute, 1978. 45 pp.

    "...this book suggests methods for adapting regular patterns and clothing...to accomodate orthopedic appliances or allow for physical deformities." It discusses fabric selection and lists companies producing functionally designed clothing and patterns for adaptive clothing. Useful to individuals with handicapping conditions, their family, and professionals working with disabled individuals and anyone involved with adapting clothing for the handicapped. The illustrations are excellent and make this a most useful resource for the seamstress. Recommended for public libraries and home economic collections.

Brattstrom, Merete. <u>Principles of Joint Protection in Chronic Rheumatic Disease</u>. Sweden: Studentlitteratur, 1973. 111 pp.

    Although this book is intended primarily for physicians, physical therapists, and occupational therapists working with patients with chronic rheumatoid arthritis, it can be quite useful to the patient. It contains excellent photographs which are arranged on a wrong-right basis. This book includes a basic explanation of the disease process, the genesis of deformities, and presentation of special rehabilitation problems. An excellent resource because it describes how to perform certain activities and identifies aids and devices to make life easier for the arthritic. Recommended for public and medical libraries.

California. Department of Public Health. Leisure Time Activities for Deaf-Blind Children. Northridge, Calif.: Joyce Motion Picture Co., 1974. 122 pp.

Although this manual is designed for relatives and friends of deaf-blind children, it would be useful to occupational and physical therapy students. The title is somewhat misleading as at least one-third of the book is devoted to activities of daily living such as eating, grooming, and dressing. Information is clearly displayed and easy to understand. Contains many illustrations and overall is a valuable resource. For each activity the purpose, necessary materials, procedures, observed behaviors, and desired behaviors are geared to give the parents a better understanding of the usefulness of the activity. Recommended for public libraries and rehabilitation collections.

Consumer's Association. Coping With Disablement. Rev. ed. London: Consumers' Association, 1976. 239 pp.

Although this monograph is published in Britain, it's usefulness is not limited to that country. It deals specifically with overcoming problems of daily living and does not offer solutions to the emotional and psychological aspects of becoming disabled. This book covers common problems, such as: sitting, walking, housework, cooking and eating, sex, and driving using special devices. The book would be most useful to recently disabled individuals or members of their family. It is well-indexed, appropriately illustrated, and easy to use. Recommended for public libraries and rehabilitation collections.

Danzig, Aaron. Handbook for One-Handers. New York: Federation of the Handicapped, 1975. 56 pp.

This handbook provides practical suggestions for accomplishing essential activities of daily living. Readers are advised that the handbook is not a substitute for a sound rehabilitation program. This manual covers the mechanical problems facing the one-hander as well as the psychological adjustment to the disability. It is written for the one-hander although it would be useful to physical and occupational therapists and family members as well. It contains very few illustrations. It is not intended to be a scholarly work but a "how to" manual. Recommended for public libraries and rehabilitation collections.

Dong, Collin H. and Banks, Jane. The Arthritic's Cookbook. New York: Bantam Books, 1973. 197 pp.

The author, an arthritic, provides an empirical method of treatment for arthritis. "The primary concept of this regieme is to consume only the basic necessary foods instead of loading the body with extras it can't handle." The diet consists of seafood, chicken and vegetables. The book contains 238 recipes to appetizers, soups, salads, breads and desserts. The book makes no claim to cure arthritis but rather how to live with it. The recipes call for readily available ingredients and are easy to follow. No one not even the arthritic could go wrong following such a diet program. Appropriate for a public library but is not a must to any collection.

Foott, Sydney, ed. Kitchen Sense for Disabled People of All Ages. London: Heinemann Medical for the Disabled Living Foundation, 1975. 218 pp.

This book was written as a result of a book Mealtime Manual for the Aged and Handicapped which was unuseable in England because of different equipment, foods, climate and eating habits. This book is intended for the disabled housewife whether male or female. Although this publication is British and requires conversion of measurement, it is well-illustrated and quite useful. The book covers: arrangement of the kitchen, equipping the kitchen, diet and menus, solutions to cooking, recipes, shopping techniques and sources of advice and help. Recommended for home economic and rehabilitation collections and public libraries.

Ford, Jack R., and Duckworth, Bridget. Physical Management for the Quadriplegic Patient. Philadelphia: F.A. Davis Company, 1974. 392 pp.

This manual is written for paramedic students, nurses and therapists working with traumatic quadriplegic patients. It provides detailed information and illustrations on the physical methods of self-care successfully used at the G.F. Strong Rehabilitation Centre, Vancouver, British Columbia, Canada. Topics which are addressed include wheelchair mobility and propelling, bed mobility and transfers, toilet transfers, bathing, dressing, bowel and bladder management, holding and manipulating, car transfers and driver training, housing, vocation, and recreation. It is well-organized and illustrated and would be extremely useful to student therapists and disabled individuals or the families of recently disabled individuals. Recommended for medical public libraries.

Gallender, Demos. Eating Handicaps: Illustrated Techniques for Feeding Disorders. Springfield, Ill.: Charles C. Thomas, 1979. 196 pp.

This is the only substantive work in the area of eating handicaps and is primarily useful to physical, occupation, and speech therapists. It is divided into two parts. Part I discusses the anatomy and physiology of the muscular, skeletal, and nervous structure involved in eating; Part II discusses the techniques and instructional materials for particular eating difficulties. The book is well-written, easy to understand, and would be quite useful to the concerned parent. Recommended for academic libraries and rehabilitation collections.

Gallender, Demos. <u>Teaching Eating and Toileting Skills to the Multi-Handicapped in the School Setting</u>. Springfield, Ill.: Charles C. Thomas, 1980. 355 pp.

    The purpose of this book is to provide a systematized approach to working with individuals having eating handicaps and/or lacking toileting skills. Multi-handicapped, as used in this book means individuals with major mental, physical and social limitations. "Mentally these students are generally classified as severely or profoundly retarded." Although the book is primarily aimed at school administrators, teachers, and health care personnel, it could be useful to many parents of multi-handicapped children. It appears to be best suited as a college text. Topics covered include a brief history of the handicapped, parents' expectations, role of the school, and physiological processes of eating and toileting. Recommended for academic libraries and rehabilitation collections.

Hoffman, Adeline M. <u>Clothing for the Handicapped, the Aged, and other People with Special Needs</u>. Springfield, Ill.: Charles C. Thomas, 1979. 192 pp.

    Attempts to cover the waterfront of clothing needs for the handicapped and aged, giving an overview of rehabilitation, description of handicaps, and clothing needs. It is <u>not</u> intended to be a "how to" book and for that reason is more useful to home economics, special education, physical and occupational therapy classes rather than to the physically disabled themselves or their families. Contains an excellent bibliography, appendices, and index, but <u>very few</u> illustrations. Recommended for home economic and rehabilitation collections.

Hotte, Eleanor Boettke. <u>Self-Help Clothing for Children Who Have Physical Disabilities</u>. Rev. ed. Chicago: National Easter Seal Society for Crippled Children and Adults, 1979. 64 pp.

    This booklet is intended for parents of physically disabled children. It is the only book which deals solely with the needs of the disabled child. The booklet not only discusses the child's clothing needs, sizing, and fabrics, but discusses the need for training the child by whom and when. Contains excellent illustrations and many helpful hints to alter ready made clothes. Is not particularly useful to a seamstress except for examples of alterations. Recommended for rehabilitation collections and public libraries.

Illinois Department of Children and Family Services. Homemaking Manual: A Reference Manual for Rehabilitation Teachers. Kalamazoo, Mich.: Western Michigan University, 1980. 43 pp.

The manual was designed for teachers "by providing her with proven techniques adapted to use by the blind homemaker..." The material has been tested and revised and should be quite useful to anyone teaching the blind homemaker. The manual is well-organized and very easy to use. It covers personal care, identification of personal and household items, cleaning, laundering, cooking, and household record keeping. Recommended for rehabilitation and home economic collections.

Jay, Peggy E. Help Yourselves: A Handbook for Hemiplegics and Their Families. 3rd ed. Hornchurch, Essex: Ian Henry, 1979. 158 pp.

Although the author describes the book as divided into four parts, it is not readily evident to the reader. The four parts include activities of daily living, working in the home, employment and recreation, and various problems associated with speech, perception, personality and sex. Its usefulness is its specificity to hemiplegies, although many of the other books in this chapter provide much the same information. It contains illustrations but again not as many as most books do. This spiral bound manual would be most useful to the individual recently disabled and to other individuals having limited experiences in the field of rehabilitation. It is useful but not a must to a rehabilitation collection.

Kernaleguen, Anne. Clothing Designs for the Handicapped. Edmonton, Alberta: University of Alberta Press, 1978. 271 pp.

"This publication is geared toward the average home sewer who can follow directions and operate a sewing machine." Discusses general information on: 1) clothing by special groups, 2) textiles, and 3) sewing instructions. Illustrates how to modify clothes and patterns, and sew miscellaneous items; such as a car slide, carrying bag for wheelchair, top tray, and for putting on socks and many other items. It contains a good bibliography on clothing for special needs and excellent illustrations. Its special binding makes it easy to refer to while sewing. This is an excellent "how-to" book. Recommended for public libraries and home economic collections.

Klinger, Judith Lannefeld. Mealtime Manual for People With Disabilities and the Aging. 2d ed. Camden, N.J.: Campbell Soup Company, 1978. 269 pp.

This easy-to-use manual is designed for individuals with physical disabilities. While it is not written for professionals, it would be quite useful to the student or novice in the field of rehabilitation. The hints for the homemaker section offer excellent advice arranging information by physical disability. It contains practical information on such things as planning, storing, selecting appliances, entertaining, and menu planning. The recipe section includes techniques for handling containers, measuring, cooking, and serving. The illustrations are both excellent and plentiful. The manual includes sources and addresses for equipment and tools which would be useful to both disabled individuals and professionals working in this field. Recommended for rehabilitation collections and public libraries.

Lawton, Edith Buchwald. Activities of Daily Living for Physical Rehabilitation. New York: McGraw-Hill Book Company, 1963. 301 pp.

The emphasis of this book is to serve as a reference for physicians, therapists, nurses, and other rehabilitation workers and as a basis for standardizing teaching and testing in the activities of daily living. The author demonstrates different techniques for the same activity carried out by various patients with the same and different disability. References are made to the author's earlier publication Physical Rehabilitation for Daily Living. It is extremely well-illustrated and contains an index and reading list. Although the publication is old and the reading list is outdated, the major portion of the book--the how-to-do various activities--remains to be useful. Recommended for rehabilitation collections, and medical and public libraries.

Lawton, Edith Buchwald. A.D.L.: Activities of Daily Living Test A New Form. Rehabilitation Monograph No. 57. New York: New York University Medical Center, Institute of Rehabilitation Medicine, 1979. 30 pp.

This booklet was designed for a one-day workshop for nurses entitled "Help the Patient Help Himself" to demonstrate evaluation of daily activities. It is the author's hope that this test be not only part of the rehabilitation program but also part of a nursing care program in a general hospital for patients with or without a disability. Activities of daily living are divided into: 1) bed activities, 2) wheelchair activities, 3) self-care activities, and 4) ambulation and traveling activities. The booklet is useful because it includes a test and examples of grading independence. Useful only to personnel evaluating activities of daily living. This publication is not a must for most libraries, but medical librarians may wish to consider it for purchase and it is recommended for rehabilitation collections.

Lieberman, Gail, ed. Daily Living Skills: (A Manual for Educating Visually Impaired Students). Springfield, Ill.: Illinois State Office of the Superintendent of Public Instruction, 1974. 2 vols.

This manual is intended to be used by parents or educators teaching activities of daily living to visually impaired children. Four areas are discussed in detail: recreational skills; practical skills; self-care skills; and social skills.

Suggestions are given with regard to age levels, objectives, instructional methods, and required materials. It is a useful publication, but is difficult to read the photocopied pages of this ERIC document and it also lacks an index. Recommended for rehabilitation collections.

Macartney, Patricia. <u>Clothes Sense: For Handicapped Adults of All Ages</u>. London: Disabled Living Foundation, 1973. 147 pp.

Although a British publication, the text is an excellent source of information for the disabled person, family, and friends. It covers the concept of clothing selection by discussing fashion versus fabrics and function. Other chapters deal with dressing techniques and aids, alterations and renovations, types of clothing, and storage. The book is extremely well-organized, provides excellent illustrations, and includes a good index and appendices to assist the user in identifying additional sources of information. This is one of the best books on the subject. Recommended for public libraries and home economic collections.

May, Elizabeth Eckhardt; Waggoner, Neva R.; and Hotte, Eleanor Boettke. <u>Independent Living for the Handicapped and the Elderly</u>. Boston: Houghton Mifflin Company, 1974. 271 pp.

A very useful how-to book for physically disabled individuals and for professional personnel in the fields of home management, rehabilitation, and child development. The work simplification techniques and principles described are useful to virtually everyone. The illustrations are in black and white and are quite old which may annoy many readers even though the written information is excellent. A new edition of this publication would be a valuable addition to any public or home economics library.

Read, Ralph. <u>When the Cook Can't Look: A Cooking Handbook for the Blind and Visually Impaired</u>. New York: Continuum, 1981. 113 pp.

The book is intended to be read aloud to individuals who are blind or visually impaired. The technique to food preparation is the central concept of the book not the recipes. The chapter entitled "For the Sighted Reader" provides many helpful suggestions on how to work with a visually impaired person. The remaining chapters are devoted to kitchen inventories, techniques for arranging, opening containers, pouring, measuring, timing, peeling, serving, cleaning, recipes and many other useful items. The Table of Contents must be used as the index to locate specific recipes and techniques, no other index exists. Recommended for public libraries and home economic collections.

Ryan, Mary. <u>Feeding Can Be Fun: Advice on Feeding Handicapped Babies and Children</u>. London: The Spastics Society, n.d. 24 pp.

This booklet deals with the feeding problems of the cerebral palsied child. It is intended for parents, health visitors, houseparents, therapists, and others associated with the daily management of handicapped children. The author emphasizes that "the child who achieves good control of his mouth for eating will be laying the foundations for speech." Topics covered include feeding, early sounds, weaning assisted feeding, independent feeding, and equipment. This is the only booklet on this subject yet identified which is aimed at parents or the layperson. Recommended for rehabilitation collections.

Sister Kenny Institute. Departments of Occupational Therapy and Nursing Education. <u>Self-Care For the Hemiplegic</u>. Rev. ed. Minneapolis: Sister Kenny Institute, 1977. 26 pp.

This booklet discussed problems common to patients with hemiplegia and teaching the hemiplegic patient activities of daily living. It covers eating, personal hygiene, dressing, and support for the involved arm. Although it is written for the health professional, this book would be useful to patients and their families. Even though it contains no index, it is easy to use and remains to be useful even with a publication date of 1970. Recommended for rehabilitation collections and public libraries.

Strebel, Miriam Bowar. <u>Adaptions and Techniques for the Disabled Homemaker</u>. Rehabilitation Monograph No. 710. 5th ed. Minneapolis: Sister Kenny Institute, 1978. 38 pp.

"A compilation of many adaptive techniques and equipment available to the disabled homemaker." The author stresses the need to evaluate the appropriateness of the aid to each individual person. Areas discussed include: work and storage areas, planning a kitchen, selecting appliances, kitchen techniques, food preparation, and general household tasks. This publication is extremely well-illustrated. The author has assisted the reader by giving the company an address from which equipment can be purchased. Recommended for public libraries and home economic and rehabilitation collections.

Utrup, Robert G. <u>Home Mechanics for the Visually Impaired</u>. Kalamazoo, Mich.: Graduate College, Western Michigan University, 1974. 96 pp.

This manual was developed in response to teaching a home mechanics course at the Michigan Rehabilitation Center for the Blind. It contains 17 lessons covering such things as: cleaning drains, faucet repairs, hand sanding, and painting, etc. The lessons are divided into six areas: the lesson, materials, tactual aids, questions and answers, procedure and safety. It is a very well-organized well-referenced and well-planned teaching manual. It would be useful to anyone developing a course for home mechanics. Recommended for vocational education and rehabilitation collections and public libraries.

Wehrum, Mary E. Techniques of Daily Living: A Curriculum Guide. Pittsburgh: Davis & Warde, Inc., 1977. 97 pp.

This curriculum guide provides the instructional outline currently employed in developing the teaching-learning strategy of the Techniques of Daily Living course at the Greater Pittsburgh Guild for the Blind. It is to be used by the instructor developing such a program for a particular blind person. Suggested learning experiences, procedures, and evaluation experiences are given for each objective. The guide is extremely easy to use and helpful and covers the areas of: table orientation and eating skills, personal grooming, special needs, and shopping and marketing. It is a useful source for professional trainers, attendant care personnel, and family members of blind individuals. Recommended for academic libraries and rehabilitation collections.

Widerberg, Lloyd C. and Kaarlela, Ruth. Techniques for Eating: A Guide for Blind Persons. Kalamazoo, Mich.: Western Michigan University, 1977. 10 pp.

As the title indicates this booklet is to be used by individuals teaching blind persons to eat. It contains no illustrations but in outline format lists techniques which should be employed by the blind individual. Techniques covered include: approaching the table, cutting meat with a fork, cutting meat with a knife, cutting a lettuce salad, pouring cream, salt and pepper and others. Should be useful to the novice teacher of blind persons. The Table of Contents tends to suffice in serving as an index. Recommended for a rehabilitation collection.

Yeadon, Anne. Toward Independence: The Use of Instructional Objectives in Teaching Daily Living Skills to the Blind. New York: American Foundation for the Blind, 1974. 96 pp.

"This book is an introduction to the use of instructional objectives in the teaching of severely visually impaired persons." The author demonstrates the methodology by using daily living skills and encourages the user to adapt this methodology to other subjects. Although the intent is to teach the methodology, the book would be quite useful to rehabilitation personnel involved in teaching activities of daily living to the blind. It is a very well-organized and easy to use publication. Recommended for rehabilitation collections and social science libraries.

Yost, Anna Cathryn; Schroeder, Stella L.; and Rainey, Carolyn. Home Economics Rehabilitation: A Selected, Annotated Bibliography. Columbia, Mo.: University of Missouri, 1977. 107 pp.

This bibliography includes home economic rehabilitation material available to the authors in July 1977. The scope of the material is limited to problems of adults. The bibliography is annotated and includes, books, audiovisual materials, Master's thesis, Doctor's dissertations, and pamphlets.

It is extremely easy to use and includes a list of publishers' addresses. It would be useful to students studying rehabilitation, physically disabled individuals and their families, and home economists. Recommended for academic and public libraries.

ANNOTATED BIBLIOGRAPHY:
Aids and Devices

Aids for Children: Technical Aids for Physically Handicapped Children. Sweden: ICTA Information Centre, 1972. 87 pp.

Although this publication is now over a decade old, it remains to be useful as a guide to the various aids available to handicapped children. This catalog is extremely well-illustrated, includes excellent descriptions for each device and gives manufacturer/supplier information. It would be useful to physiotherapists, occupational therapists and family members working with physically disabled children. This catalog represents the international work of various centers around the world, the International Cerebral Palsy Society and was financially supported by the Swedish government. Recommended for rehabilitation collections.

American Automobile Association. The Handicapped Driver's Mobility Guide. 2d ed. Falls Church, Va.: American Automobile Association, 1978. 78 pp.

For an evaluation of this work, see Chapter 11.

American Foundation for the Blind. International Guide to Aids And Appliances for Blind and Visually Impaired Persons. 2d ed. New York: American Foundation for the Blind, 1977. 255 pp.

This guide is a listing of 1500 devices of 270 distributors from 28 countries. It would be useful to the visually impaired person and professional working in this area as a means to identify manufactured devices which can be purchased for use in the home, on the job or in school. For those individuals in research, development or marketing the guide is useful in identifying products which are available. The devices are arranged by broad subject headings and cover such topics as Braille writing aids; sound equipment; clocks, timers, watches; orientation and mobility aids; and occupational aids. Each listing includes the distributor and address, the model number, and description. The guide includes a list of "Sources of Aids and Appliances," arranged alphabetically by country, and an index of "Devices." Recommended for rehabilitation collections.

Arkansas Rehabilitation Research and Training Center. Hot Springs Rehabilitation Center. Assistive Devices and Equipment for

Rehabilitation. Hot Springs, Ark.: Arkansas Rehabilitation Center, 1971. 63 pp.

A "visual catalog" of assistive devices and equipment. Some are original devices or modifications and some have been known for years. The catalog gives purpose, variations, source, and illustration for each device and would be useful to the physically disabled and their family and to professionals serving this population. Recommended for rehabilitation collections.

Bergen, Adrienne. Selected Equipment for Pediatric Rehabilitation. Valhalla, N.Y.: Blythedale Children's Hospital, 1974. 53 pp.

The equipment described in this publication was "designed and/or modified by therapists at Blythedale Children's Hospital." The purpose of and the use of this equipment is to achieve maximum function with minimal abnormal movement and to improve muscle tone and encourage more normal movement. "The equipment is not meant to replace good therapy, but to assist in the carry over of goals into all areas of daily living." Although the items were designed for use in the hospital setting, they can easily be constructed for home use. The author describes the problem, solution, and construction for each piece of equipment. The book is well-illustrated and would be useful to any parent or therapist working with physically disabled children. Recommended for medical libraries and rehabilitation collections.

The Chartered Society of Physiotherapy. Handling the Handicapped: A Guide to the Lifting and Movement of Disabled People. New York: Springer Publishing Company, 1975. 136 pp.

This guide discusses assessing the situation, rules and mechanical principles, general mobility, hoists and beds, and wheelchairs. Although it is a British publication, most all of the information is useful to an American who may wish to use another source for addresses to organizations and suppliers. Contains many fine illustrations and an index. Useful for professionals and family members of disabled persons. Recommended for rehabilitation collections.

Clark, Leslie L., ed. Proceedings of the International Congress on Technology and Blindness, New York, 1962. 2d ed. 4 vols. New York: The American Foundation for the Blind, 1963. 152 pp.

These four volumes are the results of papers and discussions of the International Congress on Technology and Blindness held in New York City in 1962. Many national, international, and private organizations were involved with the production of this work. Volume 1 deals with relationships of man and machine in the application of powers of the visually impaired. Volume 2 explores the sensory loss of the visually impaired. Volume 3 discusses the practiced applications of technology for the visually impaired.

Volume 4 is a catalog of technical devices available from over the world.

These books would be useful to any researcher working with visually impaired individuals. Articles are generally well-refererenced and illustrated. Each of volumes 1-3 are indexed. Volume 4 would be easier to use if it were also indexed. Recommended for academic libraries.

Clearfield, Daniel. Medical Devices and Equipment for the Disabled: An Examination. Washington, D.C.: Disability Rights Center, 1976. 54 pp.

This report examines the products used by individuals who are wheelchair users, mastectomy patients, and those with lung diseases. The purpose of this investigation was to examine the manufacture, design, sale, and use of selected medical devices and provide some direction for future investigations. The report includes general industry information and federal regulations and solutions and proposals for change on these medical devices. The appendices include the results of a wheelchair user survey distributed to the Capital Chapter of the National Paraplegia Foundation and a Breast Prosthesis User Survey distributed by the Reach to Recovery Program of the American Cancer Society, Washington, D.C. Chapter. This report provides an excellent overview of a very lucrative medical equipment industry which has the advantage of a captive consumer group and a third party reimbursement system.

This publication would be useful to advocacy groups, disabled individuals and anyone studying the medical equipment industry. It is well-researched and very easy to read and understand. Recommended for medical and academic libraries and rehabilitation collections.

Copeland, Keith, ed. Aids for the Severely Handicapped. New York: Grune & Stratton, 1974. 152 pp.

This publication is the result of a symposium held in 1972 by the Biological Engineering Society in association with the Committee on Research for Aids for the Disabled (CRAD) The purpose was to bring together designers and users of remote-control devices in Britain. The papers of that symposium have been supplemented and updated by eleven further contributions and now is international in scope

The book deals with communication and environmental control systems for the severely disabled individual. Each chapter discusses the technical descriptions of systems, and provides information on the needs of disabled persons and the how-to equip a patient with a particular system. Because of its technical nature it would be most useful to individuals in the field of bioengineering. Recommended for academic and engineering libraries.

Davis, Wendy, M. Aids to Make You Able. New York: Beaufort Books, 1981. 155 pp.

This simple but effective spiral bound publication will be useful to a wide variety of audiences including occupational therapists, visiting nurses, attendant care personnel, and handicapped individuals and their family. Its coverage of aids and devices is quite limited but does include the more widely used devices and for that reason this publication will be more useful to individuals new in this area. The devices are well-illustrated and the cartoons add a certain degree of humor and illustrate some difficult situations disabled individuals face everyday. One section which needs to be developed is the subject of sexuality. This is perhaps the most difficult subject for which disabled individuals can obtain information. Although the "Where to go for Help" section is limited to Canadian organizations, the book should not be ignored by Americans. Other sources can be used to identify American Manufacturers if necessary and the book does illustrate how to make your own aids and devices. Recommended for public and patient libraries.

Equipment for the Disabled, Vol. 1 - Communication. 4th ed. Compiled by E. R. Wilshere. Headington, Oxford: Oxford Regional Health Authority, 1975. 58 pp.

Describes and illustrates equipment available to assist the disabled in communication including alarm systems, telephone and telephone aids, radio and television, magnifiers, page turners, bookrests, writing frames, tables and typewriters. It provides description and information regarding manufacturer, distribution, approximate price, and export availability for each piece of equipment. Includes an index of manufacturers and an alphabetical index by type of equipment.

Its limitation is it is a British publication and equipment must be imported as is true for all volumes in this series. Is not intended to be used directly by the patient but with consultation of a professional.

Equipment for the Disabled, Vol. 2 - Clothing and Dressing for Adults. 4th ed. Compiled by E. R. Wilshere. Headington, Oxford: Oxford Regional Health Authority, 1975. 66 pp.

"...includes a variety of available clothes, a range of patterns showing different styles and features which may provide ideas for the home dressmaker and suggestions for the shopper, as well as various specially designed clothes and adaptations." It is well-illustrated and contains same type index as other volumes in the series. It includes general information such as metrication in fabrics, laundering and dry cleaning codes, fastening, foundation garments, and incontinence clothing.

Equipment for the Disabled, Vol. 3 - Home Management. 4th ed. Compiled by E. R. Wilshere. Headington, Oxford: Oxford Regional Health Authority, 1975. 80 pp.

This publication arranged by type of activity such as "opening and doing," "baking," and "washing up" describes and illustrates management techniques and equipment for the home. "Points of consideration are given throughout to help in the choice of a particular appliance" to assist the reader in purchasing appropriate equipment. Suggested equipment is well-illustrated and includes description, dimensions, manufacturers and appropriate prices. Contains an Index of manufacturer/suppliers and an Alphabetical Index of Equipment.

This publication has limited value because it is a British and and generally does not include American manufactured products. Recommended for rehabilitation collections.

Equipment for the Disabled, Vol. 4 - Outdoor Transport. 4th ed. Compiled by E. R. Wilshere. Headington, Oxford: Oxford Regional Health Authority, 1977. 43 pp.

Provides information on mobility help, insurance of electric wheelchairs and disabled drivers, childrens' mobility aids, outdoor electric wheelchairs, bicycles, car control conversions, garages, and many other areas of outdoor transports. Contains the same type of indexes as other volumes in the series as well as conversion tables for height, weight, and speed. Recommended for rehabilitation collections.

Equipment for the Disabled, Vol. 5 - Wheelchairs. 4th ed. Compiled by E. R. Wilshere. Headington, Oxford: Oxford Regional Health Authority, 1977. 101 pp.

Provides basic information and illustrations on self propelling wheelchairs, push chairs, electric wheelchairs, commodes and sanichairs, childrens' wheelchairs, children's mobility aids, prams, cushioning, restraining harnesses and accessories. Illustrations include detailed specifications for each piece of equipment. Unfortunately the equipment is limited to British manufactured products. Recommended for rehabilitation collections.

Equipment for the Disabled, Vol. 6 - Leisure and Gardening. 4th ed. Compiled by E. R. Wilshere. Headington, Oxford: Oxford Regional Health Authority, 1978. 86 pp.

This booklet illustrates "ways and means of helping the disabled person to accomplish his hobbies by suggesting simple aids and equipment to use when necessary." Major topics covered include: sewing, knitting, woodwork, stamp collecting, radio and television, reading, writing, the arts, games, travel, outdoor pursuits, sports and gardening. Recommended for public libraries and rehabilitation collections.

INDEPENDENT LIVING   131

Equipment for the Disabled, Vol. 8 - Personal Care. 4th ed. Compiled by E. R. Wilshere. Headington, Oxford: Oxford Regional Health Authority, 1979. 65 pp.

This publication is intended to be used by all people regardless of the form of disability, to assist them in washing, bathing, toileting and grooming. Each piece of equipment includes an illustration, description, manufacturer, and approximate price.

It includes Addresses of Manufacturers and an Alphabetical Index to Equipment. Disadvantage of this book is it is limited to British manufacturers. Recommended for medical and public libraries and rehabilitation collections.

Equipment for the Disabled, Vol. 9 - Housing and Furniture. 4th ed. Compiled by E. R. Wilshere. Oxford: Oxfordshire Area Health Authority, 1979. 83 pp.

This booklet provides general housing information including suggestions for design and layout. It covers topics such as garages, ramps, flooring, doors, handrails, lifts, windows, heating, and many others. Overlaps with other volumes in the series such as Personal Care. It is well-illustrated and contains the same indexes as do other volumes in the series. It is limited to British manufacturers. Recommended for public libraries and rehabilitation collections.

Equipment for the Disabled, Vol. 10 - Hoists Walking Aids. 4th ed. Compiled by E. R. Wilshere. Oxford: Oxfordshire Area Health Authority, 1980. 64 pp.

One of the most difficult problems facing the mobility impaired individual is transferring from one place to another. The booklet is intended to assist the reader by identifying hoists and other walking aids which can be used either independently or with the assistance of others. Each entry gives helpful hints on how best to use that piece of equipment. Entries are well-illustrated and include dimensions, prices, and ordering and export information. It would be extremely useful to the therapist and individual selecting equipment even though no comparison is made of equipment. However, because of its arrangement users can make their own comparison with the information this booklet provides. Recommended for public libraries and rehabilitation collections.

Equipment for the Disabled, Vol. 11 - Disabled Child. 4th ed. Compiled by E. R. Wilshere. Oxford: Oxfordshire Area Health Authority, 1980. 82 pp.

"The purpose of this booklet is to provide current ideas and information on aids and equipment available which could help a handicapped child to lead a fuller or more independent life." The book covers: wheelchairs, personal hygiene, toileting, eating and drinking, clothing and dressing, toys, communication aids, and many other devices. Caution is given to the need for a careful assessment of the individual child and his needs by experienced therapists. Entries are well-illustrated and include dimensions, export availability and excellent descriptions. Recommended for public libraries and rehabilitation collections.

Evaluating Driving Potential of Persons with Physical Disabilities. Albertson, N.Y.: Human Resources Center, 1978. 27 pp.

The purpose of this manual is to present a procedure for an interview, a functional ability, and an in-car performance assessment. The results of the evaluation are used to assess abilities and disabilities so that intelligent and realistic decisions can be made concerning the use of driving aids, vehicle adaptation, and specialized teaching methodology. It contains illustrations and evaluation charts to be used in the evaluative process. This manual is intended to be used by driver educators and examiners. Recommended for academic libraries.

Freiberger, H.; Sherrick, E. E.; and Scaddden, Lawrence. Report of the Workshop on Sensory Deficits and Sensory Aids. n.b., n.d. 37 pp.

This workshop was held at the Smith-Kettlewell Institute of Visual Sciences in San Francisco, California from March 22-24, 1977. The sponsors had hoped the workshops would provide a "fuller understanding of the present problems in sensory aids research, development, service delivery, training and interdisciplinary communication, from which, secondly, there might emerge a projection of research activities..." The principal groups addressed during the workshop were the hearing and visually impaired. This report would be useful to researchers and other persons interested in an overview of sensory aids and devices. Recommended for engineering and academic libraries and rehabilitation collections.

Garee, Betty, ed. Single-Handed: Devices and Aids for One Handers and Sources of These Devices. Bloomington, Ill.: Cheever Publishing, 1978. 25 pp.

This product-oriented pamphlet with be valuable to persons who have lost the use of one hand through birth defect, amputation, stroke, accident or disease. The pamphlet does not attempt to sell a particular product but suggests various companies offering products and suggests methods of approaching a problem which may require no special product. The pamphlet is divided into seven subject areas: Dressing; Grooming; Eating; Home Management; Communication; Recreation/sports; and Miscellaneous. In addition, the pamphlet provides the addresses to the sources of products mentioned in the text and a bibliography of "Publications of Special Interest." It would be useful to the family member or an individual who was recently physically disabled or to someone new to the field or rehabilitation therapy. Recommended for public and academic libraries and rehabilitation collections.

INDEPENDENT LIVING   133

Gilbert, Arlene E. You Can Do It From a Wheelchair. New Rochelle, N.Y.: Arlington House, 1973. 144 pp.

   This book is written from the personal viewpoint of the author and is intended to be used by wheelchair users. It would be useful to persons who were recently physically disabled who need advice on points to consider in purchasing wheelchairs and other devices to aid them to attain independent living. Newer and better materials is available today.

Green Pages Rehab SourceBook. Winter Park, Fla.: SourceBook Publications, Annual.

   Published annually this publication serves as a reference source for institutions needing access to "products and services used in the treatment, care, reeducation, personal and job accommodation of people with physical disabilities." It would be useful to educating health care practitioners and any group or individual working with physically disabled people. Information for similar products or services are grouped together to facilitate use of this publication. Not all products are illustrated, generally only an address and name is given. Therefore, it is necessary for the user to contact individual companies for a complete description of the product or service. This is a very useful publication for any individual, public library, and institution working with physically disabled individuals. Because it is annually updated it will be more useful than other guides and directories in this area. Recommended for academic, medical, and public libraries.

Gugerty, John; Roshal, Arona Fay; Tradewell, Mary D.J. and Anthony, Linda K. Tools, Equipment and Machinery Adapted for the Vocational Education and Employment of Handicapped People. Madison, Wis.: Wisconsin Vocational Studies Center, 1981. 787 pp.

   This equipment catalog serves as a guide to commercially available products. Its looseleaf format does provide for easy updating of information. The catalog contains many aids and devices to assist in performing activities of daily living but the real purpose is to acquaint vocational educators and employers with these materials to then educate and hire handicapped people. The catalog page lists the developer, contact person, where it is used, problem(s) it overcomes, Field tested, regulatory approval, warranty, for sale, how it works, and a photograph or sketch.

Hale, Glorya, ed. The Source Book for the Disabled. New York: Paddington Press, 1979. 288 pp.

   The source book is intended to be a practical guide to individuals with physical disabilities as well as a reference book for their family and friends. The information in this text is very basic and would be most useful to individuals who were recently impaired or to their family and friends. It is extremely easy to read and is formatted similar to a guide rather than a catalog of aids and devices. It covers the areas of home, personal needs, sexuality, parenting, leisure and recreation, and the child. "The Disablers" section defines specific medical conditions. "The Resources" section lists leaflets, books and periodicals, and addresses of organizations and commercial sources of aids and equipment. It is well-illustrated and indexed. Recommended for rehabilitation collections.

Hand Controls and Assistive Devices for the Physically Disabled Driver. Albertson, N.Y.: Human Resources Center, 1977. 52 pp.

This manual includes a practical evaluation of functional disabilities and describes the use and function of various hand controls and assistive devices for the disabled driver. It includes a "Guide to the Use of Hand Controls" which suggests hand controls and assistive devices for particular disabilities. It discusses the advantages and disadvantages of various devices. This very useful guide would be valuable to driver educators, rehabilitation counselors and disabled drivers. It includes many fine illustrations. Recommended for rehabilitation and driver education collections.

High, Elizabeth Codman. A Resource Guide to Habilitative Techniques and Aids for Cerebral Palsied Persons of all Ages. Washington, D.C.: George Washington University, 1979. 150 pp.

This manual is written for professionals, parents and others involved in the care and habilation of cerebral palsied individuals. It includes aids and techniques for positioning and seating, feeding, dressing, hygiene, and household and community involvement. Each of these sections begins with an overview of the subject followed by appropriate resources. The references to books and pamphlets include an annotation and all the bibliographic information necessary for the reader to obtain a copy. The references to aids and devices include simple illustrations, price and manufacturer information. This is a very handy and useful publication not only for the information between its own covers but the references it makes to other excellent publications. Recommended for public libraries and rehabilitation collections.

Hofmann, Ruth B. How to Build Special Furniture and Equipment for Handicapped Children. Springfield, Ill.: Charles C. Thomas, 1970. 88 pp.

A "how-to" manual for constructing furniture and equipment for physically disabled children. The author claims the furniture is "made with scrap wood in a limited space with comparatively few tools." The manual is well-illustrated and contains all the information necessary to construct the furniture. Explicit instructions are given to construct standing boards, standing tables, car chairs, potty chairs, slant boards and many others.

It would be useful to family and friends of a physically disabled child or to staff a rehabilitation center for children. Recommended for public libraries and rehabilitation collections.

Hurvitz, Joel and Carmen, Richard. Special Devices for Hard of Hearing Deaf, and Deaf-Blind Persons. Boston: Little, Brown and Company, 1981. 297 pp.

This publication produced by two audiologists from the Veterans Administration Medical Center in Sepulveda, California, is a compilation of products manufactured for the hearing impaired population. Because there is a large and frequent turnover of manufacturers in this area, the reader is encouraged to contact the manufacturer directly. Each product is illustrated and the description includes price, source, specification, purpose, and a code indicating to whom the product is recommended: Hard of Hearing, Deaf, Deaf-Blind, and Professional. Devices are arranged by broad subject category for ease of comparison. An index and a list of Manufacturers and their address are included. This is a very fine addition to any library attempting to serve the needs of the hearing impaired population.

Kreisler, Nancy, and Kreisler, Jack. Catalog of Aids for the Disabled. New York: McGraw-Hill, 1982. 246 pp.

Nancy Kreisler, disabled as a result of polio, does an excellent job of updating the many equipment catalogs produced during the past 15 years. She has divided the aids into the following categories: In and Out of Bed, Personal Care, Dressing, Meal Preparation, Eating, Getting Around, Household Activities, Access at Home and Elsewhere, Communication, Recreation, Travel, Accident Prevention at Home, and Safety from Crime. Greater emphasis is placed on mobility impairments than hearing and seeing impairments. Each item includes a recent photograph, description, price category, and the name of a supplier. The Appendix contains "Organizations, Agencies, and Other Sources of Help for the Disabled and Elderly," "Periodicals useful to the Disabled and Elderly," and a list of "Suppliers." A must for public libraries and rehabilitation collections.

Kwatny, Eugene, and Zukerman, Ronnie, eds. Devices and Systems for the Disabled. Philadelphia: Moss Rehabilitation Hospital, 1975. 207 pp.

This is a proceedings of a conference on "Devices and Systems for the Disabled" held in Philadelphia on April 29 and 30th, 1975. The conference was sponsored by Krusen Center for Research and Engineering at Moss Rehabilitation Hospital, Temple University Health Sciences Center. Many of the devices are commercially available others are in the research, design, and evaluation stages. This proceedings would be most useful to researchers and other individuals interested in the design of devices and systems for the physically disabled. The emphasis is on systems rather than gadget-type devices. Recommended for engineering libraries and rehabilitation collections.

LaRocca, Joseph, and Turem, Jerry S. The Application of Technological Developments to Physically Disabled People. Washington, D.C.: The Urban Institute, 1978. 117 pp.

This paper "attempts to assess the impact of technological advances...on disabled people, and the degree to which these technologies have helped disabled people..." In addition, it discusses characteristics of the disabled population in the U.S. and the effect of public policy, research, marketing, training, and funding problems associated with the development and application of these technologies. There are no illustrations. This is an excellent source of information on this topic. It would be useful to all professionals serving the physically disabled population especially advocacy and consumer groups. Recommended for academic and public libraries.

Lowman, Edward W., and Klinger, Judith Lannefeld. Aids to Independent Living: Self-Help for the Handicapped. New York: McGraw-Hill, 1969. 796 pp.

This is a catalog of aids, devices, or equipment many of which have been tested, designed or developed by the Institute of Rehabilitation Medicine of the New York University Medical Center. It includes prosthetic devices, orthosis, and adaptive devices. It is extremely well-indexed and illustrated. The "List of Sources" provides mailing information and also a brief description to the types of devices which are available through them. Although the publication date is 1969 most of the products remain to be available today. It is one of the most comprehensive books in this area and would be useful to physically disabled individuals and their families and to physical and occupational therapists. A new edition of this publication would be useful to public and academic libraries and any rehabilitation collection.

Lowthian, Peter. Portable Urinals and Related Appliances: A Guide to Availability and Use. London: Disabled Living Foundation, 1975. 108 pp.

Unfortunately the items listed are available in the United Kingdom but are not necessarily available in the U.S.A. Items are arranged alphabetically according to manufacturer's or suppliers name. This publication is intended to be used by a wide range of medical experts: physicians, nurses, occupational and physiotherapists, and by laypersons and would be particularly useful to students. It is a well-organized and easy to use guide. Recommended for medical and public libraries and rehabilitation collections.

Miller, J. D.; Foulds, R. A.; and Saunders, F. A. <u>Report of the Workshop on Communication Systems for Persons With Impaired Hearing or Speech</u> n.b. 1979. 22 pp.

This report intends to summarize the findings and the recommendations of the 1978 Workshop on Communication Systems for Persons with Impaired Hearing or Speech held at the Smith-Kettlewell Institute in San Francisco on May 8-10, 1978. It is hoped the report will "identify for scientists and engineers, the immediate needs of the handicapped; will summarize, for the handicapped, the devices currently available; and will provide, for professionals and funding agencies, certain guidelines for future activities in rehabilitation engineering." Recommended for engineering libraries and speech and hearing collections.

New York University Medical Center. <u>Environmental Control Systems and Vocational Aids for Persons With High Level Quadriplegia</u>. New York: New York University Medical Center, 1979. 124 pp.

This is an excellent examination of commercially available environmental control systems designed for persons with spinal cord injury above the level of C-5. Not only do the evaluation reports include basic product and purchasing information but also the advantages and disadvantages of the system. The most useful element to each report is actual patient comments regarding the use of the system. This publication would be used by those individuals and professionals involved in the purchase and/or development of environmental control systems. An excellent purchase for a bioengineering library.

Redford, John B. <u>Orthotics Etcetera</u>. 2d ed. Baltimore: Williams & Wilkins, 1980. 776 pp.

The title <u>Orthotics Etcetera</u> is used to cover devices attached to the external surface of the body to improve function as well as unattached assistive devices such as wheelchairs and environmental control systems. General consideration is given to orthotic devices, followed by specific applications of orthoses and other assistive devices, and special requirements of disabled persons.

This publication is an excellent reference source for anyone needing information on orthotics. It is well-referenced and illustrated. It is truly a scholarly publication. The chapter entitled "Eponymic Orthoses" will be useful to an individual trying to identify an orthotic eponym. For orthotic eponyms which do not include a full definition a reference to the original publication will be given. This publication would be useful to researchers, teachers, and clinicians in the area of orthotics. Recommended for medical and engineering libraries and rehabilitation collections.

Robinault, Isabel P., ed. Functional Aids for the Multiply Handicapped. Hagerstown, Md.: Harper and Row, 1973. 233 pp.

This not only serves as a catalog of devices but also as a how-to book. It provides information on construction of or modification of devices and basic information on methods to facilitate independent living. The aids and devices described cover infancy to maturity in the areas of mobility, personal care, communications, and recreation. The book is well-illustrated and indexed. It would be useful to family members and professionals working with the multiple handicapped. The reader is advised to select equipment specific to the individual who will be using it. The "Sources for Aids and Information" is useful to the reader to purchase many of the devices which are commercially available. The text is dated but remains to be useful. Recommended for rehabilitation collections.

Saunders, Frank A. Rehabilitation Engineering Aids and Devices for Persons with Impaired Hearing. San Francisco: Smith-Kettlewell Institute, 1979. 17 pp.

Produced as a part of 1979 Workshop on Communication Systems for Persons with Impaired Hearing or Speech and sponsored by the Rehabilitation Services Administration, this catalog describes products that are currently available under development. It gives a brief summary of the product and where to obtain additional information.

It is useful as an overview of devices for the hearing impaired such as, amplification and telephone/teletype devices, portable communicators, speech analyzers and synthesizers, architectural services, computer-based instruction, etc. It is easy to use and contains no index and no illustrations. Recommended for academic and engineering libraries.

Sloan, Louise L. Reading Aids for the Partially Sighted: A Systematic Classification and Procedure for Prescribing. Baltimore: Wiliams and Wilkins, 1977. 150 pp.

For an evaluation of this work, see Chapter 2.

Sloan, Louise, L. Recommended Aids for the Partially Sighted. Rev. 2d ed. New York: National Society for the Prevention of Blindness, 1971. 64 pp.

This manual provides a "systematic description and classification of useful optical and other aids for the partially sighted with emphasis on nonspectacle reading aids... and describes testing equipment and procedures to facilitate selections of the most suitable devices for each patient." Comparison of the reading devices were made by patients without knowledge of their costs. It contains many photographs and illustrations and would be useful to optometrists, ophthalmologists, and specialists in rehabilitation of the partially sighted. Recommended for medical libraries and rehabilitation collections.

Symington, David, C.; O'Shea, Barbara J.; Batelaan, John; and White, David A. <u>Independence Through Environmental Control Systems</u>. Toronto: Canadian Rehabilitation Council for the Disabled, 1980. 63 pp.

"This book is an outgrowth of the work of the Technical Aids Committee of the Canadian Rehabilitation Council for the Disabled." It provides basic information on such things as what is an environmental control system and where they can be used and describes 19 case studies using environmental control systems. This manual would be extremely useful to professionals and consumers considering purchasing such systems. It is very easy to use and well-illustrated. It also lists suppliers and sources of information of environmental control systems in Canada and the U.S. Recommended for engineering libraries and rehabilitation collections.

<u>Teaching Driver Education to the Physically Disabled</u>. Albertson, N.Y.: Human Resources Center, 1978. 54 pp.

This manual is intended for the driver education teacher to enable the instructor to train disabled students. The methodology presented provides detailed instruction on special driving techniques, use of driving aids, use of vans, and preparation for the road test. The manual also covers the selection of a driver education car and hints on operating a successful driver education program. Because a drivers license can change the entire life of a disabled individual any book on this topic is essential to independent living for people with physical disabilities. It is well-organized, easy to use, and contains many useful illustrations. It is intended to be used by the driver educator. Recommended for driver education collections.

<u>Technical Aids For the Speech-Impaired: An International Survey on Research and Development Projects</u>. Information Centre. Stockholm: ICTA, 1978. 60 pp.

This publication is the result of a 1976/77 survey recording studies aimed at the development of personal aids for the speech impaired. It includes project descriptions for 103 institutions. Each project description includes: title, principal investigator, type of study, type of speech defect, project result, manufacturer's address, and comments. Although the publication does not have a subject index, the author uses two tables to cluster responses by subject. It is only a catalog of projects and offers no comment or evaluation. Such a publication would be useful to researchers and designers of technical aids. Recommended for academic and engineering libraries and speech/hearing collections.

Vanderheiden, Gregg C., and Grilley, Kate, eds. Non-Vocal Communication Techniques and Aids for the Severely Physically Handicapped. Baltimore: University Park Press, 1976. 227 pp.

This publication is based upon Transactions of the 1975 Trace Center National Workshop Series on Non-vocal Communication Techniques and Aids. It is intended to be used "by teachers, clinicians and parents in trying to develop an effective means of communication in their non-vocal physically handicapped children." Emphasis is placed on communication systems to be dynamic. As children grow and develop, their communication needs will change and expand. Contains many excellent illustrations. Although the concepts may be technical in nature, the manner in which the information is conveyed can be easily understood by any adult. Recommended for academic libraries and large public libraries.

Vash, Carolyn, ed. Rehabilitation Engineering Sourcebook/ and Supplement. Falls Church, Va.: Institute for Information Studies, 1979. 84 pp.

This sourcebook is intended to be a practical aid in determining if a problem has been found to have a technological solution. The information is awkwardly organized and the user is forced to use the indexes which again are awkwardly organized. However, the publication is useful as an overview of existing technological solutions to problems which rehabilitation counselors and work supervisors confront in working with individuals with physical disabilities. The value of this publication is quite limited because of its organization and the specificity of its intended audience.

ANNOTATED BIBLIOGRAPHY:
Programs and Facilities

Baker, Bruce, L; Brightman, Alan J.; Heifetz, Louis J.; and Murphy, Diane M. Steps to Independence: A Skills Training Series for Children with Special Needs. Champaign, Ill.: Research Press, 1976.

This series contains 4 manuals: Early Self-Help Skills, Intermediate Self-Help Skills, Advanced Self-Help Skills, and Behavior Problems. Each manual was developed for and tested at Camp Freedom, "a seven-week educational residential program for children with special needs and for their families. It is a place where, every summer, each of 50 children is provided with unique and individualized programs for learning a variety of skills: from reading and writing to dressing, dance, from motor skills and mountain climbing to swimming and speech." The first three manuals are arranged in two sections. The first section, Principles and Methods, introduces parents to behavior modification techniques and specific rationales for parental responsibility in teaching. Section two, Programs, provides parents with specific steps and suggestions to follow in teaching. Behavior Problems concentrates "on the process whereby one understands and programs for petty annoyances and major disruptions alike." The authors encourage the users to use the manuals as a guide and to tailor programs for their child and to themselves. The series also contains a Training Guide. This series also contains a Training Guide. This series is an excellent resource for individuals involved in parent teaching and for parents as well. It is well-organized extremely easy to read and understand. Recommended for academic libraries and rehabilitation collections.

Baker, Bruce L.; Brightman, Alan J.; and Hinshaw, Stephen P. Toward Independent Living: A Skills Training Series for Children with Special Needs. Champaign, Ill.: Research Press, 1980. 118 pp.

Another manual in the Steps to Independence series written for parents and teachers of retarded children. This manual is for a wide range of developmentally disabled individuals from children to young adults and examines self-help skills that a child needs as he or she matures. It includes self-care skills to get the day started, home care skills to maintain a home in smooth operating condition, and information skills needed to live in a community. Again the user of this manual is encouraged to use it as a guide and to tailor a program to the special needs of the child and his family. An excellent resource for individuals involved in parent teaching. It is well-organized and easy to use. Recommended for academic libraries and rehabilitation collections.

Board, Mary Ann; Cole, Jean A.; Frieden, Lex; and Sperry, Jane C. Independent Living with Attendant Care: A Guide for the Person with a Disability. Vol. 1. Houston, Tex.: The Institute for Rehabilitation and Research, 1980. 20 pp.

This booklet is intended for use by severely disabled people for whom personal care attendants (PCA) are necessary for independant living. It discusses the interviewing and hiring of PCA's, relationships between disabled individuals and PCA's, and terminating PCA's. This is a very basic but useful and practical resource for the person with a disability. The concepts it presents are based on three years of experience in the New Options Transitional Living Project in Houston, Texas. Recommended for public and academic libraries and rehabilitation collections.

Board, Mary Ann; Cole, Jean A.; Frieden, Lex; and Sperry, Jane C. Independent Living with Attendant Care: A Message to Parents of Handicapped Youth. Vol. 2. Houston, Tex.: The Institute for Rehabilitation and Research, 1980. 12 pp.

This booklet is based on years of experience in the New Optioins Transitional Living Project in Houston, Texas and from experiences of many families dealing with a disability. This booklet attempts to help parents examine their relationship with their handicapped child and discover new options for themselves and their child. This is a very simple introduction to independent living with attendant care. It is not a must for any library collection.

Board, Mary Ann; Cole, Jean A.; and Sperry, Jane C. Independent Living with Attendant Care: A Guide for the Personal Care Attendant. Vol. 3. Houston, Tex.: Institute for Rehabilitation and Research, 1980. 24 pp.

This booklet would be useful to those individuals seeking a career as a personal care attendant. It provides very basic information in defining different categories of disability, describing interviewing techniques and where to look for jobs, and pointing out possible problems. Recommended for public libraries and career collection.

Brodsky, Carroll M., and Platt, Robert T. The Rehabilitation Environment. Lexington, Maine: Lexington Books, 1978. 157 pp.

The intent of this book is to describe how a rehabilitation unit was developed, organized, and phased out. The authors hope that by describing the system and why it failed, administrators will be able to design a rehabilitation or therapeutic unit and avoid many of the problems the authors encountered. The book does not center on unique problems of a single unit but provides insight to common problems which may exist in comparable programs.

The underlining tone of the book is pessimistic because of the time spent discussing the demise of a psychiatric and rehabilitation unit at the University of California. The book provides recommendations to the physical setting, roles, leadership, communication, patient-staff relations, patient's psychosocial needs, budgeting and community considerations. It would be useful to administrators and staff involved with the development or evaluation of a therapeutic unit. Recommended for academic libraries and rehabilitation collections.

Carnell, C. Mitchell. Development, Management, and Evaluation of Community Speech and Hearing Centers. Springfield, Ill.: Charles C. Thomas, 1976. 133 pp.

The purpose of this study is to assist communities that as yet do not have a community speech and hearing center and to encourage improvement in currently existing centers. A wide range of topics are discussed covering administration, fiscal management, records and reports, physical facilities and equipment; professional services, and professional personnel. It is well-organized and referenced and would be useful to administrators, staff members, and other groups involved with the development, management, and evaluation of the community center. Recommended for public and academic libraries and speech and hearing collections.

Casto, Marilyn Dee, and Day, Savannah S. Adaptive Housing for the Physically Handicapped. Monticello, Ill.: Council of Planning Librarians, 1975. 27 pp.

This bibliography was compiled from books, reports, bulletins and bibliographies. It includes 330 references from both national and international sources from 1946 to 1975. Citations are arranged by: 1) housing for the physically handicapped, and 2) architectural barriers. This bibliography would be useful to librarians as an acquisition source and for individuals seeking sources on housing and architectural barriers for disabled individuals. It lacks of annotations and its publication date of 1975 limits its usefulness today but would be valuable for retrospective literature searching.

Cole, Jean A., ed. Living Independently: Three Views of the European Experience with Implications for the United States. Monograph No. 10. New York: World Rehabilitation Fund, 1980. 63 pp.

This monograph represents three study trips sponsored by the International Exchange of Experts in Rehabilitation: Lex and Joyce Frieden "Observations of the Lifestyles of Disabled People in Sweden and the Netherlands" and Gini Laurie "Relationships between American and European Concepts of Independent Living." The objectives of each paper is to describe the service programs, to express the views of disabled persons, and to offer personal assessments. This publication would be useful to those interested in exchange of information to enhance the lives of disabled persons. Recommended for academic libraries.

Cole, Jean A.; Sperry, Jane C.; and others. New Options. Houston, Tex.: New Options, Institute for Rehabilitation and Research, 1979. 113 pp.

This is an introduction to the concept of independent living for disabled persons and a description of the way the New Options Transitional Living Project in Houston teaches skills necessary for independent living (decision-making, working with attendants, social skills, and sexuality). Residents live at New Options for six weeks, completing eleven courses which teach them how to live independently despite their disability. Most residents are severely mobility-impaired; many of the counselors and teachers are disabled persons. Most of the learning is by discussion, practice, and field trips into the community.

An outstanding introduction to the concept, practice and teaching of independent living skills for severely disabled persons. (See also New Options Training Manual where eleven courses are described in more detail.) The photography depicting disabled persons in a variety of learning, working, playing and social situations are excellent supplements to the text. Written for rehabilitation professionals and social science students. Recommended for appropriate special libraries and academic libraries.

Cole, Jean A.; Sperry, Jance C.; Board, Mary Ann; and Frieden, Lex. <u>New Options Training Manual</u>. Houston, Tex.: New Options, Institute for Rehabilitation and Research, 1979. 129 pp.

This manual provides additional information to <u>New Options</u> for the person or group interested in starting a program designed to improve the community living skills of physically disabled people. It outlines eleven training modules in the New Options program and includes purpose of module, requirements of group leader, a bibliography, and topics for other possible sessions in the module. Modules cover a wide range of topics such as consumer affairs, medical needs, sexuality, and time management.

It is well-organized and easy to use. Its loose-leaf format makes updating easy for the user. Should be used with <u>New Options</u> by Jean A. Cole and others. Recommended for all rehabilitation collections.

<u>Community Living Alternatives for Persons with Developmental Disabilities</u>. 4 vols. Springfield, Ill.: Illinois Governor's Council on Developmental Disabilities, 1976-.

Although these publications were sponsored by the State of Illinois, they would be useful to any individual interested in alternative living arrangements for the severely physically disabled and mentally alert cerebral palsied adult. This series is comprised "...of four studies which have been designed to encourage new types of residential services for indivuduals with developmental disabilities according to the principles of normalization." The series includes: Volume 1 - The Model System, Volume 2 - Financial Requirements, Volume 3 - Moving Ahead--The Physically Handicapped, and Volume 4 - Summary. These publications are easy to use and the chart format used throughout the series is very well done. Recommended for academic and libraries and independent living collections.

<u>Community Living for the Disabled: A Selective Annotated Bibliography</u>. South Bend, Ind.: National Center for Law and the Handicapped, 1978, 11 pp.

This publication contains annotations to 24 books and four articles on the subject of community living for the disabled. Although the subtitle indicated this is a selective bibliography, the selection criteria is stated no where in the bibliography. Most of the books annotated are for the developmentally disabled and the mentally retarded. The bibliography contains no index, table of contents, introduction, or purpose. Therefore, this publication is of limited value to anyone except for the National Center for Law and the Handicapped.

Crewe, Nancy M.; Zola, Irving Kenneth; and Associates. Independent Living for Physically Disabled People. San Francisco: Jossey-Bass, 1983. 406 pp.

The contributiong authors of this book are well known in the rehabilitation field and include such people as Bowe, Cole, DeJong, Frieden, Schawab, and Stoddard. The "book presents broad, intensified coverage of independent living as it has emerged into the present day." Its publication is a result of the interest generated from the October 1979 issue of the "Archives of Physical Medicine and Rehabilitation" on the topic of Independent Living. This is a must for any rehabilitation and/or independent living collection because it provides an excellent overview to the independent living movement.

Curtis, Bruce. How to Set up an Independent Living Program: Twenty-seven Questions and Answers. Houston, Tex.: Independent Living Research Utilization Project, 1980. 30 pp.

Designed in question-answer format this "...paper will aid planners to develop stable, flexible, effective independent living programs that are appropriate to each individual community..." The topics discussed are very basic and practical and would be useful to both the student and practitioner starting an independent living program. The appendices include a list of ILRU Technical Assistance Products and Materials which are available for purchase. Recommended for academic and public libraries.

Davidson, Roslyn. Rehabilitation Administrative Procedures for Extended Care Facilities. Springfield, Ill.: Charles C. Thomas, 1973. 124 pp.

This manual is intended to serve as a guide to establishing administrative policies and procedures for a department of rehabilitation in an extended care facility. Several procedures and programs from the Hempstead General Medical Center in New York are included. Its outline format makes it extremely easy to use. The manual is well-planned, well thought-out and well-illustrated. It is useful to physical therapists and rehabilitation personnel in extended care facilities. Recommended for rehabilitation collections.

DeJong, Gerben. The Movement for Independent Living: Origins, Ideology, and Implications for Disability Research. Boston: Medical Rehabilitation Institute, Tufts-New England Medical Center, 1978. 71 pp.

This monograph provides an overview to the independent living movement. It defines the movement as a social movement and describes its effects in disability services and its implications on disability research. It is easy to use, well-referenced and is written in the format of a dissertation. It would be quite useful to a student in the social sciences or to professionals and consumers interested in human services. Recommended for academic and public libraries.

DeJong, Gerben. The Need for Personal Care Services by Severely Physically Disabled Citizens of Massachusetts: Executive Summary. Waltham, Maine: Brandeis University, 1977. 34 pp.

This document summarizes the findings of a study conducted by the Levinson Policy Institute of Brandeis University to determine how many severely disabled people in Massachusetts are at risk of needing a personal care attendant. This publication would be useful to individuals interested in conducting a similar survey of administrators making policy decisions regarding personal care attendants. Recommended for academic and public libraries.

Fishler, Arnold L. Development of Work Programs for the Multihandicapped: Report of a Demonstration Project Directed at Broadening Vocational Opportunities for the Severely Handicapped. New York: Professional Services Program Department, United Cerebral Palsy Association, Inc., 1976. 71 pp.

A useful "how-to" manual on planning, organizing and operating an industrial oriented work activities center for the severely disabled adult. The intent is to extend the expertise developed in the demonstration projects (the UCP of Denver, Colorado and at Habilitation Inc., a UCP affiliate in Pottsville, Pennsylvania) to community based workshops and residential institutions for the retarded. It is easy to use and is well-illustrated. It includes the "American National Standard Specifications for making buildings and facilities Accessible to and usable by the Physically Handicapped, 1961 which has been updated. However, much of the information in this manual remains to be useful to vocational rehabilitation personnel.

Frieden, Lex; Richards, Laurel; Cole, Jean; and Bailey, David. ILRU Source Book: A Technical Assistance Manual on Independent Living. Houston, Tex.: Independent Living Research Utilization Project. The Institute for Rehabilitation and Research, 1979- .

This manual is intended for persons developing and/or operating independent living programs as well as persons who anticipate using such programs. The manual comes in an expensive looking loose-leaf format which allows the reader to update the material periodically. The source book contains a selected glossary of independent living terms, an annotated registry of programs in the United States, matrix identifying funding programs, a section on community involvement, and an excellent annotated bibliography.

This is a very useful source to identify current independent living programs, but the user must work at keeping it current. Recommended for public and academic libraries.

Hoffman, Sara Jeanne; Shinnick, Michael D.; and Willoughby, Mervyn, eds. Independent Living: A Resource Manual. Auburn, Ala.: Rehabilitation Services Education School of Education, Auburn University, 1980. Pagination varies.

The objectives of this manual are "1) to offer guidelines for state agency personnel and program planners in the organization and implementation of programs, 2) to provide teachers and trainers with information for the development of an Independent Living Curriculum, and 3) to present an annotated bibliography of Independent Living materials that may assist in planning research, and program development."

The manual is in loose-leaf format and allows for easy updating. It includes many articles reprinted from publications in this field covering legislation; consumer involvement, program development, and housing evaluation. Because there is so little published in this area this manual would be valuable to anyone working in this area and to any rehabilitation/independent living collection. It provides excellent background material and thus, makes it quite useful to the novice. It was originally developed as a short-time training project in Independent Living for Region IV Rehabilitation Professionals.

Implementation of Independent Living Programs in Rehabilitation. Institute on Rehabilitation Issues, 1980. San Antonio, Tex.: Hot Springs, Ark.: University of Arkansas, 1980. 211 pp.

This report is from a study group of many distinguished leaders in the field of independent living from state rehabilitation agencies, Rehabilitation Services Administration, and independent living projects. During their work the study group "... attempted to provide some insights into the many problems and to provide some answers to the many questions that exist in implementation of Independent Living Programs." This report serves as both an excellent introduction into independent living and as a supplementary teaching aid on this subject. The chapter on staff training describes activities, objectives, and lists the necessary materials and equipment to provide the user with information to implement an independent living program. The bibliography and appendices are exceptionally well done providing the user with job descriptions, guidelines for grant getting, sources of information, and addresses for the total Study Group. Recommended for academic and public libraries and independent living collections.

Independent Living Skills for the Severely Handicapped Deaf Person Preparing to Enter Gainful Employment. Monograph No. 5. Silver Spring, Md.: American Deafness and Rehabilitation Association, 1980. 103 pp.

This publication is a compilation of articles and materials presented at a national workshop held in Knoxville, Tennessee on August 13-16, 1979 and sponsored by the University of Tennessee and the Rehabilitation Services Administration. The purpose of workshop was to increase competency in independent living skills training to severely handicapped deaf individuals and focused on eight areas: Basic assessment of Independent Living Skills; Health/Hygiene; Social/Interpersonal Behavior Patterns; Job Practices; Money Management/Budgeting; Family Responsibilities; Community Awareness; and Legal Awareness. This proceedings would be useful to both the student and practitioner working in the area of independent living because the material and information is very practical and has actually been used by the workshop contributors.

Laker, Mark. Nursing Home Activities for the Handicapped. Springfield, Ill.: Charles C. Thomas, 1980. 81 pp.

"The purpose of this book is to improve the quality of life for handicapped persons living in nursing homes." The book would be useful to activity coordinators, recreation therapists, and activity aids working in nursing homes. It is divided into five chapters: 1) The Stroke Patient; 1) The Bedridden Patient; 3) The Wheelchair Patient; 4) The Visually Handicapped Patient; and 5) The Confused Patient. The name of the activity, the procedures, the benefits, and the supplies and equipment are discussed under each specific activity. A brief bibliography of books and films is included. It is a very easy to use and basic book for planning and adapting activities for the handicapped. Recommended for public libraries and rehabilitation collections.

Larson, Maren R., and Snobl, Daniel E. Attendant Care Manual: Rehabilitation Services. Marshall, Minn.: Southwest State University, 1978. 81 pp.

Although this manual was developed for individuals providing attendant care to physically disabled students at Southwest State University, it would be useful to anyone who attends to the daily needs of a disabled individual. The manual provides very basic and introductory information about the various types of disabilities and the attendant care needs they require. It is well-illustrated, well-organized, and easy to use. Recommended for academic and public libraries and rehabilitation collections.

Laurie, Gini. Housing and Home Services for the Disabled: Guidelines and Experiences in Independent Living. Hagerstown, Md.: Harper & Row, 1977. 432 pp.

This publication covers topics such as adaptations to housing, independent living experiences, California Attendant Programs, apartment living, HUD-Assisted Housing Projects, legislation, and international experiences. It is an extremely useful reference for disabled persons, organizations of disabled per- sosons, government agencies and professionals such as architects, occupational and physical therapists, counselors, social workers to name only a few. The book gives many examples of housing arrangements and services which will assist readers in creating solutions for their own particular situation. It contains an excellent index and bibliographies. Recommended for academic and public libraries.

Means, Bob L., and Roessler, Richard T. Personal Achievement Skills Training Package. Fayetteville, Ark.: Arkansas Rehabilitation Research and Training Center, 1976. 4 vols.: Instructor's Manual; Participants's Manual; Instructor's Supplement; and Discussion Paper.

Although these publications were developed by a rehabilitation research and training center, they would be useful to any group involved in a general personal adjustment training program. The Personal Achievement Skills Training is designed to teach communication and goal setting skills and to facilitate personal growth in a two step process. First, the problem behavior is identified. Then, effective alternative behaviors are identified to replace the undesired or ineffective behavior. Users of these publications are encouraged to complete a training program prior to conducting a Personal Achievement Skills group. Such training would make these publications more understandable to the user. This type of training would be extremely valuable to anyone involved in a rehabilitation program. Recommended for academic libraries and rehabilitation collections.

National Workshop on Rehabilitation Centers. Rehabilitation Centers for the Blind and Visually Impaired: The State of Art, 1975. Final Report. New York: American Foundation for the Blind, 1975. 72 pp.

The Workshop, sponsored jointly by the Rehabilitation Services Administration and the American Foundation for the Blind, was developed in response to the many developments and changes in work with the visually impaired in recent years. This final report is a result of many dedicated workshop participants. The report discussed the rehabilitation center's goals, structure, standards, evaluations, financing, staff, services and activities. It would be useful to a student, an administrator, and family members of visually impaired individuals in determining how a rehabilitation center should operate. The publication would be more useful if it included a bibliography or at least a list of sources used to compile this report. It appears the report is a result of first hand experiences only. Recommended for academic libraries and rehabilitation collections.

Petal, Maria. Independent Living and Deafness: Incorporating Deaf Clients into the Independent Living Network. Issues in Independent Living Series, Houston, Tex.: Independent Living Research Utilization Project, 1980. 30 pp.

The purpose of this study is to facilitate the inclusion of deaf persons into the independent living movement by identifying the minimum services they require to live independently. This report includes a description of five programs located in Texas and California that provide such services to deaf persons. This publication would be useful to individuals involved in setting up or evaluating independent living programs to ensure equal consideration be given to deaf persons. Recommended for independent living and speech and hearing collections.

Pflueger, Susan Stoddard. Independent Living. Emerging Issues in Rehabilitation Series. Washington, D.C.: Institute for Research Utilization, 1977. 78 pp.

This publication serves as a review of independent living services. It covers such topics as legislation, defining the population, alternatives for delivery of services, cost/benefits of independent living, and pragmatic features of the consumer model of independent living. It contains reports of independent living programs at California, Massachusetts, Texas, and Colorado. It includes a "Checklist for Developing Independent Living Projects" and an annotated bibliography. Extremely useful as an overview in independent living for the novice. Recommended for independent living collections.

Rice, B. Douglas, and Roessler, Richard T. Introduction to Independent Living Rehabilitation Services. Hot Springs, Ark.: Arkansas Rehabilitation Research and Training Center, 1980. 34 pp.

This publication provides the very basic introduction to the concept of independent living answering such questions as what is it, what is its history and what are the trends in independent living? Primarily it would be useful to new students in the field of rehabilitation only. Recommended for public libraries.

Royse, Richard E. The CIL: Design for Success. Lawrence, Kan.: Kansas Center for Mental Retardation and Human Development, UAF, The University of Kansas, 1980. 113 pp.

This manual outlines a Center for Independent Living (CIL) model by combining various components from CIL's in California at Berkeley, San Diego, Long Beach; Boston, Massachusetts; Madison, Wisconsin; and Mount Clemens, Michigan. It is to be used as a guide and the user is encouraged to blend existing service systems to the needs of the people in the community. It addresses center development, housing, attendant care, transportation, employment, funding, and accountability. This publication would be extremely useful as an introduction or overview to those individuals involved in setting up a CIL. The chapter on funding is extremely valuable because it identifies funding sources and considerations about those sources. The information is basic to developing a CIL and the manual is extremely well-written. It is a must for any independent living collection.

Schwab, Lois O. Independent Living Assessments for Persons with Disabilities. Lincoln: University of Nebraska, 1981. 55 pp.

The author presents 1) a Self-Assessment of Needs for Independent Living, 2) an Observer Checklist for Need in Independent Living Services, 3) Independent Living Assessment, and 4) A Demonstration Project Using Independent Living Assessment. The University of Nebraska's special project funded by the Developmental Disabilities Office of HEW made use of this program in a study of 70 persons with cerebral palsy. The assessment charts and questionnaires would be extremely useful to rehabilitation counselors and independent living evaluators. This manual is spiral bound and very easy to use. Recommended for rehabilitation collections.

Schwab, Lois O. Rehabilitation for Independent Living: A Selected Bibliography. Washington, D.C.: President's Committee on Employment of the Handicapped, 1982. 60 pp.

Now in its sixth edition this bibliography provides a list of basic materials in the field of independent living. It primarily covers the subjects of clothing, home management, homes and furnishings and cookbooks. The bibliography includes books, pamphlets, motion pictures, filmstrips and slides. Material cited includes an abstract, price information, and a reference to a section of publishers' addresses.

This excellent bibliography is easy to use and the materials cited are very inexpensive, many of them are free to under $20. This bibliography would be useful for an individual who was recently injured, individuals providing attendant care services, and for teachers of home economics. Recommended for public libraries and independent living collections.

Simkins, Jean. The Value of Independent Living. Monograph No. 4. International Exchange of Information in Rehabilitation Services. New York: World Rehabilitation Fund, 1979. 86 pp.

This work examines independent living from a cost-benefit viewpoint within the United Kingdom and suggests approaches which may be useful in the United States. It emphasizes the impossibility of assigning dollar values to the benefits of independent living. It would be extremely useful for individuals such as administrators and politicians needing to justify independent living programs for disabled individuals. Recommended for academic and public libraries and independent living collections.

Sioux Vocational School. Independent Living Evaluation - Training Program. Reprint Series No. 16. Menomonie, Wis.: Materials Development Center, Stout Vocational Rehabilitation Institute, 1979. 98 pp.

This program is used initially to evaluate an individual during the first 30 days of enrollment in a residential training center. It is used again annually where the client's total training program is evaluated. This publication would be extremely useful to residential instructors and program managers of independent living programs. The accompanying pretests and task analysis can be easily modified and adapted for other programs. This is an extremely well-planned, well-organized, and well-illustrated publication. Recommended for rehabilitation and professional collections.

Trela, James E., ed. The Role of Facilities in Training Rehabilitation Personnel. Cleveland, Ohio: Vocational Guidance and Rehabilitation Services, 1972. 79 pp.

This publication is the abstracted papers of a three day conference on "The Role of Facilities in Training Rehabilitation Personnel" held on April 4-6, 1972, and sponsored by the Vocational Guidance and Rehabilitation Services and the Rehabilitation Services Administration of the U.S. Department of Health Education and Welfare. It was developed to make the proceedings immediately available in abstract form until all conference papers can be revised, edited, and printed. This publication would be useful for educators and individuals interested in rehabiltitation training as it examines the role of facilities in meeting expanding training needs of the future and ways of strengthening this role. Recommended for academic libraries.

Walls, Richard T.; Zane, Thomas; and Thvedt, John E. The Independent Living Behavior Checklist. Morgantown, W. Va.: West Virginia Rehabilitation Research and Training Center, 1979. 218 pp.

This publication is a list of 343 independent living skills objectives arranged into six categories: Mobility Skills, Self-Care Skills, Home Maintenance and Safety Skills, Food Skills, Social and Communication Skills, and Functional Academic Skills. Each chapter lists skills, behaviors, and standards which can be easily modified to suit a particular client and trainer. It includes a Skill Summary Chart to be used as an overall record for initial assessment and later training. It is a well-organized and easy to use publication and would be useful to rehabilitation counselors, occupation and physical therapists and others involved in teaching independent living skills to individuals with mobility impairments or multiple handicaps. Recommended for academic and medical libraries and independent living collections.

Walton, Kathy M.; Schwab, Lois O.; Cassatt-Dunn, Mary Ann; and Wright, Virginia K. Independent Living Techniques and Concepts: Level of Use vs. Importance to Independent Living as Perceived by Professionals in Rehabilitation. Lincoln, Nebr.: The Nebraska Agricultural Experimental Station, Department of Human Development and the Family College of Home Economics, University of Nebraska, 1978. 74 pp.

This publication describes a research project conducted by the rehabilitation staff of the Department of Human Development and the Family, University of Nebraska - Lincoln, in Spring 1978. The study indicated "that a definite gap exists related to the techniques and concepts listed in terms of importance to independent living, and the level at which these techniques and concepts are used in the field." The authors believe that if the techniques and concepts important to independent living as perceived by professionals are incorporated into the curriculum of the independent living specialist the new professional will be better prepared to deal with the individual problems of clients. This publication especially the tables and appendices would be very useful to those professionals involved in designing curriculum or teaching independent living specialists. Recommended for academic and education libraries and independent living collections.

6 COMMUNICATION FOR THE DEAF AND HEARING IMPAIRED

ROBERT E. KRETSCHMER/Coordinator of the Program in Hearing Impairment and Associate Professor of Special Education, Teachers College, Columbia University, New York, New York

INTRODUCTION

The communicatively disabled, as a group, constitute a large segment of the handicapped population. In fact, it may be argued that all but a few of the existing disabilities, particularly if incurred early in life, have as concomitant side effects altered and/or disrupted communication abilities. For example, blind or partially sighted individuals not only have difficulty with reading normal print but they may also have difficulty in developing referential meanings for words and in dealing with certain aspects of conversation. Similarly, other disabled and handicapped individuals may demonstrate communication and language deficiencies.

Among those who may be counted as having significant communication problems are hearing impaired individuals. It has been estimated that one in ten individuals possess a hearing loss. This is not to suggest, that all these individuals are profoundly deaf or that they have been deaf since birth. Rather, this generic group is comprised of individuals with varying degrees of hearing loss (ranging from a mild to a profound loss), sustained at various times of their lives (anywhere from birth to the senior years). This 10% figure also includes those individuals who at any given moment may have a significant but yet temporary (conductive) hearing loss as well as those who have a more permanent (sensorineural) loss. As a result, this generic population is a very heterogeneous one and is termed hearing impaired.

The general public's use of the term deaf often refers to those who were born severely or profoundly hearing impaired, or are "educationally deaf." This group of individuals comprise a relatively small percentage of the population at large. Estimates as to the percentage of educationally deaf individuals in the school age population range from .01 to .05%.

Because of the heterogeneity of this group, the rehabilitative needs of its constituent members are quite varied and are the result of a number of medical, genetic, and/or environmental factors. The following annotated bibliography is a respresentative and not an exhaustive listing of publications dealing with these processes, factors, and issues. More particularly, the bibliography annotates a series of texts concerned with identification, diagnosis, and (re)habilitation of communicationally disabled individuals, particularly the hearing impaired.

To begin with, a number of the texts reviewed concern themselves with a general overview of the diagnostic-remediation process with regard to hearing impairment and its impact upon the individual. As a result, they serve as professional introductions to the fields of audiology, speech and hearing sciences, deaf education, and the psychology and sociology of deafness. The text Hearing and Deafness, edited by Davis and Silverman, has long been considered a classic with respect to these notions. It provides an overview of topics ranging from acoustics and psychoacoustics to medical aspects, diagnostic concerns, and to various remediation and psychosocial concerns. For a more advanced overview of these topics see the Handbook of Clinical Audiology by Katz. This book's strength lies in the technical areas associated with differential diagnosis, audiological and medical aspects, and hearing aids as related to hearing impaired individuals.

There are a number of other texts annotated in the bibliography which too stress primarily information relating to the adequate audiological evaluation of individuals and on adequate hearing aid fittings. The most detailed of these is the text <u>Hearing Assessment</u> by Rintelmann. For a relatively current coverage of the broader scope of hearing, language, and speech diagnostic procedures the reader is referred to Singh and Lynch's <u>Diagnostic Procedures in Hearing, Language, and Speech</u>.

Finally with respect to audiological notions, three texts of a highly specialized nature deal with various aspects of the auditory processing abilities of hearing impaired adults Danhauer and Singh's <u>Multidimensional Speech Perception by the Hearing Impaired</u>; of hearing impaired children Stark's <u>Sensory Capabilities of Hearing-Impaired Children</u>; and of the development of a specially designed speech and hearing test for hearing impaired children Bench and Bamford's <u>Speech-Hearing Tests and the Spoken Language of Hearing-Impaired Children</u>. One reference text which may be useful to both lay persons and professionals is Delk's <u>A Comprehensive Dictionary of Audiology</u> which is a complete and encyclopedic dictionary of speech and hearing terms.

While some of the above texts address issues relating to prosthetic devices (hearing aids), there are a number of other texts which specialize in this topic. The text <u>The Hearing Aid: Its Operation and Development</u> by Berger discusses in detail the historical development of hearing aid technology. Other texts cover current aspects of hearing aid technology, hearing aid fittings and the role of hearing aids in the (re)habilitation process, e.g., Hodgson and Skinner's <u>Hearing Aid Assessment and Use in Audiologic Habilitation</u>, Rubin's <u>Hearing Aids: Current Developments and Concepts</u>, and Miller's <u>Hearing Aids</u>. The last text is fairly nontechnical in nature. A well-written text, especially prepared for parents and other lay individuals, is <u>Your Child's Hearing Aid</u> by Craig, Sins, and Ross. Two publications specially designed for hearing impaired individuals (particularly congenitally deaf persons) are Craig's <u>Hearing Aids and You</u> designed for children and Gauger's Orientation to Hearing Aids written for a college or adult level population. Extreme care, however, must be exercised in using these two texts, and the reader is referred to the actual bibliography for further comments. For an in-depth, but very readable, text on the electro-acoustical and operational properties of different hearing aids, the reader is referred to Staab's Hearing Aid Handbook.

(Re)habilitative programming for hearing impaired individuals is not restricted to the prescriptive use of hearing aids. As a result, a number of texts have been written outlining various positions and methodologies regarding this issue. Among these texts are Sander's Aural Rehabilitation (a general text in the area), Schow and Nerbonne's Introduction to Aural Rehabilitation (which also presents a number of case studies), and Oyer and Frankmann's The Aural Rehabilitation Process: A Conceptual Framework Analysis (which is very client oriented and emphasizes the psychological processes involved in adjusting and coping to the disability and rehabilitation).

The above mentioned texts address several aspects of the rehabilitative process, but only discuss them in relatively general terms. The text A Workbook in Auditory Training for Adults written by Smith and Karp, on the other hand, provides specific exemplar lessons in auditory training for use with deafened adults and the texts Visual Communication of the Hard of Hearing by O'Neill and Oyer and Speechreading (Lipreading) by Jeffers and Barley review the scientific and pedagological study associated with the phenomenon of speechreading with both adults and children. One publication which should be very useful in the affective management of deafened individuals in helping them to come to grips with their disability and to answer many of their initial queries is Helleberg's Your Hearing Loss: How to Break the Sound Barrier.

Although several of the rehabilitative audiology texts above addressed issues concerned with children, they do not do so intensively. Likewise, the general audiologic assessment and medically oriented texts do not stress these issues. There exists a number of texts on the market, however, that were written specifically with these topics in mind. One group of such texts are concerned with issues specifically related to infants, e.g., Gerber's Audiometry in Infancy and Gerber and Mencher's Early Diagnosis of Hearing Loss. Other texts, are concerned with a wider age range of children. The most notable of these are: Hearing Loss in Children: A Comprehensive Text edited by Jaffe; Hearing Disorders written by Northern; Auditory Management of Hearing Impaired Children edited by Ross and Giolas; and The Hard of Hearing Child: Clinical and Educational Management edited by Berg and Fletcher. The text Auditory Management of Hearing Impaired Children is particularly good, though technical. It may well become a standard text. There are two other important texts reviewed which are specific in nature and focus on various audiologic and medical screening procedures, i.e., Harford's Impedence Screening for Middle Ear Disease in Children and Detection of Hearing Loss and Ear Disease in Children by Gerwin and Glorig.

All of the above texts, while briefly addressing (re)habilitative issues, primarily stress medical and audiological assessment concerns. The following texts, on the other hand, are good examples of texts stressing the various kinds of oral/aural management techniques and approaches that are available and certain oral/auditory habilitative issues. These texts are Mencher and Gerber's Early Management of Hearing Loss; Principles of Aural Rehabilitation by Ross; and Aural Habilitation by Ling and Ling. There is one text of particular note that should be mentioned and that is Your Child's Hearing and Speech: A Guide for Parents by Miller et al. This publication requires special notation in that it is specifically written for uninformed lay individuals, such as parents, and it does so in a nonthreatening informative manner.

At a macro systems level, with respect to habilitation, there are several texts which attempt to outline methods of establishing, organizing, and maintaining entire (re)habilitative programs on a group rather than an individual basis. This is done, sometimes, by describing actual model programs. Examples of these texts are: A Guide to Clinical Services in Speech-Language Pathology and Audiology by the American Speech-Language-Hearing Association and Residential Facility Programs for the Hearing Impaired Developmentally Disabled: The ATPC Sensory Training Unit Model by Stewart et al.

Should the reader be more interested in a general overview of the fields of the education of the hearing impaired, the psychology of deafness, and the sociology of deafness, he is referred to Moores' Educating the Deaf: Psychology, Principles, and Practice, Quigley and Kretschmer's The Education of Deaf Children: Issues, Theory, and Practice or Levine's Ecology of Early Deafness. These three texts cover a wide range of topics, including the use and development of manual communications and general pedagogy. For other texts of this nature and more specific to the psychology of deafness, the reader is referred to Chapter 3 "Deafness and Hearing Impairment."

In addition to the above, there are two other groups of texts which were written specifically to acquaint their audiences with the language behavior of deaf children and the various educational practices used to remediate it. The first group of books is primarily of historical interest only. Those include Harris' Language for the Preschool Deaf Child, Streng et al. Hearing Therapy for Children, Whitehurst's Teaching Communication Skills to the Pre-School Hearing Impaired Child, Hart's Teaching Reading to Deaf Children, and Dale's Language Development in Deaf and Partially Hearing Children. The second group of texts reflect contemporary practices emphasizing psycholinguistic notions. These books are Blackwell et al's Sentences and Other Systems, Kretschmer and Kretschmer's Language Development and Intervention with the Hearing Impaired and Streng et al's Language, Learning and Deafness.

Another pedagogical area in which there has been several texts written is that of teaching speech to deaf children. Two of the most widely used are: Speech and the Hearing-Impaired Child: Theory and Practice by Ling and Speech and Deafness by Calvert and Silverman. The first entry, in particular, is being widely read and used by educators of the hearing impaired.

Among the most rapidly expanding areas of publication within the field of hearing impairment is that of texts dealing with various aspects of manual communication. Not all of these texts, however, deal with exactly the same subject matter in the same manner. With regard to those texts defined as dictionaries, there are a number of such books, each with their own idiosyncracies. The text A Basic Course in Manual Communication by O'Rourke, for example, was one of the first such books published and is still widely used. Riekehof's text Joy of Signing is fairly new on the market but is useful because it provides mnemonics which the text states are the "origins" of these signs. While many of these "origins" may be questionable, they are still useful in remembering how to form or recognize a certain sign. In addition to these general dictionaries, a number of others exist appealing to specific interest groups. For example, the text Manual Communication: A Basic Text and Workshop with Practical Exercises by Christopher was written with the speech and hearing clinicians in mind. Thus, it provides special signs for clinical purposes; whereas, A Basic Vocabulary: American Sign Language for Parents and Children by O'Rourke, as the title suggests, was written for parents and emphasizes common words peculiar to a deaf child's environment. The text by Christopher also has an unusual, but yet unproven, feature of receptive practice lessons consisting of pictures of signs printed in a left to right sequence corresponding to sentences. The following two texts, too, cover specialized vocabularies, as is obvious from their titles: Signs of Drug Use: An Introduction to Drug and Alcohol Vocabulary in American Sign Language by Woodward, Signs of Sexual Behavior: An Introduction to Some Sex-Related Vocabulary in American Sign Language by Woodward.

For those interested in texts attempting to acquaint the student with the grammer of American Sign Language (ASL) via a patterning approach, the reader is referred to any of the following: three texts by Fant Ameslan: An Introduction to American Sign Language, Sign Language, and Intermediate Sign Language and Madsen's Conversational Sign Language II; an Intermediate-Advanced Manual. These texts do not approach the grammer of ASL in systematic fashion. However, they do present a number of individual signs. Alternatively, Hoemann's Communicating with Deaf People and Baker and Cokeley's American Sign Language: A Teacher's Resource Text on Grammar and Culture attempt to sensitize the reader to linguistic principles of ASL while blending the explanation of these principles with actual practice in their use. Both of these texts presume that the student already possesses a basic vocabulary in manual communication. The Baker and Cokley text is very detailed and quite well-organized.

The scholarly reader interested in the scientific study of ASL will want to peruse Stokoe et al's A Dictionary of American Sign Language on Linguistic Principles, which inaugurated the modern study of ASL, and Wilbur's American Sign Language and Sign Systems, which is the most comprehensive text on the subject matter to date. Another fairly comprehensive, scientific coverage of the topic is Klima and Bellugi"s The Signs of Language. Other very important and useful texts dealing with various ASL topics are Friedman's On the Other Hand: New Perspectives on American Sign Language, and Schlesinger and Namir's Sign Language of the Deaf: Psychological, Linguistic and Sociological Perspectives.

In addition to the texts dealing with manual communication itself, a number of other texts have been written providing the theory and/or rationale behind the pedagogical movement of total communication (which advocates the use of all communication modalities in the education of deaf children) or behind specific pedagogical signing systems which are currently in use and are different from ASL. Many of these publications discuss the research conducted in this area but they also review and engage in the politics surrounding its use. Some of these texts are Pahz and Pahz's Total Communication: The Meaning Behind the Movement to Expand Educational Opportunities for Deaf Children. Bornstein et al's A Guide to the Selection and Use of the Teaching Aids of the Signed English System, Gustason et al's Signing Exact English, and Savage et al's Psychology and Communication in Deaf Children.

In the past few years a few publications have been written reflecting concerns and issues, related to the expanding subspecialty of manual communication interpreting. The four texts annotated in this chapter concerning these matters are: Yoken's Interpreter Training: The State of the Art, Johnson et al's Proceedings of the Third Biennial Registry of Interpreters for the Deaf, the International Symposium on Interpretations of Sign Languages, The Development of Interpretation as a Profession, and Dicker's Facilitating Manual Communication for Interpreters, Students, and Teachers.

Finally, there are a few, but only a few, texts dealing with the needs of a very low incidence disabling condition, i.e., the blind, and the deaf-blind. Kramer et al's text Audiological Evaluation and Aural Rehabilitation of the Deaf-Blind Adult is very interesting and useful in that it describes the modes of communication, the hearing evaluation techniques, prosthetic considerations, rehabilitation, and prognosis associated with all possible combinations and permutations of a certain number of variables associated with deaf-blindness. Bergman et al's text Auditory Rehabilitation for Hearing Impaired Blind Persons describes a model demonstration speech and hearing program designed for deaf-blind persons. Dinsmore's book entitled Methods of Communication with Deaf-Blind People provides a very interesting description of eight different manual spelling and letter coding systems used internationally. Finally, Leavitt's Oral-Aural Communication (OAC); A Teacher's Manual presents a review of the types and various uses of different oral/aural communication aids available for use with blind persons.

As can be seen there are a number of texts available which cover a variety of evaluative and (re)habilitation concerns of hearing impaired persons. The interested readers, regardless of their level of sophistication, should be able to find several references within this chapter to satisfy their curiosity or needs.

ANNOTATED BIBLIOGRAPHY

Alpiner, Jerome G. Handbook of Adult Rehabilitative Audiology. Baltimore: Williams & Wilkins, 1978. 267 pp.

A text written for students in speech pathology and audiology and practicing audiologists to acquaint them with the rehabilitation process for adults with a hearing loss. The topics covered are the present status of aural rehabilitation, client input regarding the rehabilitative process, evaluation of communication functioning, hearing aid use related to rehabilitation, the remediation process, psychological and counseling aspects, the geriatric client, the adult-deaf client, the role of auxillary personnel, community aural rehabilitation programs and research aspects. Well-written and organized. A number of useful communication scales and assessment forms are provided in appendices. A number of topics are covered which are not usually included in other texts or are covered much less comprehensively, e.g., the evaluation of communication functions, counseling aspects, and providing for the congenitally deaf adult. Recommended for special education, rehabilitation and professional libraries.

American Speech-Language-Hearing Association. Guide to Clinical Services in Speech-language Pathology and Audiology. 9th edition. Rockville, Md.: The American Speech-Language-Association, 1979. 215 pp.

Contains detailed information on accredited service programs, certified private practitioners, nonaccredited service programs and state resource personnel. Information is arranged by state and city. The guide is to be used as a reference source for people needing service and also as a referral source for professionals. The information was gathered from a 1978 survey. It is not indexed. However, the arrangement by state and city makes it very easy to use. This reference work should be purchased for collections serving users with the above information needs.

Baker, Charlotte, and Ballison, Robin. Sign Language and the Deaf Community. Silver Springs, Md.: National Association for the Deaf, 1980. 267 pp.

COMMUNICATION FOR THE DEAF 165

A compendium of sixteen essays and articles written by individuals influenced by and dedicated to William Stokoe, father of modern sign language studies. Each essay/article was to describe the individual's "own involvement" in the field and their personal/professional association with Stokoe. The topics covered include sign language systems in other countries and the personal/professional life of Stokoe. They range from scientific presentations to testimonials.

The book presents the field of sign language studies as both a science and a social movement. As a result, at times, it is emotionally charged. It is valuable as an overview of various aspects of sign language studies. Recommended for special education, rehabilitation, linguistic, social science, and professional libraries.

Baker, Charlotte, and Cokely, Dennis. American Sign Language: A Teacher's Resource Text on Grammar and Culture. Silver Springs, Md.: T. J. Publishers, 1980. 469 pp.

A teacher's resource manual overviewing and providing guidance in the use of a series of three texts designed to teach students American Sign Language. It provides a brief explanation of what ASL is and a discussion of the use of English in the education of deaf children. Each of the 17 lessons covered in the three student texts are repeated in this text, along with a verbal description of the linguistic notions of ASL being taught. The three student texts present all of the known ASL linguistic structures in a spiraling curricular format.

The text and the program it explains is a sophisticated presentation of ASL which blends both theory and practice. It is superior to any other text of its kind. The text presupposes some knowledge of signs at least in terms of a vocabulary.

Baker, Charlotte, and Padden, Carol, eds. American Sign Language: A Look at its History, Structure, and Community. Silver Spring, Md.: T. J. Publishers, 1978. 22 pp.

A pamphlet briefly defining what American Sign Language is, how it's organized, and its history. It also briefly describes the deaf community. Its primary purpose is to briefly sensitize the reader to what American Sign Language is and to demonstrate its complexity to legitimize it as a language.

Very useful for anyone wanting a cursory understanding of what ASL is and how it differs from spoken English. Particularly useful to parents, professionals other then deaf educators and the lay public. Recommended for social science education, high school, and public schools.

Bench, John, and Bamford, John. Speech-Hearing Tests and the Spoken Language of Hearing-Impaired Children. New York: Academic Press, 1979. 528 pp.

A detailed technical description of the development of several new tests of hearing using connected speech devices for hard-of-hearing children. These tests were devised from a detailed analyses of the spoken language of these children. The text is written in a scientific format for other professionals.

An extremely lengthy, detailed and technical but significant volume of interest primarily to professionals. Much normative data on the spoken language of hard-of-hearing children is provided. Recommended for special education and professional libraries.

Berg, Frederick S. <u>Educational Audiology: Hearing and Speech Management</u>. New York: Grune & Stratton, 1976. 312 pp.

A book written for university students and professionals outlining and delimiting the field of educational audiology which deals with the clinical and educational management of hard-of-hearing children. It incorporates eight chapters of practical information, which focuses on basic considerations, hearing and speech management, and models of delivery of services at the infant through university levels. Specific topics covered are definition of terms, audiometry, spectrography, communication, auditory trainees and hearing aids, programming during infancy, communication training in special classes, speech technology, technology in listening training, and support services.

A well-written text. Although reported to be geared toward "education audiologist" much, if not most, of the information is applicable to the oral/aural instruction of deaf children as well. Recommended for special education, rehabilitation and professional libraries.

Berg, Frederick S., and Fletcher, Samuel G., eds. <u>The Hard of Hearing Child: Clinical and Educational Management</u>. New York: Grune & Stratton, 1970. 363 pp.

A collection of topics and chapters relating to the identification, diagnosis and education of the hard-of-hearing child. In addition to specific information concerning techniques in obtaining case history information, differential diagnosis, psychological evaluation procedures, educational programming, educational audiology, auditory training and the role of language and reading in educational process of hard-of-hearing children. Basic information regarding definitions and incidences, the auditory mechanisms, linguistics, and language development, acoustic phonetics and behavioral analysis are included.

A number of very useful chapters to professionals are included, such as those on linguistic acoustic phonetics, functional analysis of behavior, case history interviewing; differential diagnosis, and educational audiology. Although the book is intended to focus on the hard-of-hearing child, much of the information is also applicable to deaf children. It is difficult to determine what is specific to hard-of-hearing children. Recommended for special education, rehabilitation, professional and possibly public libraries.

Berger, Kenneth W. The Hearing Aid: Its Operation and Development. Livonia, Mich.: National Hearing Aid Society, 1974. 258 pp.

A fairly comprehensive historical and technical account of the development of hearing aids, earmold-receivers, and batteries, beginning with pre-electric versions, progressing through the first electric hearing aids, the vacuum tube models, the transitor models and the use of integrated circuits. Chapters are also devoted to hearing aid organizations, hearing aid legislation and codes and acoustical descriptions of hearing aids. Appendices enumerating hearing aid battery numbers and sizes, periodicals pertaining to hearing aids, the National Hearing Aid Society Code of Ethics and several state and national codes, and tours are provided. As an addendum, all the hearing aid manufacturers brands and their individual models which were available at the time of print are provided with appropriate descriptions.

A very interesting and complete presentation of the history of hearing aid technology and overview of the acoustical description of hearing aids. Particularly useful are the sections on hearing aid organizations and legislation and the extensive listing of hearing aid manufacturers and models which is in need of updating. Recommended for special education, rehabilitation, professional and public libraries.

Bergman, Moe; Rusalem, Jerbert; Malles, Irwin; Schiller, Vera; Cohan, Helen; and McKay, Evelyn. Auditory Rehabilitation for Hearing Impaired Blind Persons; ASHA Monograph, no. 12. Washington, D.C.: American Speech and Hearing Association, 1965. 98 pp.

A description of a pilot speech and hearing demonstration project at the Industrial Home for the Blind in Brooklyn. The history of the project is provided as are the audiologic evaluative procedures, hearing aid evaluative procedures and the follow-up procedures used. A number of audiological research studies having to do with localization, lateralization and other phenomenon are reported as well as a study on the social impact of special speech and hearing services for hearing impaired blind persons. Appendices containing various forms used in the project are also provided.

Useful description of the organization and operation of an exemplar speech and hearing program for hearing-impaired deaf persons. The research projects provide technical, but relevant information regarding the auditory abilities of hearing-impaired blind persons. Recommended for special education, rehabilitation and professional libraries.

Bess, Fred H., ed. Childhood Deafness: Causation, Assessment, and Management. New York: Grune & Stratton, 1977. 341 pp.

An edited volume of twenty-five chapters providing a current comprehensive text on childhood deafness generated from the International Symposium on Childhood Deafness in 1976. The chapters deal with various aspects of causation, assessment, and management of childhood deafness. The papers presented generally are well-written and present the current state of the art.

A broad based up-to-date technical portrait of the state of the art and written for professionals. Some areas not included, however, are manual communication approaches to communication and teaching psycho-social aspects of deafness and the availability of various mainstreaming options and plans. Recommended for special education and professional libraries.

Blackwell, Peter M.; Engen, Elizabeth; Fischgrund, Joseph E.; and Zarcadoolas, Christina. Sentences and Other Systems: A Language and Learning Curriculum for Hearing-Impaired Children. Washington, D.C.: Alexander Graham Bell Association for the Deaf, 1978. 190 pp.

A presentation and explanation of the curriculum used at the Rhode Island School for the Deaf. A brief history regarding the evolution of scientific thought at the Rhode Island School for the Deaf is provided as well as brief overviews of the theoretical positions of Bruner, Piaget, Vygotsky, Chomsky, and Brown. The bulk of the text describes the process of curriculum design and an explanation of the thematic content (which is social sciences oriented) and sequence of syntactic language forms in their curriculum. Particular emphasis is placed on the role of reading in the curriculum; the relationship between literature, reading and writing, and grammar and interdisciplinary programming. Written for professionals.

Very useful to those interested in the application of linguistic data and concept formation to the teaching of deaf children and in the development of curricula. Very topical and stimulating. Somewhat behind the times in terms of semantics, discourse cohesion and schema theory particularly with reference to written text. Still, very useful. Takes primarily a syntonic, structured approach to teaching. Recommended for special education, rehabilitation, curriculum, and professional libraries.

Bornstein, Harry; Saulnier, Karen Luczak; and Hamilton, Lillian B. A Guide to the Selection and Use of the Teaching Aids of the Signed English System. Washington, D.C.: Gallaudet College Press, 1976. 20 pp.

Provides the rationale behind and an annotation of a series of books and teaching aids designed to teach a deaf child to read Signed English, a signing system, designed by the principle author and print by setting up a sign to print correspondence. An explanation as to the series organization and purpose is discussed.

Valuable reference for parents and educators who wish an overview of the teaching aids available in this area and a descriptive summary of them. It also contains a useful description of the Signed English system itself. Recommended for special education and public libraries and media and curriculum centers particularly for deaf children.

Calvert, Donald R., and Silverman, S. Richard. Speech and Deafness: A Text for Learning and Teaching. Washington, D.C.: Alexander Graham Bell Association for the Deaf, 1975. 243 pp.

A basic text outlining the rudimentary anatomy associated with speech production, the factors affecting speech development, the speech science behind speech perception, and general and specific approaches to teaching and developing speech. The approach taken is somewhat analytic and structural. An extensive bibliography and suggested readings are provided.

This is a very good basic text in speech teaching and development geared toward upper division and graduate level students. Its advantages, which could also be its disadvantage if used as a cookbook, are the instructional analyses of each of the speech phoneme elements. Recommended for college courses, special education, rehabilitation, and professional libraries.

Charlip, Remy; and Ancona, Mary Beth and George. Handtalk: An ABC of Finger Spelling & Sign Language. New York: Four Winds Press, 1980. 40 pp.

An artistic presentation of the manual alphabet written for the general public. On each page a separate letter is present with a photograph of the hand formation along with an exemplar word which is spelled and depicted visually in the form of photography of the individual fingerspelled letters and a photograph of the American Sign Language sign analog.

An artistic introduction to finger spelling and sign. The photography is excellent. Recommended for public libraries.

Christopher, Dean A. Maunual Communication: A Basic Text and Workshop with Practical Exercises. Baltimore: University Park Press, 1976. 530 pp.

A dictionary of approximately seven hundred signs and letters on general use as well as those associated with clinical contexts. They are organized and presented in 48 lessons. For each lesson visual illustrations of each letter or sign are presented as are written descriptions of the signs. Also practice material to help encode and decode these signs are provided. The encoding materials are written in English sentences while the decoding material are sequences of illustrated sign drawn in a left to right order along with answer key. The sign, depicted is a combination of American Sign Language and Seeing Essential English signs and word ending signs. The last three lessons give practice material pertaining to conducting a hearing, language, and speech evaluation.

The illustration and verbal explanation for the most part are well-expressed and clear. The communication format used is one which approximates Manual English. The use of SEE Signs, may not be appropriate when communicating with many deaf persons. The most unique and desirable features is the decoding exercises which make them almost a totally self instructive manual. Recommended for special education, rehabilitation, foreign language, linguistic, professional and public libraries.

Cohen, Lillian Kay. <u>Communication Aids for the Brain Damaged Adult</u>. Minneapolis: Sister Kenny Institute, 1977. 32 pp.

A listing and the definition of various communication aids and techniques that can be used with nonvocal individuals or those with verbal communication problems due to brain damage. Each aid, e.g., communication board, is explained and an example is given. The neuropathologies of aphasia, apraxia, and dysarthria are briefly explained.

A good nontechnical description of alternative communication systems and techniques for nonvocal brain damaged adults or those without a communication system. Very useful for allied professionals and relatives of brain damaged individuals. Recommended for special education, rehabilitation, social service, professionals and public libraries.

<u>Communication: Everybody's Business</u>. Chicago: National Easter Seal Society for Crippled Children and Adults, 1977. 52 pp.

A compendium of scholarly papers defining and discussing the nature of American Indian hand signs and the use of alternative communication systems such as the Bliss symbols and communication boards with nonvocal individuals. Written as an introductory explanation to these systems.

The three papers dealing with Bliss symbols and communication boards are a good overview of these methods and systems and should prove valuable as adjunct readings for professionals in preparation for patients interested in the fundamentals of these approaches. Recommended for special education, rehabilitation, and professional libraries.

<u>Communicative Skills Program. A Basic Course in Manual Communication</u>. Silver Spring, Md.: The National Association of the Deaf, 1973. 161 pp.

Forty-five lessons of approximately 10-20 signs each, with corresponding practice sentences at the end of the book. The sentences include words previously learned and words not yet taught; the latter must be finger spelled. Illustrations are drawings and are rather small; facial expressions are not shown. No explanatory notes accompany the signs. The book seems to have little coherence as regards the choice of signs taught in each lesson. (They do not seem to be related to other signs taught in the same lesson. Total number of signs taught is 734).

Annotated bibliography of books and audiovisual materials which teach sign language, and a select list of books about deafness. Its size, makes it readily portable, an advantage the larger manuals don't have. Might be useful to some individuals, but most libraries will want to purchase a larger, more comprehensive book. Alphabetical index of signs taught is useful.

Cozad, Robert L., ed. The Speech Clinician and the Hearing Impaired Child. Springfield, Ill.: Charles C. Thomas, 1974. 219 pp.

Discussion of the role of speech pathologist in working with the hearing impaired child particularly the hard-of-hearing child. Written for professionals. Covers such topics as how to establish and organize a hearing conservation program, medical aspects of hearing impaired children; psychological considerations of hard-of-hearing children; speech and language problems of the hearing impaired; and therapeutic approaches to speech, language, speech-reading, auditory training and the application and use of hearing aids with hard-of-hearing children.

Good text describing the organization and execution of a hearing conservation program. The chapters on hearing conservation programs, speech problems and language are particularly interesting. The chapter on medical implications emphasizes conductive etiology and has a good nontechnical discussion of otitis media. Recommended for special education, professional, and public libraries.

Craig, Helen B.; Sins, Valeria A.; and Rossi, Sandra L. Hearing Aids and You. Beaverton, Ore.: Dormac, 1976. 118 pp.

Workbook type teaching aid designed to teach deaf youngsters basic hearing aid maintenance. Numerous cartoons, illustrations and review questions are included. No preface is provided to explain the nature and use of the text.

Although an attempt obviously was made to control the complexity of the language used, this was not done on a systematic basis. Given the nature of the subject matter and the language used, it is recommended that the teaching aid be used with upper elementary and secondary level deaf children with fairly good language skills and elementary age hard-of-hearing children. This should not be used as a self-instructional manual. Recommended for special education, curriculum and public libraries.

Craig, Helen B.; Sins, Valerie A.; and Rossi, Sandra L. Your Child's Hearing Aid. Beaverton, Ore.: Dormac, 1976. 42 pp.

A nontechnical explanation of the parts, function and maintenance of hearing aids geared to the needs of parents and other nonprofessionals.

Excellent nontechnical initial introduction to this topic. Recommended for special education, social services, curriculum, professional and public libraries.

Dale, Dion Murray Crosbie. Applied Audiology for Children. 2d ed. Springfield, Ill.: Charles C. Thomas, 1967. 159 pp.

A basic text on the application of audiological principles to the assessment of children. Topics covered are the basic physics of sound and sound amplification; basic principles and procedures in air, bone, and speech audiometry; audiometric test interpretation; basic principles in speech and accoustic science; hearing aid fitting; the problem of recruitment; auditory training; and habilitation considerations.

Although dealing with basic information this text is in need of revision in many respects, particularly in the areas of habilitation and the tympanometry. Recommended for special education libraries.

Dale, Dion Murray Crosbie. Language Development in Deaf and Partially Hearing Children. Springfield, Ill.: Charles C. Thomas, 1974. 259 pp.

A basic introduction text written for students and professionals attempting to outline the language instructional process with deaf and hard-of-hearing children. The first five chapters attempt to cover teaching methods and practices by identifying and defining the major approaches, pathologies, and communication modalities currently in use, the role of parents and house parents in language development, the use of visual aids, the role of pets and animals in language instruction and the integration of hearing impaired children into schools. The bulk of the text outlines numerous possible language topics that can be used for instructional purposes at different ages.

Another disjointed collection of chapters and topics lacking theoretical importance. The treatment of the subject is superficial and ignores current research data in deafness, linguistic and psycholinguistics. The collection of possible language topics based on current practices and intuition may still be useful to students and professionals in the field. Recommended for special education libraries.

Danhauer, Jeffrey L., and Singh, Sadanand. Multidimensional Speech Perception by the Hearing Impaired. Baltimore: University Park Press, 1975. 130 pp.

The book investigates a theory of speech perception, based upon distinctive features by focusing on the research on different groups of sensori-neural hearing impaired subjects and the perception of speech stimulae. A brief overview of distinctive feature theory is provided as is a detailed review of the research literature in the application of the theory to the hearing impaired population. The authors present the design and results of a series of experiments they conducted in this area. The results are discussed in terms of their pedogological and theoretical implications.

Excellent review and presentation of data in this area of study. The book is basically a forum for the presentation of a series of studies the authors have conducted. Written in quasi-journal style. Contains technical material geared toward the professional. Recommended for special education and professional libraries.

Davis, Hallowell, and Silverman, S. Richard. Hearing and Deafness. 4th ed. New York: Holt, Rinehart and Winston, 1978. 552 pp.

A classic general introductory survey text of the field of audiology and deaf education written for students and professionals. Topics covered are acoustics and psychoacoustics, anatomy and physiology, abnormal hearing and deafness, conservation and prevention of hearing loss, medical treatment, puretone and simple speech audiometry, standards for hearing and medicolegal rules, hearing aids, counseling, auditory training, speech reading, conservation and development of speech, manual communications, historical developments, early and elementary education, post secondary education, the psychology of deafness and the deaf community.

A well-written and organized introductory text. Considered a classic in the field. Recommended for special education, rehabilitation, professional and public libraries.

Delk, James H. A Comprehensive Dictionary of Audiology. Sioux City, Iowa: Hearing Aid Journal, 1973. 175 pp.

A complete and encyclopedia dictionary of terms relating to audiology and speech and hearing. In addition to the dictionary of terms, twenty five pages of illustrations relating to the anatomy of the ear and various hearing aids, ear molds, audiometrics, hearing aid battery changeable stock numbers, and other audiologically related items are provided. The appendices and agenda provide various audiological word lists, tests, various languages, guidelines for audiometric symbols and descriptions of various CROS hearing aid systems.

An excellent and comprehensive dictionary of terms related to speech and hearing sciences and audiology. Useful to parents and professionals alike. Recommended for special education, rehabilitation, social science, professional and public libraries.

Dicker, Leo. <u>Facilitating Manual Communication for Interpreters, Students, and Teachers</u>. Washington, D.C.: National Registry of Interpreters for the Deaf, 1978. 299 pp.

A manual designed to assist in translating ideas in English into either American Sign Language or a manually coded English system of signs. The first parts of the manual are suggested activities, multiple meaning of cards (15 lessons) English idioms (31 lessons), finding alternate signs (16 lessons) and an article on interpreter training. Each lesson presents a series of sentences containing English idioms or words with multiple meanings. The students are to brainstorm possible translations or interpretations in ASL.

This is not a self-teaching device and presumes that the student has a basic knowledge of the grammar and vocabulary of ASL. The student must have access to someone fluent in ASL. Recommended for advance manual communication courses and special education, rehabilitation and professional libraries.

Dinsmore, Annette Bockee. <u>Methods of Communication with Deaf-Blind People</u>. New York: American Foundation for the Blind, 1959. 48 pp.

Verbal and pictorial description of eight manual spelling and letter coding system used with deaf blind individuals in the United States and internationally. Brief descriptions of other systems are also presented.

An excellent descriptive reference for a number of fingerspelling systems often mentioned in other texts but not presented. Recommended for special education, education, social science, rehabilitation, and public libraries.

Fant, Louie J. <u>Sign Language</u>. Northridge, Calif.: Joyce Media, 1977. 165 pp.

Basic signs in American Sign Language format in 15 lessons with accompanying explanations of signs and practice sentences. Fingerspelling is not taught. The language of Ameslan is presented as a series of symbols (signs) in its own grammer rather than as a visual reproduction of the English language. Approximately 340 signs are introduced.

Illustrations are photographs (single or in series), which is rare in books on sign language; the photographs are valuable chiefly because many show the facial expressions which often accompany the signs in actual conversation. Has index. The emphasis is on Ameslan, rather than on signing exact English, thus it does not prepare hearing people to talk to deaf persons who sign in exact English. Recommended for courses in ASL using conversation method and special education, foreign language, rehabilitation, and public libraries.

Fant, Louie J., Jr. Ameslan: An Introduction to American Sign Language. Northridge, Calif. Joyce Media, 1972. 101 pp.

An introduction to the grammar of American Sign Language. Fourteen lessons are presented in a conversational format. Numerous pictures illustrating the signs and English glosses and grammatical notes are provided. A vocabulary of 375 signs is used and periodic review and practice items are provided. A bibliography is provided and film demonstrating the sentences can be obtained to accompany the text.

Not a self-teaching device. One must have access to a fluent signer. Not as comprehensive as the Baker and Cokely series but has an advantage (photographs) over the Hoemann, The American Sign Language text. Considered a classic in that it is the first popular attempt to teach the grammar of ASL via conversational method. Has a brief introduction distinguishing ASL from English. Recommended for special education, rehabilitation, social science, foreign language and public libraries and courses in ASL.

Fant, Louie J., Jr. Intermediate Sign Language. Northridge, Calif.: Joyce Media, 1980. 242 pp.

Second in a series of books designed to teach American Sign Language by practicing it directly rather than studying its principles. It builds upon the author's previous book Sign Language. 370 new vocabulary items are presented accompanied by photographs, explanation of the meaning of the sign, and exercise sentences and stories.

Well-organized and presents a number of signs often not included in other instructional texts. Most valuable for those who learn a language using the conversational method. Recommended for special education, rehabilitation, foreign language and public libraries.

Fiedler, Miriam Forster. Developmental Studies of Deaf Children. ASHA Monographs, no. 13. Washington, D.C.: American Speech and Hearing Association, 1969. 172 pp.

Report of a longitudinal research of twenty children in a residential oral school for the deaf. Both development and school progress were followed over a period of seven years by means of periodic testing, observations of behavior, teacher's reports and other school records. The resultant data are presented as case histories and are organized for discussion on the basis of school achievement. Thus, the best, poorest, and average learners are discussed separately as are the hard-of-hearing students in terms of their met and unmet psychological and educational needs.

A scientific report primarily of interest to professionals. The study itself has methodological flaws but the findings and implications are still of interest. Recommended for special education and rehabilitation libraries.

Fine, Peter J., ed. <u>Deafness in Infancy and Early Childhood</u>. New York: Medcom, 1974. 232 pp.

For an evaluation of this work, see Chapter XII.

Friedman, Lynn A., ed. <u>On the Other Hand: New Perspectives on American Sign Language</u>. New York: Academic Press, 1977. 245 pp.

A compendium of eight scholarly chapters dealing with various topics and issues of interest regarding the linguistics of American Sign Language. The text is an out-growth of a course in the structure of ASL and covers topics as the role of iconicity and visual imagery in ASL, its grammatical and semantic devices used in establishing verb/agreement relationships. The issue of subordination and certain issues regarding time expressions and eye movements in turn taking.

The book does not and is not intended to be a thorough treatise on the structure of ASL, but rather address specific issues and topics within this area. For a more comprehensive overview see Wilbur or Baker and Cokley . This text will be difficult reading for those not familiar with the writings and notions of linguists and linguistics. Recommended for special education, linguistics, social sciences and professional libraries.

Gauger, Jaclyn. S.; Clymes, E. William; Young, Marsha; and Woolever, L. Dean. <u>Orientation to Hearing Aids</u>. Rochester, N.Y.: National Technical Institute for the Deaf, 197?. Numerous pagings.

An individualized introductive learning packet designed to orient deaf adolescents and young adults to the proper use and maintenance of hearing aids. The packets consist of an audiologist manual; a student manual; five instructional manuals covering the explanation of what a hearing aid is and what it does, the different types of ear molds and batteries, hearing aid maintenance, troubleshooting and basic consumer information; a hearing aid record; standardized examinations; performance checklist; hourly charts; achievement stickers; and storage and distribution suggestions. The packets are designed to motivate hearing aid usage. An attempt was made to control and simplify the vocabulary and syntax.

This program is meant to be interactive and completed in conjunction with a program of hearing aid evaluation and thus should be completed under the supervision of a qualified audiologist. It is not self-instructive. It is well-organized and designed and potentially useful to a segment of the hearing impaired population, hard-of-hearing and higher verbal deaf adolescents and young adults. Recommended for special education, rehabilitation and professional libraries.

Gerber, Sanford E., ed. <u>Audiometry in Infancy</u>. New York: Grune and Stratton, 1977. 362 pp.

An edited volume of sixteen contributions outlining the problem in terms of the epidemiology of a hearing loss, their pathologies, high risk conditions and auditory development; the methods available for audiometric evaluation including behavioral impedance, respiratory, cardiovascular, electroencephelic, evoked cochlear potential, and evoked brain potential measurements; and the eventual consequences of hearing loss in terms of sensory deprivation communication development, articulatory development, social and educational development, and public health considerations.

A well-organized systematic presentation and delimitation of the current knowledge in the area of infant audiology and the subsequent effects of a hearing impairment are generally informative and current. Recommended for special education, rehabilitation, and professional libraries.

Gerber, Sanford E., and Mencher, George T. Auditory Dysfunction: A Text By and For Audiologists. Houston, Tex.: College-Hill Press, 1980. 256 pp.

A book written to offer the beginning audiology student an introduction to hearing disorders and to provide the framework from which advanced students may proceed. The book is medically and clinically oriented and outlines audiological as well as otologic procedures and methods. The book is divided into four parts: disorders of sound conduction mechanism, disorders of the sensory end organ, disorders of the neural transduction system, and the assessment of the handicap.

The medical descriptions and associated audiological and medical considerations of these disorders, although technical are well-presented. Of particular interest are the periodic case studies presented. Recommended for special education, rehabilitation, and professional libraries.

Gerber, Sanford E., and Mencher, George T., eds. Early Diagnosis of Hearing Loss. New York: Grune and Stratton, 1978. 377 pp.

Proceedings of the Saskatoon Conference on Early Diagnosis of Hearing Loss. The series of papers concentrated on medical aspects of differential diagnosis including the need to expand the high risk register, problems of middle ear infusion, and the need to upgrade the information provided in medical schools; the relative merits of early identification and diagnosis, reviewing the studies in visual response auditometry; the strength and weaknesses of various types of electric response therapy and outlining the programmatic organization of exemplar programs.

The issues and concerns associated with this topic are well-addressed and discussed and should be particularly useful to those interested in early identification and diagnosis. The emphasis, as might be expected, is on the identification process and not the habilitative process per se. Recommended for special education, social sciences and professional libraries.

Gerwin, Kenneth S., and Glorig, Aram. Detection of Hearing Loss and Ear Disease in Children. Springfield, Ill.: Charles C. Thomas, 1974. 190 pp.

Presents the results of a study comparing the validity of various types of screening tools for the detection of hearing loss and ear disease. The tools compared are the verbal auditory screening for Children (VASC), medical questionnaires, medical history, pure tone sweep check, and pure tone threshold. A review of literature related to causes of ear disease, identification audiometry, hearing conservation and the VASC approaches is provided.

Useful for those interested in a comparative study of the effectiveness of various auditory screening tools. Requires careful reading and knowledge of research design to effectively evaluate the findings and recommendations offered. Recommended for special education and professional libraries.

Giffiths, Ciwa, ed. Proceedings of the International Conference on Auditory Techniques. Springfield, Ill.: Charles C. Thomas, 1974. 240 pp.

Proceedings of the first International Conference on Auditory Techniques or the Auditory Approach. A wide variety of papers are included ranging from auditory testing techniques, to issues related to integration, to various training techniques, and organization schemes currently in use to provide auditory training. Information regarding the effects of early sensory deprivation in animals and the relationship between audition, blindness, and spatial behavior is provided.

Particularly useful in that a number of exemplary auditorially based programs and research projects are described in one volume. A few of the chapters provide more technical information than others. Recommended for special education and professional libraries.

Gustason, Gerilee; Pfetzing, Donna; and Zawolkow, Esther. Signing Exact English. Los Alamitos, Calif.: Modern Signs Press, 1980. 455 pp.

The latest edition of the authors' own particular signing system sometimes referred to as SEE II. An explanation of the system's rationals is given as well as an extensive dictionary of all the signs developed thus far. Also included is a bibliography relating to the system. Line drawings of how the signs are to be made are provided along with a verbal description of how they are to be executed. Since a one to one correspondence is set up between a sign and an English word, the English equivalent is simply printed underneath the picture. The dictionary is alphabetized according to English orthography.

This is a reference dictionary intended for anyone who is using this particular signing system. Although it shares its vocabulary with American Sign Language and other sign systems, it is not identical to them. This system is thought to be the most widely used system in educational settings to date. Recommended for special education, rehabilitation, professional and public libraries and curriculum laboratories.

Harford, Earl R.; Bess, Fred H.; Bluestone, Charles D.; and Klein, Jerome O., eds. <u>Impedence Screening For Middle Ear Disease in Children</u>. New York: Grune and Stratton, 1978. 303 pp.

Proceedings of a symposium on impedence screening. Topics covered were middle ear diseases in children, including epidemiology of otitis medici; morbidity complications and sequealae of otitis medici; and the impedance screening of infants, preschool, school age and special populations.

Most complete and comprehensive text on the subject of impedence testing with infants and children available to date. Recommended for special education and professional libraries.

Harris, Grace M. <u>Language for the Preschool Deaf Child</u>. 3rd. ed. New York: Grune and Stratton, 1971. 346 pp.

A presentation of general and specific methodological concerns and techniques associated with utilizing an oral/aural approach to deaf children. Much of the information regarding various teaching activities and the children's responses to them are drawn from personal experiences and knowledge of child development. A combination of the natural and the analytic approach is presented. Specific activities relating to language, auditory training, speech development and readiness skills are covered.

This is a fairly representative text of the era before the advent of total communication and before the influence of developmental psycholinguistics and cognitive psychology. It explores an oral/aural teaching philosophy and discusses the teaching process heavily from intuition and experiences, which at times is consistent with and at other times at odds with scientific knowledge and study. Good for those interested in insights and thinking of an experienced teacher, though it must be tempered by scientific knowledge, e.g., Kretchmer and Kretschmer. Recommended for special education and professional libraries.

Hart, Beatrice Ostern. <u>Teaching Reading to Deaf Children</u>. Washington, D.C.: Alexander Graham Bell Association for the Deaf, 1978. 221 pp.

An outline of reading skills and activities for preschool to junior and senior high deaf children. Basically, the text is a curriculum outline utilized by the Lexington School for the Deaf. Reading is viewed as a language activity and little distinction is made between language and functional reading development. A traditional taxonomy and outline of recalling skills are presented. Appendices outlining major developmental goals, reading skills checklists, reading problems checklist and example materials are provided.

This is a useful text for those interested in traditional approaches to the teaching of reading. Many of the activities and approaches may still be useful when viewed in light of current information processing and reading theories. Recommended for special education, rehabilitation, curriculum, and professional libraries.

Hartbauer, R. E. Aural Habilitation. Springfield, Ill.: Charles C. Thomas, 1975. 82 pp.

An introductory text designed to expose students to a particular philosophy of aural/oral habilitation. Topics covered are definition of terms, the sense modalities of vision and hearing, hearing aids, communication development, auditory training and language development, lipreading, manual education, motivational aspects, educational placement, and re-evaluation techniques.

This is a very superficial somewhat biased text. It is biased in that its treatment of manual communication is somewhat inaccurate and slanted. Recommended for special education libraries.

Helleberg, Marilyn. Your Hearing Loss: How to Break the Sound Barrier. Chicago: Nelson-Hall, 1979. 257 pp.

A "self improvement", self educating type of book designed to help the consumers come to grips with their hearing loss and to provide them with basic information regarding the different types of losses, their remediation, and rehabilitation. Although a great deal of technical information is covered it is done so in layman's terms and in a question answer format so as to follow as popular style and to anticipate questions raised by the consumer.

Although the book covers a fair amount of technical material, it does so in a very palatable nonthreatening way. Additionally it anticipates and addresses many affective and pragmatic questions that an individual recently involved with deafness, at least of an acquired nature, might ask. Care should be given to not recommend the book to parents who recently have discovered that their infant or child is deaf since much of the information may not be appropriate. Recommended for special education, rehabilitation, professional and particularly public libraries.

Hodgson, William R., and Skinner, Paul H., eds. Hearing Aid Assessment and Use in Audiologic Habilitation. Baltimore: Williams and Wilkins, 1977. 188 pp.

A basic text written for university students and professionals covering the basic elements of hearing aid assessment and use in the habilitation process. Topics covered are the role of audiology, the history of the development of the hearing aid, the physical characteristics of hearing aids and their accessories, electroacoustic characteristics, speech acoustics and intelligibility, relationship of electro and psycho acoustic measures, clinical measures of hearing aid performance, hearing aids for children, special types of hearing aid assessment, learning to use the hearing aid, aural rehabilitation, classroom amplification, and hearing aid delivery systems.

The title of the book is somewhat of a misnomer in that it covers rehabilitation aspects as much if not more than habilitative aspects. The majority of the text deals with various technical aspects of hearing aids. It provides practical information regarding hearing aid use and maintenance. Recommended for special education, rehabilitation, and professional libraries.

Hoemann, Harry W. American Sign Language. Silver Spring, Md.: National Association of the Deaf, 1976. 122 pp.

Ten lessons using a patterning approach teaching American Sign Language are presented. In each lesson a paragraph written in English is presented followed by the English gloss of how the same paragraph would be said in American Sign Language. Following each of these, each lexical item or phrase unit is explained in terms of how the sign is produced, its meaning and its grammatical function. Finally, exercise sentences written in ASL format are provided for practice and interpretation.

The book is not a self teaching device but it requires the assistance of someone knowledgable in ASL. The primary method of acquainting the student with the grammar of ASL is via imitation, patterning and the explanation of the grammatical function of specific items within specific sentences. Recommended for advanced courses in ASL and special education, rehabilitation, foreign language, and professional libraries.

Hoemann, Harry W. Communicating With Deaf People: A Resource Manual for Teachers and Students of American Sign Language. Baltimore: University Park Press, 1978. 124 pp.

A text written for teachers and students of American Sign Language, combining both information about the linguistic structure of the language as well as practice in its use. It is superior to the author's previous work in that the grammatical principles are presented in a systematic fashion. The introduction defines what ASL is and twenty-one chapters briefly describe aspects of the grammer of ASL.

An excellent introduction to the grammar of ASL written, for the most part, in nontechnical terms. The reader does need to be familar with some linguistic principles and concepts. Although a very good text of theory and practice, it does not teach individual signs. To complete the exercises the reader must already know the signs or use one of the many dictionaries available. Recommended for a basic course in ASL using a format approach and special education, rehabilitation, linguistic, social science, professional and public libraries.

Huffman, Jeanne. Talk With Me: Communication With the Multi-handicapped Deaf. Northridge, Calif.: Joyce Media, 1975. 276 pp.

A dictionary of maps for teaching sign language to children, deaf (including deaf children with other handicaps) or hearing. Fifteen chapters with over 400 signs, well-organized. Chapter 16 presents suggested activities such as cooking, sorting and matching various items in which signs can be incorporated and taught. A unique feature is practice sentences which show the sign for each word in the sentence, following in English word order. Illustrations are drawings. Very short written explanations of signs are given.

Appropriate for teachers and parents who wish to learn sign language in order to teach. Has some advantage in that it has teaching activities geared to teaching children. A very short introduction, which means that readers should already be somewhat familiar with deafness and sign language. Recommended for special education libraries, foreign language and public libraries.

International Symposium on Interpretation of Sign Languages. The Development of Interpretation as a Profession. S.L.: s.n., between 1977 and 1980. 84 pp.

This book is a transcription of the proceedings of an international conference on interpreter services. Papers describe the interpreter services and the effort to educate interpreters and consumers in various countries, as well as position papers to determine the need for a world federation of interpreters.

Interesting and informative monograph regarding the state of the art in this country via the National Interpreter Training Consortium and other countries. Of particular interest was the similarity in form of the various sign language systems described and the manner in which they deviate from their respective parent languages. Recommended for special education, rehabilitation, social science, and professional libraries.

Jaffe, Burton, F., ed. Hearing Loss in Children: A Comprehensive Text. Baltimore: University Park Press, 1977. 784 pp.

For an evaluation of this work, see Chapter III.

Jeffers, Janet, and Barley, Margaret. Look, Now Hear This: Combined Auditory Training and Speechreading Instruction. Springfield, Ill.: Charles C. Thomas, 1979. 204 pp.

The bulk of the book provides numerous auditory training and speechreading exercises for children and adults ranging from quick recognition exercises, to comprehending connected discourse and stories, to playing various games and quizzes. An introductory chapter provides an organizational framework for these activities.

Gives example lessons and activities for those teachers and therapists following a highly structured approach to speechreading and auditory training. Recommended for special education, rehabilitation, social science, and professional libraries.

Jeffers, Janet, and Barley, Margaret. Speechreading (Lipreading). Springfield, Ill.: Charles C. Thomas, 1971. 392 pp.

An in-depth review and discussion of the phenomenon of speechreading and the research associated with it up to 1971. Topics covered are principles of speechreading, the visibility of speech, factors affecting the ability to speech read, the historical development of speechreading methodologies, example lessons, and speechreading tests.

This is a more detailed but less current treatment of the subject than that of O'Neill and Oyer. It is intended for the professional interested in the science and possible application of the speechreading process. Recommended for special education, rehabilitation, social sciences, and professional libraries.

Johnson, Mildred; Minkin, Marilyn; and Husted, Judie. Proceedings of the Third Biennial Registry of Interpreters for the Deaf, Inc. National Workshop/Convention. Washington, D.C.: Registry of Interpreters for the Deaf, 1978. 128 pp.

Proceedings of a convention consisting of verbatim transcripts of five workshops, a summary of the organization's business meeting and two luncheon meetings. Workshop and luncheon topics covered sensitivity training and value clarification, the legal rights of interpreters, the role and ethics associated with interpreters, conducting interpreter training classes, and the relationship of rehabilitation services, the federal government, and television to interpreter services.

Valuable to those interested in the issues, concerns, ethics and values associated with the Registry of Interpreters of the Deaf and being an interpreter of the deaf. Recommended for special education, rehabilitation, social science, and possibly public libraries.

Katz, Jack. ed. Handbook of Clinical Audiology. 2d. ed. Baltimore: Williams and Wilkins Co., 1978. 623 pp.

An attempt to summarize the current state of the art of clinical audiology in forty-nine chapters. The general topics covered are: medical aspects of a hearing loss; hearing conservation; basic evaluation techniques; differential techniques for diagnosing cochlear, retrocochlear, central and pseudohypoacoustic dysfunctions; special physiological testing including impedance testing; the evaluation of young children and the elderly; the management of the hearing impaired; hearing aids; and communication training.

The book is well-written, concise overview of the general field of clinical audiology. The chapters concerned with various aspects of audiological evaluations are superior to, more detailed than, and more informative than those dealing with management and training techniques.

Keith, Robert W., ed. Audiology for the Physician. Baltimore: Williams and Wilkins, 1980. 327 pp.

An edited volume intended to serve as a complete audiology text written for the physician. Primary emphasis is put on explaining various audiological medical evaluative procedures, though topics relating to hearing aids and the habilitative process are presented.

Valuable as a general reference for understanding the various types of audiological and medical diagnostic procedures in use in this area. The sections on habilitation and rehabilitation are good and general in nature. Notably absent are discussions of etiologic factors and the role of the physician as an effective case manager and his effect on the first person to confirm the parents' suspicions. Recommended for special education, rehabilitation, social science, and professional libraries.

Keith, Robert W., ed. Central Auditory and Language Disorders in Children: Diagnosis and Remediation. Houston: College-Hill Press, 1981. 198 pp.

An edited volume addressing the problems of an ill-defined group of handicapped children, i.e., those possessing central auditory processing difficulties or those with learning-language disorders. The problem is discussed from the point of view of speech and hearing personnel. This volume is the result of a symposium on the topic. Topics covered are neurological consideration, psychoeducation considerations, the evaluation of central auditory functioning, audiological and auditory-language tests the pediatrician view of this disorder, the delimitation of the term, perceptual motor deficits in the population, the testing and training of phonemics synthesis, and the description of language processing disorders.

A well-written and scientifically referenced work oriented toward professionals. The work on central testing and general processing abilities is particularly good. Recommended for special education and professional libraries.

Klima, Edward S., and Bellugi, Ursula. The Signs of Language. Cambridge, Mass.: Harvard University Press, 1979. 417 pp.

A scholarly discussion of various aspects of the linguistics and psycholinguistics of American Sign language. The relationship between formal signs, gestures, and language in terms of the iconic and structural properties and historical evolution and development are explored. Particular emphasis is given to psycholinguistic data and the expressive use of signs as exemplified in with, humor, poetry, and song.

Explores and provides data and information concerning American Sign Language not typically covered in other scholarly treatments of this topic. Valuable to students and scholars interested in the linguistics and psycholinguistics of ASL. Recommended for graduate courses on the topic and special education, linguistic, foreign language, social science, professional, and public libraries.

Kramer, Lynne Chadwell; Sullivan, Roy F.; and Hirsch, Linda Marshall. Audiological Evaluation and Aural Rehabilitation of the Deaf-Blind Adult. Sands Point, N.Y.: Helen Keller National Center for the Deaf-Blind Youths and Adults, 1979. 240 pp.

An attempt is made to describe the modes of communication, the hearing evaluation techniques, prosthetic consideration, rehabilitation, and prognosis associated with all the possible combinations and permutations of the variables of total and partial, adventious and congenital, hearing and visual impairment. Additional information regarding various communication methods and suggestions for working with deaf-blind persons is included. Several appendices dealing with auditory evaluation and hearing aids are included as are a glossary of terms, a bibliography, and suggested readings.

Well-organized description of the various functional types of deaf-blindness and the evaluative rehabilitative process and prognosis associated with them. The glossary and bibliography suggested readings are particularly useful for both lay persons and professionals. Recommended for special education, rehabilitation, and professional libraries.

Kretschmer, Richard R., Jr.; and Kretschmer, Laura W. Language Development and Intervention with the Hearing Impaired. Baltimore: University Park Press, 1978. 358 pp.

A professional text summarizing the current thinking regarding the language acquisition process as applied to hearing impaired children. It overviews the nature of language and normal child acquisitions of language. Comprehensive coverage of traditional and current research in the language of hearing impaired children. Discusses language assessment and education procedures appropriate for this population.

Excellent text for anyone wanting an overview of language and normal language acquisition and an in-depth coverage of the language acquisition of hearing impaired childern. Well-organized and written but reviews technical material. Curricular matters should be of particular interest to professionals. Recommended for graduate course work, special education, rehabilitation, social science, professional, and public libraries.

Larson, Vernon D.; Egolf, David P.; Kirlin, R. Lynn; and Stile, Stephen W., eds. Auditory and Hearing Prosthetics Research. New York: Grune and Stratton, 1979. 456 pp.

A professional and graduate level technical text dealing with aspects and problems associated with researching, designing, evaluating, and fitting conventional and nonconventional hearing aids. It begins with a description of the fundamentals of the auditory mechanism but then rapidly moves into more technical aspects of acoustical and hearing aid sciences.

Excellent text dealing with aspects of hearing and hearing aid research. Deals with current knowledge and work in the area of hearing science. Highly technical and requires a strong background in audiology and acoustical science. Recommended for graduate level courses and professional libraries.

Leavitt, Glen Sheffield. Oral-Aural Communications (OAC); A Teacher's Manual. Springfield, Ill.: Charles C. Thomas, 1974. 125 pp.

A review of the types and various uses of different oral/aural communication aids available for use with blind persons. Numerous resources are cited and a useful glossary of technical terms is provided.

A useful reference for those not familiar with the technology of communication aids for blind persons. Recommended for special education, rehabilitation, public, and professional libraries.

Leshin, George. Speech for the Hearing Impaired Child. Tucson: University of Arizona, 1975. 151 pp.

A text designed to provide information regarding the development and teaching of speech to deaf children. It reviews the major historical approaches to teaching speech, describes and outlines the most common speech errors associated with deafness and presents the major orthography systems used to represent speech. The anatomy and physiology of speech is briefly covered. The bulk of the text deals with describing the formation and characteristics of individual speech elements. General overall goals are provided and discussed too.

This is an elemental approach to the teaching of speech, not unlike other such approaches and texts, e.g., Calvert and Silverman. Its strength lies in its emphasis on the various orthography systems available and an in-depth description of the Northhampton charts. Recommended for special education and professional libraries.

Levine, Edna S. The Ecology of Early Deafness. New York: Teachers College Press, 1981. 422 pp.

This is more than an up-date of her earlier text the Psychology of Deafness, though large sections of that manuscript are repeated in this one. In addition to her repeated discussion regarding suggested psychometric evaluation procedures to be used with hearing impaired children and adults and her "sketches" from life and from research, the text also provides new information regarding early environmental influences, language environments, and educational environments-options and issues. Recommended for special education, rehabilitation and professional libraries.

Ling, Daniel. Speech and the Hearing-Impaired Child: Theory and Practice. Washington, D.C.: Alexander Graham Bell Association for the Deaf, 1976. 402 pp.

A text written primarily for students and professionals outlining a particular system and approach to the teaching of speech to deaf children based upon research findings and on information processing notions.

The book is quite detailed and technical but extremely useful in that it provides a rationale for speech teaching and provides a rational curriculum. It is rapidly becoming a classic. Recommended for college courses and special education, rehabilitation, and possibly public libraries.

Ling, Daniel, and Ling, Agnes H. Aural Habilitation: the Foundations of Verbal Learning in Hearing-Impaired Children. Washington, D.C.: Alexander Graham Bell Association for the Deaf, 1978. 324 pp.

The description of a particular aural/oral approach to teaching deaf children. Topics covered are the general description of communication and the development of spoken language, the organization of speech sounds and their acoustic properties, audiological assessments, hearing aids, the use of residual hearing, the role of vision and touch in speech reception and speech production, speech assessment and teaching, parent-infant communication, language assessment, the relationship between language and reading, program designs for individual needs, and the preparation of professional personnel.

Although the title suggests an emphasis on the aural approach to teaching, the actual content stresses both an oral and an aural approach. It is an excellent example of the position taken by current oral/auralists. Recommended for special education, professional, and public libraries.

Lowell, Edgar L., and Stoner, Marguerite. Play It By Ear: Auditory Training Games. Los Angeles: John Tracy Clinic, 1960. 187 pp.

A collection of 36 lessons and auditory training activities devised for profoundly deaf children. An introduction is provided explaining the complexity of listening processes and some practical suggestions in how-to conduct these activities. Three appendicies are a guide to the phonemic symbols used in the book. The activities revolve around being aware of sounds, discriminating environmental sounds, discriminating certain speech sounds, words, discourse and suprasegmental patterns, and distancing and lateralization. Written for professionals.

A useful collection of structured auditory training activities which have the potential of being abused and treated in cookbook fashion since they are not cast with the context of a theoretical framework of auditory processing or the teaching/learning process. Recommended for special education and professional libraries.

McPherson, David L., and Thatcher, John W. Instrumentation in the Hearing Sciences. New York: Grune and Stratton, 1977. 181 pp.

A basic introduction to the concepts and principles in the operation, development and configuration of experimental and clinical instruments and professional audiological equipment. Written for students and professionals. Topics covered are the physical parameters of sound, the fundamentals of electrical currents, units of measurement, signal generation and control, acoustic transducers, the measurements of sound, recording devices, and electrodes.

The material, although presented in an introductory manner, covers technical material and necessitates that the reader be familiar with basic algebra, and a number of other basic concepts such as impedance, resistance, and reactive inducance. Recommended for special education, engineering, and professional libraries.

Madsen, Willard J. Conversational Sign Language II; an Intermediate-Advanced Manual. Washington, D.C.: Gallaudet College, 1972. 220 pp.

A course text designed to teach manual communications, divided into three parts. The first part covers 750 signs and provides sentences for practice following straight English syntax, the second part deals with interpreting English idioms into the language of signs. The third part deals with translating deaf idioms (syntactic structures) into English.

A disadvantage of the text is that the execution of all the signs is described in print rather than pictorially. Like many other self-teaching books in sign language this book tends to be a dictionary of sign-English equivalents with structured sentence level exercises. Recommended for advanced sign language courses and special education, rehabilitation, social science, foreign language, and professional libraries.

Martin, Frederick N. Introduction to Audiology. Englewood Cliffs, N.J.: Prentice-Hall, 1975. 443 pp.

A text designed to be an introduction to the study of audiology and thus was written for students. Topics covered are the elements of hearing and sound, basic audiometric procedures, special tests for sites of lesions, the anatomy and physiology of hearing, and the delimitation of special problem groups encountered in audiometric testing.

A well-written standard text designed to acquaint the reader with the basic principles of audiology. Recommended for special education, rehabilitation, and professional libraries.

Mencher, George T., and Gerber, Sanford E. eds. Early Management of Hearing Loss. New York: Grune and Stratton, 1981. 468 pp.

Proceedings of the third Elks International Conference held in Winnepeg, Manitoba in 1980. A major portion of the Conference dealt with its audiological and medical management of hearing impaired children in the form of papers from pediatric, otologic, audiologic, and multidisciplinary perspectives. Also considered were issues concerning family-child management with respect to counseling psychosocial development, communication methodology, and the habilitative process.

An excellent and broad, but not comprehensive, review of issues and scientific knowledge relating to the early management of hearing impaired children. Of particular interest are the thirty-six pages of recommendations offered in the form of resolutions generated from the Conference. Of particular note and importance is the preface to the text outlining the strengths and limitations of the text. Recommended for special education and professional libraries.

Methods of Communication Currently Used in the Education of Deaf Children. London: Royal National Institute for the Deaf, 1976. 158 pp.

A collection of papers presented by twenty professionals from the British Commonwealth and the United States at a seminar held in London in 1975. The proceedings were designed to provide a forum for advocates of "oralism" and "manualism" to present their cases. Issues, practices, and approaches to the oral-manual debates are presented from the perspective of a wide variety of professionals and consumers.

The monograph presents a fairly representative overview of the various philosophies, positions, and sub-issues associated with the overall issue regarding the educational methodological oral/manual controversy. It also exposes the reader to much of politics associated with the debate. Recommended for special education, rehabilitation, social science, professional, and public libraries.

Miller, Alfred L.; Rohman, Barbara Farrel; and Thompson, Frances Vena. Your Child's Hearing and Speech; A Guide for Parents. Springfield, Ill.: Charles C. Thomas, 1974. 89 pp.

A text intended to answer parents' questions regarding various aspects of speech and hearing problems. It is written in a question-answer format in understandable terms.

Well-written readable book appropriate for answering many of the questions often raised by parents. It is similar to the book Your Hearing Loss, though written for a different population and is less comprehensive. Recommended for special education, rehabilitation, professional, and public libraries.

Miller, James B.; Foulds, Richard A.; and Saunders, Frank A. Workshop on Communication Systems for Persons with Impaired Hearing or Speech. Washington, D.C.: NARIC, 1979. 22 pp.

Proceedings summary of a workshop on Communication Systems for Persons with Impaired Hearing or Speech. Two separate lists of recommendations and immediate needs were generated.

Useful resource for those interested in doing applied research in this area. Recommended for special education, rehabilitation, and engineering libraries.

Miller, Maurice H. Hearing Aids. Indianapolis, Ind.: Bobbs-Merrill, 1972. 47 pp.

A basic relatively nontechnical introduction to the components of a hearing aid, their function, their types and how they are fitted.

A good text for those beginning in professions associated with hearing impaired people and parents wanting a more in-depth but not comprehensive understanding of hearing aids. Recommended for special education, rehabilitation, social science, professional, and public libraries.

Moores, Donald F. Educating the Deaf: Psychology, Principles, and Practice. Boston: Houghton Mifflin Co., 1978. 347 pp.

For an evaluation of this work, see Chapter 3.

Newby, Hayes A. Audiology, 4th ed. Englewood Cliffs, N.J.: Prentice-Hall, Inc., 1979. 514 pp.

A basic introductory text in the field of audiology. The text presents a brief history of the field of audiology and some basic speech and hearing science. Other topics included are elementary pure tone and speech audiometry, special problems in hearing testing, the development and maintenance of a hearing conservation program, industrial audiology, the impact of a hearing impairment, the (re)habilitation of hearing impaired individuals, and audiology as a profession.

Well-written and easy to read. A good general introduction to the field. As with most texts of this nature, the sections on (re)-habilitation are very general.

Northern, Jerry L., ed. Hearing Disorders. Boston: Little, Brown, 1976. 306 pp.

An edited volume of twenty-five chapters covering five different aspects of hearing impairment designed to provide a comprehensive review of the clinical evaluation of the hearing process, medical aspects of a hearing loss, habilitation and rehabilitation processes, and future directions. Written for students and parents alike.

This is a clinically oriented text and thus the section on habilitation is limited. Otherwise, the text is thorough and informative. Recommended for special education, rehabilitation, and professional libraries.

O'Neill, John J., and Oyer, Herbert J. Visual Communication for the Hard of Hearing: History, Research, and Methods. 2d ed. Englewood Cliffs, N.J.: Prentice-Hall, 1981. 211 pp.

Overview of information and approaches related to assessing and teaching hard-of-hearing adults and children to speechread. Although alternative visual communication systems, e.g., signs, are mentioned their treatment is very brief. Aspects of constructing a speechreading test, factors effecting speechreading performance, visual perceptual training, the experimental study of speechreading, its role of television in the instruction of speechreading and the sociological manifestation of having a hearing impairment are addressed.

This is a brief treatment of the definition, history, and science of the phenomenon of speechreading and is intended as an introductory text for professionals. It might be useful to others who wish to have a better understanding of what speechreading is, how its assessed, factors effecting performance and traditional and historical approaches to teaching it. The relationship between speechreading and the acquisition of language is not sufficiently explored. Recommended for special education, rehabilitation, social science, and professional libraries.

O'Rourke, Terrance J. A Basic Course in Manual Communication. Silver Spring, Md.: The National Association of the Deaf, 1973. 161 pp.

Forty-five lessons of approximately 10-20 signs each, with corresponding practice sentences at the end of the book. The sentences include words previously learned and words not yet taught; the latter must be fingerspelled. Illustrations are drawings and are rather small; facial expressions are not shown. No explanatory notes accompany the signs. The book seems to have little coherence as regards the choice of signs taught in each lesson. (They do not seem to be related to other signs taught in the same lesson.) Total number of signs taught is 734.

Contains an annotated bibliography of books and audiovisual materials which teach sign language, and a select list of books about deafness. Its size, makes it readily portable, an advantage the larger manuals do not have. Alphabetical index of signs taught is useful.

O'Rourke, Terrence J. A Basic Vocabulary: American Sign Language for Parents and Children. Silver Spring, Md.: T. J. Publishers, 1978. 228 pp.

A dictionary of approximately 1000 American Sign Language word signs selected from a number of basic word lists and basic words peculiar to a deaf child's environment. It is intended as a resource for both parents and educators. Simple but very graphic line drawings are provided.

Because a basic vocabulary is presented a great deal of overlap with other dictionaries, reviewed here, exists. Recommended for special education, rehabilitation, foreign language, linguistic, and professional libraries.

Oyer, Herbert J., ed. Communication for the Hearing Handicapped: An International Perspective. Baltimore: University Park Press, 1976. 537 pp.

A text designed to provide professionals with a systematic comparative description of the manner in which habilitation and rehabilitation programs in hearing impairment are carried out around the world. Reports and position papers outlining representative philosophies, programs, methods, and research were obtained from the U.S., Canada, Argentina, Ireland, France, Spain, Sweden, Switzerland, Poland, the Arab world, Israel, India, Malaysia, and Japan.

A very imformative and comparative look at the habilitative process in different countries. Particularly interesting to students of comparative education. Recommended for special education, education, and rehabilitation libraries.

Oyer, Herbert J., and Frankmann, Judith P. The Aural Rehabilitation Process: A Conceptual Framework Analysis. New York: Holt, Rinehard and Winston, 1975. 260 pp.

A review and critical evaluation of research literature that deals directly or indirectly with the aural rehabilitation process. The conceptual framework consists of six major concepts: handicap recognition including self-recognition and identification procedures, motivational aspects including role performance, self concept, and value need relationship; the identification and acquisition of professional assistance by hearing handicapped including information dissemination, selection of services and continuation of services, measurement and evaluation of auditory deficients, rehabilitative methods and clinical milieui/pattern of sessions, and the effects of training and counseling. The process described relates to the deafened adult propulation and is intended for students and professionals.

This is a unique volume in that it is research-based and addresses issues and topic often not adequately treated in other similar texts, e.g., self-recognition of the handicap, motivational aspects, and the effects of training and counseling. One of the advantages of this text is that the monograph is written only by two authors and thus a consistent style and approach is maintained. Recommended for special education, rehabilitation, and professional libraries.

Pahz, James Alon, and Pahz, Cheryl Suzanne. Total Communication: The Meaning Behind the Movement to Expand Educational Opportunities for Deaf Children. Springfield, Ill.: Charles C. Thomas, 1978. 115 pp.

A description of the history of deaf education set within the framework of the oral/manual debate, beginning in ancient and medieval times to the currently popular use of total communication. Various audiological and communication systems are defined. A significant portion of the book is devoted to providing a justification for the rationale behind the use of total communication.

The book probably outlines as well as any other source the historical anticedents of the total communication movement as well as much of the philosophy and politics associated with it. It attempts to justify the movement on rational rather than empirical grounds and does so from a particular point of view. Recommended for special education, rehabilitation, and social science libraries.

Pollack, Michael C., ed. Amplification for the Hearing-Impaired. 2d ed. New York: Grune and Stratton, 1980. 456 pp.

An edited monograph outlining the history and development of hearing aids, their electroacoustic characteristics, earmold technology and acoustics, various practical and philosophical considerations in hearing aid use, hearing aid selection for adults and children, special application of amplifications, speech signals, and hearing aids, hearing aid orientation and counseling, business aspects of hearing aid dispensory and the maintenance of professional relationships. Written for professionals.

A good technical survey of amplification systems and their use with hearing impaired individuals. Covers the area broadly but with sufficient depth to be useful. Recommended for special education, rehabilitation, and professional libraries.

Prescod, Stephen V. Audiological Handbook of Hearing Disorders. New York: Van Nostrand Reinhold Co., 1978. 273 pp.

The book explores the auditory systems, specifying major problems ranging from the outer ear to the control mechanism of hearing. Each chapter begins with a general consideration of the problem to be discussed and then examines such areas as etiology, symptomatology, otological and audiological management of the disorders involved and ends with a comprehensive bibliography and suggested reading lists for the disorder. The final chapter deals with the importance of differential audiology in testing for site of lesion and the intensive limitations of the special tests used for this purpose.

Has the advantage over other audiological texts in that it is organized according to disorders subdivided by types of etiologies for quick reference and thus it tends to be medically oriented. The style is simple and comprehensible by anyone in the field of aural rehabilitation, and will equip the reader with the basic knowledge he needs to recognize the numerous hearing problems that might be encountered. Recommended for special education, rehabilitation, professional, and public libraries.

Quigley, Stephen P., and Kretschmer, Robert E. The Education of Deaf Children: Issues, Theory and Practice. Baltimore, Md.: University Park Press, 1982. 127 pp.

A concise review of the major issues within the field of deaf education. Topics covered include: basic definitions and the various educational options available; the use of various language and communication methods and modalities; the role of various learning environments; the cognitive and intellectual development of deaf children; the reading and writing achievement of deaf children; and the social, affective and occupational status of hearing impaired individuals.

This is a well-organized readable introduction to the field of deaf education and the deaf population. It approaches the task in an objective, non-emotional basis, relying as much as possible on research evidence. Recommended for general as well as professional libraries.

Quigley, Stephen P.; Steinkamp, Marjorie W.; Power, Desmond J.; and Jones, Berry W. Test of Syntactic Abilities: A Guide to Administration and Interpretation. Beaverton, Ore.: Dormac, 1978. 114 pp.

Presents the rationale and overview of the Test of Syntactic Abilities as well as the technical data associated with it. A significant proportion of the text is devoted to test interpretation.

A well-organized presentation of necessary technical and practical information associated with a well-constructed and technical sound test of syntax for deaf children. An indispensible reference for anyone using the test. Recommended for special education, rehabilitation, social science, and professional libraries and curriculum and materials laboratories or centers.

Riekehof, Lottie L. The Joy of Signing. Revised and Enlarged Edition. Springfield, Mo.: Gospel Publishing House, 1978. 336 pp.

Twenty-five chapters logically organized. Illustrations are small drawings with accompanying explanations of origin, usage and written explanation of how to make the sign. Introductory chapters discuss Ameslan as a language, fingerspelling and the history of sign language. Meaning of terms commonly used in talking about deafness and communication (e.g., total communication) is also given.

Annotated bibliography of books on sign language and deafness. Good index. Book is well-organized. Many signs, adequate illustrations, good explanations and applications for the signs are given. No practice exercises, but the usage of each sign is indicated in sentence form. One of few sign language books in hard cover. Recommended for libraries with an interest in sign language manuals.

Rintelmann, William F., ed. <u>Hearing Assessment</u>. Baltimore, Md.: University Park Press, 1979. 616 pp.

This is an edited book intended to serve as a text for graduate level audiology courses concerned with the assessment of the peripheral and central auditory mechanism. Several chapters present basic concepts and others deal with specific topics. Topics covered are threshold measurement methods, pure tone audiometry, clinical masking, otoneurologic evaluations, speech audiometry, auditory adaptation, differential intensity discrimination, recruitment, impedance measures, central auditory processing, assessment of central auditory lesions, pseudohypoacusis, electrocochleography and brain-stem-evoked responses, assessment of hearing in animals, test battery interpretation and instrument calibration.

An excellent but somewhat technical introductory survey type course text dealing with the broad spectrum of hearing assessment. Recommended for special education, rehabilitation, and professional libraries.

Rose, Darrell E., ed. <u>Audiological Assessment</u>, 2d ed. Englewood Cliffs, N.J.: Prentice-Hall, 1978. 550 pp.

An edited text of 14 chapters covering the following topics: the physics of sound; the anatomy and physiology of the auditory system; otologic assessment and treatment; psychological aspects of a profound hearing loss; the organization of a school hearing conservation program; pure tones (unclear word), speech, pediatric, geriatric differential, impedance and neuroelectric audiometry; the audiological management of environmental noise; and hearing aids. Written for students and professionals.

A standard, well-written, for the most part, up-to-date survey text emphasizing the clinical evaluation and management of hearing impaired individuals, particularly children. Recommended for special education, rehabilitation, and professional libraries.

Ross, Mark. <u>Principles of Aural Rehabilitation</u>. Indianapolis: Bobbs-Merrill, 1972. 50 pp.

A brief manual written for students and professionals discussing the application of aural rehabilitation principles to young children. A rationale is offered as well as suggestions for developing and maintaining a home management program, preschool programs, and school age programs. Particular problems associated with speech reading and auditory training are also discussed.

A brief but useful introduction to the oral/aural approach. As with most manuals or texts of this nature, little attention is paid to the developmental psycholinguistic process. Recommended for special education and professional libraries.

Ross, Mark, and Giolas, Thomas G., eds. Auditory Management of Hearing Impaired Children: Principles and Prerequisites for Intervention. Baltimore: University Park Press, 1978. 376 pp.

A text designed to provide graduate university students in training and practitioners with basic information necessary to manage the auditory and educational needs of hard-of-hearing children, and is the result of a symposium on this subject. Topics covered are the role and primacy of the auditory channel in speech and language development; the acoustics of speech production, speech perception and the sensory-neural hearing loss; classroom acoustics; auditory coding and recoding; signal processing, compensatory electroacoustic processing of speech, issues, and exposition.

Well-organized, very informative, but technical. Text is useful not only to those interested in the hard-of-hearing, but the deaf as well. Recommended for special education and professional libraries.

Rubin, Martha, ed. Hearing Aids: Current Developments and Concepts. Baltimore, Md.: University Park Press, 1976. 293 pp.

A collection of 22 independently authored chapters resulting from a conference held in 1975 at the Lexington School for the Deaf. The areas covered are current developments in hearing aid technology; hearing aid dispensement and instruments for speech discrimination; developments in electroacoustic standards; developments in fitting hearing aids to children; and developments in general hearing aid evaluations, such as prescriptive fitting of master hearing aids, signal processing for hearing aids and the fitting of children. Periodic verbatim discussion sections are included. Appendices on legislation relating to hearing aid standards and the proposed American National Standards Institute (ANSI) standards are provided.

A current review of the state of the art in hearing aid technology and fitting. The sections and subsequent discussion on the fitting of infants and general hearing aid fitting procedures are particularly interesting and useful, though at times somewhat technical and presupposing of basic audiological information. Recommended for special education, rehabilitation and professional libraries.

Sanders, Derek A. Aural Rehabilitation. Englewood Cliffs, N.J.: Prentice-Hall, 1971. 374 pp.

A general text designed to acquaint the reader with the principles of adult aural rehabilitation. Topics covered are human communication systems, acoustic aspects of speech, the visual aspects of speech, auditory and visual perception, amplification and hearing aids, auditory training, visual communication training, the integration of vision, and audition and case management.

A well-written and organized general introduction to the topic which has almost become a standard text in many university courses. Recommended for special education, rehabilitation, professional, and possibly public libraries.

Savage, R. D.; Evans, L.; and Savage, J. F. Psychology and Communication in Deaf Children. New York: Grune and Stratton, 1981. 307 pp.

A description of the issues and problems encountered in undertaking a research investigation entitled, "A Developmental Study of the Use of One-handed Fingerspelling in Teaching Deaf Children." The first two sections of the text overview the history of fingerspelling and manual communication within the context of the education of the deaf in Britain and a discussion of various cognitive functions and research as they relate to deaf children and their education. They also discuss some of the general findings of the study. The last three sections describe the general procedures used and other findings of the study which tend to support the use of fingerspelling.

This is a highly specific and technical presentation of a study. The chapters on the history of fingerspelling and manual communication may have general appeal.

Schlesinger, I. M., and Namir, Lila, eds. Sign Language of the Deaf: Psychological, Linguistic, and Sociological Perspectives. New York: Academic Press, 1978. 380 pp.

A compendium of ten scholarly-written chapters dealing with aspects of phylogeny, ontogeny, linguistics, psychology, sociology, and educational aspects of American Sign Language and other signing systems. Written for students and professionals.

Well-written and well-organized scholarly book which requires some familiarity with ASL. Recommended for special education, rehabilitation, linguistics, social science, professional, and public libraries.

Schow, Ronald L., and Nerbonne, Michael A., eds. Introduction to Aural Rehabilitation. Baltimore, Md.: University Park Press, 1980. 450 pp.

An edited volume designed for undergraduate students who have limited background in communication disorders. It attempts to provide a comprehensive coverage of topics bearing on the rehabilitation process. Fundamentals of aural habilitation and rehabilitation, approaches to aural habilitation and rehabilitation, and case studies are presented.

An up-to-date but general review of the habilitative rehabilitative process. The case studies are particularly useful. Recommended for special education, rehabilitation, professional and possibly public libraries.

Schubert, Earl D. Hearing: Its Function and Dysfunction. New York: Springer-Verlag, 1980. 184 pp.

A technical overview of the anatomy and physiology of the auditory system, psychoacoustics (including auditory sensitivity, frequency analysis, loudness, temporal patterns, spectrum analysis, and binaural hearing), the differential types of hearing losses and audiometric tests used to diagnose them, threshold shift, and various types and fitting of hearing aids.

This book was intended for allied professionals such as physicians, psychologists, physicists, engineers and the like. As a result, certain technical background information, e.g., the physics of sound, basic physiology and neurophysiology, and experimental psychology is presumed. Recommended for graduate courses and special education and professional libraries.

Singh, Sadanand, and Lynch, Joan, eds. Diagnostic Procedures in Hearing, Language, and Speech. Baltimore: University Park Press, 1978. 647 pp.

A compendium of 17 chapters dealing with hearing, language, and speech evaluative procedures and processes written for professionals. The ten chapters dealing with language and speech do not deal with hearing impaired children, but rather, bilingual children, language disordered children and adults, and general articulatory processes and evaluative techniques. The section on hearing covers the diagnostic process from birth to adulthood, hard to test children, the fitting of hearing aids, auditory screening and a disordered-functions approach to audiologic analysis which stresses audiologic habilitation and an information processing approach to audition.

In general, the text provides current and useful information in each of the areas discussed. The chapter on Disordered Functions Approach to Audiologic Diagnosis is particularly interesting. Although the chapters on Language and Speech Evaluation do not directly relate to the assessment of hearing impaired children, many of the issues and information provided, particularly in the area of bilingualism, may be of interest and benefit to those interested in hearing impaired persons. Recommended for special education, rehabilitation, and professional libraries.

Smith, Clarissa R., and Karp, Adrienne. A Workbook in Auditory Training for Adults. Springfield, Ill.: Charles C. Thomas, 1978. 103 pp.

A series of 21 auditory training sessions stressing phonetic contrastive listening drills, word and sentence recognition drills and discrimination, and information giving and attitude development.

These lessons are preceded by sections dealing with general principles of auditory training and the organization of auditory training sessions.

Well-constructed lessons and text provide useful information about chronically ill patients. Unusual in that it is a text developed to provide auditory training exercises for deafened adults. Recommended for special education, rehabilitation, and professional libraries.

Staab, Wayne J. *Hearing Aid Handbook*. Blue Ridge Summit, Pa.: G/L Tab Books, 1978. 334 pp.

An in-depth, detailed presentation of the types, component parts, electroacoustical properties, operation and maintenance of hearing aids and other amplification devices. Written for individuals who have more than a passing interest in this topic.

Although technical in nature and technically written, it presumes little prior knowledge of the subject matter on the part of the reader. Excellent for anyone wanting a working knowledge of hearing aids. Recommended for graduate level courses and special education, rehabilitation, and professional libraries.

Stark, Rachel E., ed. *Sensory Capabilities of Hearing-Impaired Children*. Baltimore, Md.: University Park Press, 1974. 302 pp.

Proceedings of a symposium designed for practitioners in the field outlining the sensory capacities of hearing impaired children. Topics covered include the state of the art from reports with verbatim accounts of subsequent discussions of sensory capabilities, perceptual and cognitive strategies, and language processing.

Highly technical but informative text geared toward professionals. Many issues and questions were raised through discussions of the topics. Recommended for special education, rehabilitation, and professional libraries.

Stewart, Larry; Overbeck, Daniel; and Miller, Donna. *Residential Facility Programs for the Hearing Impaired Developmentally Disabled: The ATPC Sensory Training Unit Model*. Tucson: University of Arizona, 1978. 110 pp.

A description of the growth, developmnent, and operation of a model demonstration program for developmentally disabled deaf children, including client assessment and program evaluation procedures, philosophical considerations, and staff and facility modifications and concerns.

A detailed description of the development and organization of a demonstration program for developmentally disabled deaf persons which is not normally available through typical print media and sources. Much pragmatic information regarding program development and organization is presented. Written for professionals. Recommended for special education, rehabilitation, curriculum and professional libraries.

Stokoe, William C.; Casterline, Dorothy C; and Croneberg, Carl G. A Dictionary of American Sign Language on Linguistic Priniciples. Silver Spring, Md.: Linstok Press, 1976. 346 pp.

A reissue of a classic piece of work published in 1965 with an expanded preface and bibliography on the linguistics of American Sign Language. The introduction outlines the elements of ASL and introduces the scientific orthography used to describe the formation of a sign and various aspects related to the linguistics of ASL and the book. The dictionary itself describes and gives the meaning of several hundred signs. Four appendices briefly describe ASL syntax, sign variation and the deaf community.

This is a very sophisticated, highly technical description of the lexicon of ASL with grammatical notes. It is intended for professionals interested in the linguistics and lexicon of ASL. There are no photographs or pictures; rather, the reader must master a complex orthography system. Recommended for special education, social science, and professional libraries.

Streng, Alice; Fitch, Waring J.; Hedgecock, LeRoy D.; Phillips, James W.; and Carrell, James A. Hearing Therapy for Children. New York: Grune and Stratton, 1958. 353 pp.

A classic text describing the traditional approach to the oral/aural method in a time prior to the influences of linguistics. Topics covered are the history of deaf education, the general impact of a hearing impairment on the development of the individual, basic audiology and types of hearing impairments, and the educational management of hard-of-hearing and deaf students. Emphasis is put on particular problems these individuals typically encounter and various teaching techniques and sequences of activities that can be used in teaching them language and various oral/aural skills. Written for students and professionals.

Although some of the technical information is still adequate, some is antiquated. This text is historically valuable in providing a glance at the state of the teaching art in the 1950's. Recommended for special education libraries.

Streng, Alice H.; Kretschmer, Richard R., Jr.; Kretschmer, Laura W. Language, Learning and Deafness: Theory, Application, and Classroom Management. New York: Grune and Stratton, 1978. 232 pp.

A general, basic text describing the teaching of language to deaf children using a natural experiential approach. The book briefly recounts the history of various educational methodologies and then discusses the impact of P.L. 94-142. The various theories accounting for language development are reviewed, including S-R, cognitive, developmental and information processing theories, as are various linguistic theories and some of the literature in the cognitive abilities of deaf children. The bulk of the text deals with how language is organized and acquired, how communication is normally maintained, how language can be developed and stabilized via an experience-based curriculum, the role of reading and writing in the curriculum, and assessment and planning procedures.

This is an up-to-date, though introductory, treatment of the subject matter. It presents a good blend between theory and practice in that the practical applications are grounded in theory and research. In addition to the practical suggestions regarding language teaching, a scope and sequence chart of language behavior is provided which is particularly useful. Recommended for special education, rehabilitation, curriculum, and professional libraries.

Studebaker, Gerald A., and Hochberg, Irving. Acoustical Factors Affecting Hearing Aid Performance. Baltimore: University Park Press, 1980. 450 pp.

A highly technical compendium of 18 chapters outlining the current state of the art in the acoustic areas of hearing aid performance, resulting from a conference held in 1978. The chapters are divided into 4 general areas, including; the acoustic effects of the environment, such as reverberation, room acoustics, noise and microphone location; the acoustical effects, both actual and simulated, associated with the external ear, ear molds, and earphones; modeling techniques; and the use of frequency-response selection techniques in the fitting of hearing aids.

A technical, but very useful and current, overview of the research in hearing aid research. The section in frequency selection techniques as an alternative hearing aid fitting procedures should be useful and interesting to various social service personnel, rehabilitation workers and educators. Recommended for special education, rehabilitation, and professional libraries.

Vorce, Eleanor. Teaching Speech to Deaf Children. 2d ed. Washington, D.C.: Alexander Graham Bell Association for the Deaf, 1974. 111 pp.

A curricular guide on the teaching of speech to deaf children from the Lexington School for the Deaf. An organizational plan with general goals and objectives for preschool to secondary levels is provided, along with exemplar activities. Written for students and professionals.

This is a traditional treatment of the subject matter which was developed in large measure out of personal experience and intuition. Recommended for special education, curriculum and professional libraries.

Ward, Jill. Ward's Natural Sign Language Thesaurus of Useful Signs and Synonyms. Northridge, Calif.: Joyce Media, 1978. 393 pp.

An attempt to provide a cross-indexed dictionary/thesaurus of American Sign Language signs presented via photographs and English words. The lexical items are presented in alphabetical order according to English spelling. If a specific sign does not exist for an English word or one of its meanings, the reader is referred to the appropriate signed synonym. Since a one-to-one correspondence does not exist between American Sign Language signs and English words, the book attempts to provide the reader with the cross-indexed relationship of the meaning of these words. Approximately 2,500 signs and many more English words are covered.

Although an attempt is made to show how the signs are made, this is not always well done. It is not clearly explained that the printed English equivalent of a sign follows and does not precede the photograph of the sign. The monograph must be used in conjunction with other sign language books if the objective is to learn signs. It also can be misleading to all but sophisticated users of signs in that it gives the false impression that if a deaf person knows a particular sign, e.g., surrender, they will know all of the English equivalents, e.g., abdicate.

Whitehurst, Mary Wood. <u>Teaching Communication Skills to the Pre-School Hearing Impaired Child: A Manual</u>. Washington, D.C.: Alexander Graham Bell Association for the Deaf, 1971. 45 pp.

A series of ten auditory training and language lessons using an oral/aural approach, designed to be used with preschool deaf children who have little or no language by teachers and parents alike. The lessons, although structured in nature, were developed to capitalize on natural play-like activities and music in the form of action songs, using a limited vocabulary. Other traditional auditory training techniques are also provided.

A cookbook presentation of language and auditory training without providing an adequate methodological rationale for the activities. While the lessons may be useful to some in showing how play, music and language/auditory training can be combined, some of the vocabulary and methodologies and procedures utilized run counter to what is know about language development. Recommended for special education libraries.

Wilbur, Ronnie B. <u>American Sign Language and Sign Systems</u>. Baltimore: University Park Press, 1979. 312 pp.

A scientific overview and presentation of the current research in the area of the linguistics and psycholinguistics of American Sign Language. The topics covered are: the cheremic structure of signs; the syntax of ASL; the psycholinguistic research related to ASL; sociolinguistic aspects of ASL; the definition of pedagogical sign systems; and the use of these systems with deaf and other disabled populations.

The single most complete text on the subject matter to date. Because the field of ASL research is expanding so rapidly, the reader of this text is advised to supplement the text with a personal review of the research in this area since 1979.

Woodward, James. Signs of Drug Use: An Introduction to Drug and Alcohol Vocabulary in American Sign Language. Silver Springs, Md.: T. J. Publishers, 1980. 83 pp.

A dictionary of signs for drug related terms, such as pills, alcohol, caffeine, tobacco, illegal drugs such as marijuana, and their effects. Signs for new drugs such a qualludes and angel-dust are also given. The introductory chapter discusses data collection and reasons for variant signs (regional, ethnic, and age variations). Index and bibliography of books and articles on American Sign Language are included

An important reference tool for medical libraries where communication with deaf patients or drug-users may be essential. Illustrations of signs are clear and origins or regional variations for many signs are given. Very comprehensive coverage of the necessary terms.

Woodward, James. Signs of Sexual Behavior: An Introduction to Some Sex-Related Vocabulary in American Sign Language. Silver Spring, Md.: T. J. Publishers, 1979. 81 pp.

Chapters illustrate common ASL signs for sexual organs and sexual activities. An introductory chapter discusses the importance of learning and disseminating this information, and cautions about regional differences in signs and the fact that different signs for the same thing may carry difference connotations (e.g., one may be for polite conversation, another only for intimate conversation). The author is a hearing person, Linguistics and English professor at Gallaudet College. Extensive research among deaf persons was necessary to identify these signs. Index and bibliography of books and articles on sign language included.

Illustrations of how to make the signs are well done. Implications of different signs are explained (e.g., 3 different signs for penis, 3 for vaginal), and when different signs for the same thing are used in different regions, all known to the author are given. A good reference tool for special education, medical and legal libraries, where communication with deaf people about sexual topics may occur.

Yanick, Paul , Jr., ed. Rehabilitation Strategies for Sensorineural Hearing Loss. New York: Grune and Stratton, 1979. 222 pp.

Proceedings from the second symposium on the Application of Signal Processing Concepts to Hearing Aids. The specific papers deal with the influence and role of otolaryngology in the hearing rehabilitation process, signal processing and hearing rehabilitation, the history of electrostimulation of the cochlea, real-ear measures of hearing aid performance, binaural hearing advantages, otomandibular syndrome, digital approaches to speech discrimination testing, auditory training, counseling, the audibility and intelligibility of speech for listeners with sensorineural hearing loss, and hearing aid selection and fitting.

The papers presented are fairly technical with limited appeal for the general public, but of particular interest to professional audiologists. Recommended for special education, rehabilitation, and professional libraries.

Yoken, Carol., ed. <u>Interpreter Training: The State of the Art</u>. Washington, D.C.: National Academy of Gallaudet College, 1979. 64 pp.

A summary of the proceedings of a conference on interpreter training held in Atlanta. Attitude and practices related to administration, ethics, evaluation, levels and types of training of interpretors and interpreter trainers are summarized. A listing of available and forthcoming research and materials relating to the teaching of acquisition of sign language as well as an annotated bibliography on the subject are included.

Of particular value to anyone interested in teaching or researching aspects of sign language instruction or acquisition are the lists of studies, materials and annotations on the subject. In this request, it is an excellent reference and resource. Recommended for special education, rehabilitation, social science, foreign language and professional libraries.

Yost, William A., and Nielsen, Donald W. <u>Fundamentals of Hearing</u>. New York: Holt, Rinehart and Winston, 1977. 240 pp.

An up-to-date text outlining the basics of audition at an introductory level, requiring little prior knowledge of the auditory process or mathematics. The book is divided into three parts: a) the physics of sound b) auditory anatomy and physiology c) psychophysics and auditory perception. Primarily written for students. Recommended for special education, rehabilitation and professional libraries.

7 MEDICAL ASPECTS OF REHABILITATION

CAROL A. KLINK/Assistant Head of Acquisitions, Library of the Health Sciences, University of Illinois at the Medical Center, Chicago, Illinois

DIANNE C. OLSON/Catalog/Acquisitions Librarian, Loyola University Medical Center, Maywood, Illinois

INTRODUCTION

As is the case in many other fields, texts on rehabilitation for medical and allied health professionals are increasing in number. In the past the emphasis in medicine was on the treatment of a given disease: rehabilitation was seen as a part of that treatment. Many texts dealing with a specific field of medicine, for example orthopedics or neurology, included sections on rehabilitation as it is related to that field. Today, there is a trend to see rehabilitation as a specialty in itself, so more texts are being written on rehabilitation in general.

Many texts try to approach the topic of rehabilitation in a comprehensive fashion. Others approach the subject from the viewpoint of a specific disability or class of disabilities. Texts have been written on the rehabilitation of multiple sclerosis, cancer, cerebral palsy, scoliosis, heart attack, and stroke patients. Others deal with the rehabilitation of conditions such as amputation, spinal cord injury, speech difficulties, and orthopedic problems.

Much of the medical literature on rehabilitation has been written for physicians and nurses, because these professions are most involved in treating diseases of or conditions causing disability. However, texts have also been written specifically for dentists, physical therapists, speech therapists, psychologists, and rehabilitation counselors. Many texts attempt to cover rehabilitation from the viewpoint of several different health professionals. Texts written specifically for a certain class of professionals such as physicians and nurses, may vary from an elementary text intended for students to an advanced work for the specialist. Certain works may be written for the clinician, others for the researcher. Some texts emphasize the practical approach to rehabilitation, while others take a more theoretical approach.

An important aspect of a rapidly changing field such as medicine is the currency of publication. In fact, much of the medical literature is found in periodicals, which are outside the scope of this bibliography. Texts in this chapter were for the most part written in the last five years. Older titles have been included where no other current title is available, or if it has considerable research value.

Evaluation of professional rehabilitation monographs raises some complex problems. What is considered essential for some libraries and professionals may be of little or no interest to others. Although we may divide libraries into general categories such as hospital, medical school, and research, all libraries of one particular type may not be the same. For example, hospital libraries vary in size and may serve different teaching programs such as residency training, nursing schools, or other allied health education. Medical schools too vary in size and may emphasize specific training areas. Many community colleges offer courses in allied health education and would have need of some of the texts included here. In addition, there is a growing interest among the general public in health care and health-related topics. Laypersons who themselves have a disability or who have a close friend or family member who is disabled want to find out as much as possible about that condition. Many of the books written for allied health professionals would be useful for that purpose, because there continues to be a lack of materials on health problems written for the general public. For those reasons only the individual reader can decide what is most appropriate to his particular situation. Therefore, we have provided recommendations only as general guidelines to what is available.

General works can be defined as those which discuss more than one condition or disability and are meant to be applicable to all physicians and students rather than a specialized audience. <u>Guides to the Evaluation of Permanent Impairment</u> by the American Medical Association is a "must" for any practicing and future physician who will eventually have to evaluate the degree of a patient's disability so he may qualify for private and public disability funds. Tips on testifying in court and giving testimony are included. <u>Rehabilitation Medicine</u> by Nichols is an excellent overview of all disabilities and their rehabilitation. However, it lacks illustrations and photographs and should not be utilized as a main text, but would serve well as a supplementary and introductory guide. An overall text is Abreu's <u>Physical Disabilities Manual</u>. It contains excellent tables and illustration and is very comprehensive in its coverage, as well as being up-to-date. Since it was published in 1981 Kenedi's <u>Disability</u> is a "state of the art" monograph to which over 252 international seminar participants contributed. Coverage may not be as complete as Abreu's, but it does offer an international perspective on rehabilitation. Basmajian's <u>Therapeutic Exercise</u> deals with a more specific subject in a comprehensive manner. It contains exercise for a variety of specific diseases and disabilities and is a good working and teaching text for the entire medical rehabilitation community.

Some conditions are seldom written about in monographic form, but rather are handled in serial format. Mulder's <u>Diagnosis and Treatment of Amyotrophic Lateral Sclerosis</u>, Longacre's <u>Rehabilitation of the Facially Disfigured</u>, Morrison's <u>Management of Sensorineural Deafness</u>, and Feller's <u>Reconstruction and Rehabilitation</u>

of the Burned Patient are four such titles. Each title is a very excellent source of information for specialists and general physicians. Although Longacre was published in 1973, it is still useful because of its discussion of the psychological and socioeconomical effects of facial disfigurement on the patient. None of these titles are suitable for a layperson or as patient education material. The vocabulary is extremely specialized.

Very little has been written about dentistry and the physically disabled. Rosentein's Dentistry in Cerebral Palsy and Related Handicapping Conditions is a "must" for all dentistry libraries. Practicing dentists as well as students can learn valuable information on treating their special patients. The 1973 Symposium on "Dental Management of the Handicapped Child" may be considered outdated, but may be of some historical and research value.

Monographs dealing with amputation, spinal cord injury and orthopedics fall into three categories: management, the interdisciplinary approach, and adjustment to the condition. The management books seem to be written with the surgeon in mind. Friedmann's The Surgical Rehabilitation of the Amputee and Moberg's The Upper Limb in Tetraplegia: A New Approach to Surgical Rehabilitation are two surgical titles dealing with amputation. Pierce's Total Care of the Spinal Cord Injuries and Early Therepeutic, Social, and Vocational Problems in the Rehabilitation of Persons with Spinal Cord Injuries by Weiss are two surgical books dealing with spinal cord injury. Two excellent titles for orthopedic surgeons are Lehman's The Clubfoot and Menelaus' The Orthopedic Management of Spinal Bifida Cystica. Each provides a comprehensive treatment of a specialized subject area.

The interdisciplinary or team approach is utilized in the second category of titles. Bleck's Orthopaedic Management of Cerebral Palsy, Cull's Physical Medicine and Rehabilitation Approaches in Spinal Cord Injury, and Eisenberg's Treatment of the Spinal Cord Injured: An Interdisciplinary Perspective all advocate treatment of

MEDICAL ASPECTS   209

the patient as a whole and the importance of team work by all professionals involved in the rehabilitation of an individual.

Friedmann's The Psychological Rehabilitation of the Amputee and Trieschmann's Spinal Cord Injuries: Psychological, Social, and Vocational Adjustment constitute the last category of titles. Neither title can be used as a source of patient education, but are rather professional tools to help the physician help the patient toward acceptance and adjustment to his disability. Friedmann's text is written specifically for physicians, whereas Trieschmann's is intended for all health professionals.

Of course there are always titles which defy categorization. Pearman's The Urological Management of the Patient Following Spinal Cord Injury, Constantian's Pressure Ulcers: Principles and Techniques of Management, and Miller's Evaluating Orthopedic Disability: A Commonsense Approach are three such titles. Pearman's and Constantian's book are highly specialized and are invaluable in the survival of the spinal cord injured patient. Miller's title will be of interest to all physicians in preparing a medical report or giving legal testimony about the orthopedic disabled individual.

In the rehabilitation of heart attack, cancer, and stroke patients the rehabilitation professional must be aware of the patient's viewpont and outlook in order to affect appreciable rehabilitation. Unlike any other disabling condition discussed before there seems to be more books dealing with the patient-physician inter-relationship and inter-dependency available in these areas than the other areas. Brown's Physiological and Psychological Considerations in the Management of Stroke, Hardy's Counseling and Rehabilitating the Cancer Patient and Monteiro's Cardiac Patient Rehabilitation: Social Aspects of Recovery are three such monographs. These books can also be utilized as self-help and patient education materials to help patients understand their conditions, limitations, and potentials toward recovery.

Nutritional information is always difficult to locate and controversial at times. A Comprehensive Cardiac Rehabilitation Program explains the cardiac rehabilitation program practiced at the Archbishop Bergan Mercy Hospital in Omaha, Nebraska, contains diets, and is a self-help instructional manual. Cancer Rehabilitation: An Introduction for Physiotherapists and the Allied Professions by Downie is one of a few monographs with nutritional information for the rehabilitation of cancer patients.

There are also unique titles such as: Licht's Stroke and Its Rehabilitation which is the only book examined which contains a chapter on assistive electrical devices for the stroke patient. A discussion on drugs and their use in rehabilitation is contained in Rossi's Functional Evaluation and Rehabilitation of Cardiac Patients. Dietz's Rehabilitation Oncology has a section on the employment of the recovered cancer patient.

Texts written in the field of orthotics and prosthetics are aimed at audiences ranging from the specialist in the field to the nonprofessional and rehabilitation counselor. Texts aimed at the specialist discuss the evaluating of new prosthetic and orthotic devices. These include Total Hip Prosthesis, the Rehabilitation Engineering Center's Lower Limb Orthotics, Wannstedt's Evaluation of the Limb-Load Monitor, and Wilson's Manual for an Ultralight Below-Knee Prosthesis.

Other texts are written as an aid in prescribing a suitable orthosis or prosthesis for a given condition. These are most helpful to the medical student or beginning clinician. These include Bunch and Keagy's Principles of Orthotic Treatment and Vitali's Amputations and Prostheses. Redford's text Orthotics, Etcetera is a very comprehensive text meant for clinicians in the field yet useful to all health care personnel. Blount's text, The Milwaukee Brace describes a specific type of treatment in terms understandable by all health care personnel. Malick's text Manual on Management of the Quadriplegic Upper Extremity: Using Available Modular Splint and Arm Support Systems again describes specific disorders and their treatment for the use of all health care personnel. Mastro's Selected Readings: A Review of Orthotics and Prosthetics is a useful review of current developments for the practitioner. Wilson's text entitled Limb Prosthetics is meant for nontechnical personnel, while his text Limb Prosthetics for Vocational Rehabilitation Workers is meant primarily for rehabilitation counselors and emphasizes what the amputee can and cannot do.

The books written for nurses approach the subject of rehabilitation in a variety of ways. A few texts try for the comprehensive approach, covering all aspects of rehabilitation, such as Martin's Comprehensive Rehabilitation Nursing or Stryker's Rehabilitative Aspects of Acute and Chronic Nursing Care. Their approach differs: Stryker limits her discussion to rehabilitation in general, while Martin discusses specific disorders as well. Riffle's Rehabilitative Nursing, Case Studies is meant as a self-study guide, giving specific cases covering different types of disorders and study questions related to each case. Preston's The Dilemmas of Care takes a highly philosophical approach to the care of the disabled. Conference proceedings such as the Nursing Clinics of North America's Rehabilitation Nursing are meant to update the working nurse's knowledge in the field. Murray's Current Perspectives in Rehabilitation Nursing has the same purpose. Walsh's The Expanded Role of the Rehabilitation Nurse covers the changing and varied aspects of rehabilitation nursing. Rehabilitation Nursing and Related Readings: A Bibliography, although somewhat out of date, provides an excellent starting point for the study of any topic related to rehabilitation nursing.

Other texts written for nurses and/or physiotherapists discuss the subject of rehabilitation from the standpoint of a specific disorder. Comoss's Cardiac Rehabilitation: A Comprehensive Nursing Approach, Fardy's Cardiac Rehabilitation: Implications for the Nurse and Other Allied Health Professionals, and Garcia's Rehabilitation After Myocardial Infarction are all intended as teaching texts and include such features as case histories and review questions to aid the student. Texts on stroke care are written by both nurses and physiotherapists and are intended for the use of professionals in both fields. These include Dardier's The Early Stroke Patient: Positioning and Movement, Johnstones's two texts The Stroke Patient: Principles of Rehabilitation and Restoration of Motor Function in the Stroke Patient, and O'Brien's Total Care of the Stroke Patient. Hardy's text Practical Management of Spinal Injuries: A Manual for Nurses and Krenzel's Paraplegic and Quadriplegic Individuals each covers nursing care in a specific area. Wallace's Staff Manual for Teaching Patients About Rheumatoid Arthritis was written to aid the health professional in patient education.

Texts written specifically for the nonprofessional health care worker emphasize bedside techniques such as patient positioning and transfers. Rantz's text Lifting, Moving and Transferring Patients: A Manual would be an excellent training manual for health care personnel. Providing Early Mobility, although written primarily for nurses and physical therapists, is an especially valuable text because of its recent publication date (1980) and its excellent illustrations, especially demonstrating use of transferring and positioning equipment.

Speech therapy after stroke and speech therapy after laryngectomy involve two very different problems. Aphasia resulting from stroke may affect the ability to comprehend and the ability to write as well as the ability to speak. The aphasic patient may need to learn to speak all over again, whereas the patient who has lost his larynx must learn a whole new way of speaking, perhaps involving mechanical aids or surgery. Both problems have been extensively discussed in the literature.

Stryker's Speech After Stroke and Ross' Aphasia Rehabilitation follow a similar approach. Both are written for the speech therapist and include exercises geared to the adult patient. Because instructions for use are also included these texts could be used by family members as well as by the speech therapists. Aurelia's Aphasia Therapy Manual is slightly different in that it discusses the disorders that may be involved in stroke in greater detail while

MEDICAL ASPECTS 213

many of the therapeutic techniques are not covered in such detail, instead references are given to other texts. Hayne's <u>Understanding Aphasia</u> is intended for nurses and allied health personnel, to help them understand the behavior of these patients. Chapey's <u>Language Intervention Strategies in Adult Aphasia</u> attempts to evaluate different methods of aphasia treatment and is rather technical. This evaluative approach, plus its recent publication date (1981), makes it important reading for the speech pathologist.

Changes in the field of medicine will require revision and updating of many of the texts in this bibliography, and new texts will continue to be written. More emphasis will be placed on patient education, and texts written for professionals to be used for this purpose are needed. For a view of what is currently available in the field of patient education see **Chapter 9 entitled** "Health Education."

ANNOTATED BIBLIOGRAPHY

Abreu, Beatriz Colon, ed. <u>Physical Disabilities Manual</u>. New York: Raven Press, 1981. 360 pp.

Twenty-six authorities in their various fields of rehabilitation contributed to this volume. Divided into two section: 1) Systems, and 2) Disabilities, it accomplishes its objective of defining "the theoretical and clinical basis for evaluation and intervention procedures" and provides a very comprehensive coverage to the field. Chapter references for further study, subject index, and excellent tables and illustrations make this a fine supplementary textbook for occupational and physical therapists. Recommended for medical school and nursing libraries.

American Medical Association. Committee on Rating of Mental and Physical Impairment. <u>Guides to the Evaluation of Permanent Impairment</u>. Chicago: American Medical Association, 1977. 164 pp.

This practical guide assigns percentage ratings to the physical impairment of the patient. Written for the physician it explains permanent impairments and permanent disability. It also has a combined value chart for evaluating multiple impairments. A good ready reference index is included. This work is a must for all physicians evaluating patients for public and private disability funds. Recommended for large and small libraries and personal office collections. Not recommended for layperson usage.

Anderson, Miles H.; Bray, John J.; and Hennessy, Charles A. Manual of Above-Knee Wood Socket Prosthetics, rev. 2d printing. Springfield, Ill.: Charles C. Thomas, 1980. 286 pp.

Revision of a 1960 text, which is justified by the author since wood is still being used extensively in prosthetists, despite the advent of plastics. It is meant as a training manual for prosthetists and deals primarily with the fabrication of the prosthesis. Introductory material covers the anatomy of the hip, thigh, and knee, and principles of locomotion. The text is extensively illustrated as step-by-step procedures are discussed for fitting the prosthesis, making adjustments, etc. It could be read by all health care personnel and even the layperson if interested in such a detailed discussion of prosthesis fabrication. Recommended for larger medical libraries, especially those involved in prosthesis fabrication.

Aurelia, Joseph C. Aphasia Therapy Manual, 2d ed. Danville, Ill.: Interstate Printers and Publishers, 1970. 79 pp.

Meant as a guide for the speech therapist in the treatment of the adult aphasic, this text explains several different disorders that may be part of aphasia and may affect its treatment. Among these are muscular disorders such as apraxia and dysarthria, reading difficulties, writing difficulties, comprehension problems, synaptic and syntactic difficulties. Each disorder is discussed, along with references to other texts in discussing therapeutic techniques and a bibliography of these works is included. The text is fairly technical, so it is more useful to the professional in the field than to the layperson. Recommended for larger medical libraries.

Barnerjee, Sikhar Nath, ed. Rehabilitation Management of Amputees. (Rehabilitation Medicine Library) Baltimore, Md.: Williams and Wilkins, 1982. 456 pp.

This text tries to encompass all aspects of amputee care, including physiological, psycho-social, environmental, and vocational problems. It is sequentially organized to go along with the different phases of amputee treatment. Subjects covered include the causes and prevention of amputation, preoperative care, prosthetic fitting, adaptive devices, stump complications and management, reintegration into society, and current trends. The authors of this text come from many disciplines and include physicians, surgeons, physical and occupational therapists, and social workers, and the text is intended for all health care professionals. It is useful as an introductory text and as a resource for current information. Well-illustrated, each chapter contains references, and there is an index. Recommended for hospital and medical school libraries.

Basmajian, John V., ed. Therapeutic Exercise, 3rd ed. Baltimore, Md.: Williams and Wilkins, 1978. 600 pp.

This contributed publication which covers all forms of therapeutic exercise is an excellent working and teaching text for the whole medical rehabilitation community. Included are unique and specialized exercises for specific diseases and conditions not found in other publications examined. References at the end of each chapter are included as well as many informative charts and drawings. Intended for the medical professional and not the layperson this title is recommended for purchase by teaching hospitals and academic medical institutions.

Bauer, Helmut Johannes. A Manual on Multiple Sclerosis. Vienna, Austria: International Federation of Multiple Sclerosis Societies, 1977. 84 pp.

For an evaluation of this work, see Chapter 1.

Beasley, Robert W., ed. Symposium of Management of Upper Limb Amputations. (Orthopedic Clinics of North America, vol. 12 no. 4, October 1981) Philadelphia: Saunders. 261 pp.

Based on a seminar held in Paris in June 1980, with chapters by "internationally recognized authorities." Subjects covered include general considerations in management of upper limb amputations, traditional surgery, reattachment surgery, and upper limb prosthetics. This is a comprehensive discussion of new developments in the field and is meant for the practicing professional rather than the student. Each chapter includes references and is well-illustarated. An index is included. Recommended for medical school and hospital libraries.

Bleck, Eugene E. Orthopaedic Management of Cerebral Palsy. Philadelphia: Saunders, 1979. 266 pp.

Divided into three classic areas of cerebral palsy: hemiphegia, diplegia and total body involvement. This text is intended for all those who deal with cerebral palsied individuals, both adults and children. Included are chapters on orthopedic assessment, neurobiology, prognosis and structural changes, and goals and methods of treatment. A very good appendix on rehabilitation devices, as well as many photographs, illustrations, graphs, and charts make this monograph an excellent teaching tool for students who are especially interested in cerebral palsy. The text is too complicated for layperson usage and is recommended for special and medical school libraries.

Blount, Walter P., and Moe, John H. The Milwaukee Brace, 2d ed. Baltimore, Md.: Williams and Wilkins, 1980. 252 pp.

Meant for the orthopedic surgeon and his paramedical team, this text discusses the nonoperative treatment of scoliosis as used by the developers of the Milwaukee Brace. It covers the principles and techniques of treatment, exercises used in conjunction with treatment, complications that may occur, and end results of treatment. It includes a chapter on making the Milwaukee Brace and sample instructions for patients. Well-illustrated, includes bibliographies and an index. This is the authoritative text on this particular method of treatment and essential reading for any physician using the Milwaukee Brace. It might also be of interest to other members of the health care team involved in this treatment. Fairly technical but might be of some use to patients or family members undergoing this treatment. Recommended for all medical libraries.

Bowker, John H., ed. "Symposium on Special Problems in Orthopedic Rehabilitation." (Orthopedic Clinics of North America. vol. 9, no. 1. April 1978) Philadelphia: Saunders. 351 pp.

This is a contributed work by specialists in the field of orthopedics and related fields. Topics included are spinal cord injury, hemiplegia stroke, locomotor disabilities, spina bifida, myclo-meningocele, muscular dystrophy, brain injury, hemophilia, and juvenile rheumatoid arthritis. The management, rehabilitation, and evaluation of most of these listed areas are covered. An index to illustrations is included. An attempt to update the field is made, and with fairly good results. Because this is a symposium, it is more likely to be utilized by the researcher than the teacher. Recommended for large medical libraries.

Bromley, Ida. Tetraplegia and Paraplegia: A Guide for Physiotherapists, 2d ed. Edinburgh: Churchill Livingstone, 1981. 256 pp.

Based on the author's experiences at Stoke Mandeville (England) Spinal Centre, this text emphasizes the team approach and the importance of the spinal injuries unit. Among topics discussed are an outline of medical treatment, the physical reeducation of the patient, self-care, and use of wheelchairs. Intended as a practical manual for physiotherapists, the text gives step-by-step procedures and illustrations of various techniques of moving, lifting and exercising. The text is more technical than others available on this topic, and therefore is most useful to those already having some basic knowledge in the field, such as physiotherapists and nurses. Includes a bibliography, index, and a list of useful addresses including organizations and manufacturers (English only). Recommended for hospital and medical school libraries.

Brown, Arnold. Physiological and Psychological Considerations in the Management of Stroke. St. Louis, Mo.: Warren H. Green, 1976. 83 pp.

For an evaluation of this work, see Chapter 1.

Bunch, Wilton H., and Keagy, Robert D. Principles of Orthotic Treatment. St. Louis, Mo.: C. V. Mosby, 1976. 144 pp.

Intended for the resident or student as an aid in prescribing orthoses, this book discusses the principles of fit, cosmetics and function, rather than the specific materials or methods used. It covers the basics and applications of upper and lower extremity orthotics, spine treatment, wheelchairs, and braces. A well-illustrated text which includes a chapter on terminology as well as references and an index. Although meant for the medical student, this text could also be useful to other health care personnel desiring basic knowledge on orthotic treatment. It is a rather technical text for the layperson. Recommended for medical libraries.

Cailliet, Rene. Scoliosis: Diagnosis and Management. Philadelphia: F. A. Davis Company, 1975. 121 pp.

This introductory text is aimed at all professionals and nonprofessionals who work with children. It is hoped that the general education offered by this text will make individuals aware of the early manifestations, identification, and treatment of scoliosis, and thereby reduce the large percentage of affected children and disabled adults. Definition and natural history of scoliosis, normal spinal column anatomy, glossary of scoliosis terms, types of scoliosis, recognition and diagnosis, treatment, adult scoliosis and cardio-pulmonary functions are aspects of the disability which the book covers. A bibliography and index as well as many fine illustrations are included. An excellent basic text for medical school libraries.

Chapey, Roberta. Language Intervention Strategies in Adult Aphasia. Baltimore, Md.: Williams and Wilkins, 1981. 383 pp.

A comprehensive critical review of the major approaches to treating language impairments of the adult aphasic. Theory and research data relating to various methods of treatment are discussed, as well as the clinical application of these methods. An attempt is made to evaluate the various approaches to language intervention. The text is divided as follows: part one -- Basic considerations -- includes such subjects as the role of the aphasiologist, medical management, assessment of language disorders; part two -- seven language intervention strategies classed as simulation approaches; part three -- other approaches to therapy; part four -- remediation of specific deficits; epilogue -- future issues for graduate students in speech pathology or as an update for practitioners. Also useful to other health professionals, but too technical for the average layperson. Illustrated, and includes bibliographies and an index. Recommended for medical libraries, especially those with programs in speech pathology.

Comoss, Patricia McCall; Burke, E. Ann Smith; and Swails, Susan Herr. Cardiac Rehabilitation: A Comprehensive Nursing Approach. Philadelphia: Lippincott, 1979. 334 pp.

Intended for nursing personnel, this text discusses the four different phases of cardiac rehabilitation as outlined by the American Heart Association. Each phase covered includes chapters on the background and basics of that phase, assessment, planning, implementation, and evaluation pertinent to that phase. A sample case is followed throughout, with sample charts and forms. Each chapter begins with behavioral objectives and a general introduction and ends with references for further study. The format lends itself well to self-study. Especially useful as a text for the nursing student or the nurse wanting further knowledge in this area. The information provided might also be useful to other members of the health care team, or even to interested laypersons, if not put off by the format. Illustrated, and includes an index. Recommended for medical libraries.

A Comprehensive Cardiac Rehabilitation Program. St. Louis, Mo.: The Catholic Health Association of the United States, 1980. 61 pp.

This booklet explains the Cardiac Rehabilitation Program practiced at the Archbishop Bergan Mercy Hospital in Omaha, Nebraska. It is designed specifically for physicians and specialists treating cardiac recovery patients. The book has many charts, diets, medications, progress records, and some references. Basically, it is intended as a reference tool for doctors and other medical professionals, or as a manual for patient recovery for the physician. It serves as a good daily reference guide to diets for cardiac patients and as a good teaching or self-instructional manual. This manual has some fill-in-the-blank areas, probably should not be owned by a library unless the selection policy includes the purchase of such materials. Recommended for hospital and medical libraries.

Constantian, Mark B., ed. Pressure Ulcers: Principles and Techniques of Management. Boston: Little, Brown and Company, 1980. 308 pp.

Intended for surgeons this title attempts to "separate fact from fiction about pressure ulcers and distill all the vast literature of information into one manageable book that surgeons can use repeatedly for treatment advice." Specialists in plastic surgery and neurosurgery contributed to this pioneering volume. The author intended the book to be a symposium rather than a text, but because of the rarity of a separate text in this area, and its currentness, it would be a fine supplementary text. An index, references, and many good photographs and illustrations are included. Recommended for medical libraries.

Cull, John G., and Hardy, Richard E., eds. Physical Medicine and Rehabilitation Approaches in Spinal Cord Injury. Springfield, Ill.: Charles C. Thomas, 1977. 324 pp..

Various professionals contribute to the rehabilitation of a spinal cord injured individual. The purpose of this book is to detail those contributions. The authors are specialists from the fields of orthopedics, surgery, urology, counseling, physical therapy, allied health, clinical nursing, psychology, and occupational therapy. The title covers the entire rehabilitation of the spinal cord injured individual very completely. It includes references at the conclusion of each chapter and an index and could be utilized as a supplementary text on the rehabilitation of spinal cord injury. Recommended for medical school libraries.

Dardier, Esme L. The Early Stroke Patient: Positioning and Movement. London: Balliere Tindall, 1980. 116 pp.

Although written by a physiotherapist and based on her work at Chedoke Hospital and the McMaster Medical Centre in Hamilton, Ontario, this text is intended for the nurse as well as the physiotherapist. The physical effect of a stroke on the patient, and the use of positioning and movement as a method of restoring mobility are discussed. Emphasis is on the early period in patient rehabilitation as this is often neglected in other tests. Because this text is fairly technical and assumes a basic knowledge of anatomy and physiology, it is most useful to experienced health care personnel. Well-illustrated and includes a bibliography and an index. Recommended for hospital and medical school libraries.

Dietz, J. Herbert. Rehabilitation Oncology. New York: John Wiley and Sons, 1981. 180 pp.

This title is an explanation of the Oncology Rehabilitation program in operation at the Memorial-Sloan Kettering Cancer Center in New York, which, it is hoped, can serve as a prototype for more programs throughout the United States. This is an important book in a field where not much has been written. An example of its importance is the section on employment, which is not included in other works which were evaluated for this chapter. Intended for physicians, therapists, and students interested in cancer care. Chapters on methodology, general support and evaluation of the patient are included. A bibliography is also included as a general index. Recommended for hospital libraries in which such a program has been proposed, as well as special and academic research medical libraries.

Downie, Patricia A. Cancer Rehabilitation: An Introduction for Physiotherapists and the Allied Professions. London: Farber and Farber, 1978. 205 pp.

Originally written as a dissertation for the Fellowship of the Chartered Society of Physiotherapy, this British work is written by a physiotherapist for physiotherapists and other professionals. It is meant to be a brief introduction to the types of cancer treatment and of the physiotherapists' role in patient care. One of the few titles which contains nutritional information for the rehabilitation of cancer patients. It also contains a list of useful organizations, homes, and hospices in the United States and Canada. Because the chapter on nutrition is so worthwhile this title should be updated. Recommended for medical school libraries.

Eisenberg, M. G., and Falconer, J. A., eds. Treatment of the Spinal Cord Injured: An Interdisciplinary Perspective. Springfield, Ill.: Charles C. Thomas, 1978. 127 pp.

This work is derived from the Spinal Cord Injury Conference held at the Cleveland Veterans' Hospital in November 1977, and is primarily written for nurses, physical and occupational therapists, social workers, and psychologists. It stresses the importance of interdisciplinary team work and involving patients in planning. Name and subject indices are included, as well as references at the conclusion of each chapter. It is a good work giving a general overview of the subject and should be of interest to the audience for which it is intended. Because it is a collection of papers given at a conference, this work is primarily recommended for large medical research libraries.

Eldridge, Priscilla B. Caring for the Disabled Patient: An Illustrated Guide. Oradell, N.J.: Medical Economics Co., 1978. 133 pp.

This book was written by a physiotherapist for the use of nonprofessionals in nursing homes or in home treatment, and covers a variety of topics including emergency procedures, routine exercises, positioning, ambulation, transfers, activities of daily living, the patient's emotional and speech problems, recreational and work activities, costs, and nutrition. It includes a glossary and also a list of commercial and community sources that sell or donate equipment. It is a humorous, yet practical, treatment of the subject, with cartoon illustrations covering a variety of techniques necessary in dealing with the disabled. Especially useful to those with little or no previous background in health care. Recommended for all medical libraries and also for larger public libraries.

Evans, C. D. Rehabilitation After Severe Head Injury. Edinburgh: Churchill Livingstone, 1981. 218 pp.

Contributors to this text all worked at two leading rehabilitation centers in England. The material was accumulated over about a 10 year period and represents observations on some 1000 patients. Emphasis is on the long term management of patients with severe head injuries. Some of the more severe and common problems are discussed, as well as methods of treatment. This text emphasizes the importance of the involvement of all members of the rehabilitation team. Each chapter is written by a different member of that team -- the physician, the physiotherapist, the speech therapist, the occupational therapist, the remedial gymnast, the nursing staff, and the educational therapist. The text thus would be of interest to all members of the health care team. References are given for each chapter, and illustrations and an index are included. Recommended for all medical libraries.

Farber, Shereen D. Neurorehabilitation: A Multisensory Approach. Philadelphia: Saunders, 1982. 282 pp.

MEDICAL ASPECTS 221

Although edited by a professor of occupational therapy, this text is intended for all health professionals. Contributors are from the fields of medicine and physical therapy as well as from occupational therapy. Among the subjects covered are an overview of functional neurology, principles of neurorehabilitation, therapeutic relaxation, and adaptive equipment. The text is illustrated and includes bibliographical references and an index. This text is fairly technical and would be useful primarily to professionals in the field. Recommended for larger medical and hospital libraries.

Fardy, Paul S.,; Bennet, James L.; Reitz, Norma L; and Williams, Mark A. Cardiac Rehabilitation: Implications for the Nurse and Other Allied Health Professionals. St. Louis, Mo.: C. V. Mosby, 1980. 283 pp.

Written by thirteen authors from diverse areas of expertise and meant as a "broad-based multidisciplinary reference for professionals involved in cardiac rehabilitation." Primarily directed to the nurse, but would also be useful to other health professionals involved in cardiac rehabilitation. The book is divided into four main sections: 1) identifying a need, 2) concepts and procedures for exercise, 3) approaches to behavioral modification; and 4) planning and establishing a program. Unique chapters include those on cardiac medications, patient motivation, and nutrition. Case studies are included, and references are given with each chapter. Appendices include a sample continuing home exercise program, and a beginning fitness program. Illustrated, with an index. A comprehensive text, emphasizing the practical approach to cardiovascular rehabilitation. It is especially useful for health care personnel involved in developing and implementing a cardiac rehabilitation program, and is also useful for increasing the knowledge of those currently working in the area, including the involved layperson. Recommended for hospital and medical school libraries.

Feller, Irving, and Grabb, William C., eds. Reconstruction and Rehabilitation of the Burned Patient. Ann Arbor, Mich.: National Institute for Burn Medicine, 1979. 423 pp.

Multiauthored by specialists in the burn care field for burn care teams in hospitals. This is a very comprehensive treatise of new methods of burn care for the entire patient. It is divided into nineteen anatomical sections and then short chapters, with author and subject indices and historical illustrations also included. This is a unique book that would serve well as a comprehensive "state-of-the-art" text on burn patient rehabilitation. A must for all large teaching institution libraries.

Field, Ephraim J. Multiple Sclerosis in Childhood: Diagnosis and Prophylaxis. Springfield, Ill.: Charles C. Thomas, 1980. 111 pp.

This work is a collection of essays by thirteen neurologists and microbiologists. It is intended to answer questions about multiple sclerosis for the general physician and points out the difficulty of diagnosis of MS and conflicting laboratory tests and data results. Some of the essays deal with MS from an epidemiological viewpoint, while others deal with the variety of laboratory tests performed to determine MS and the future outlook of the disease. No information on the rehabilitation of multiple sclerosis is included. Recommended for general physicians and medical libraries.

Flaherty, Patricia Toohey, and Larson, Corrine W. Range of Motion Exercise: Key to Joint Mobility. Minneapolis: Sister Kenny Institute, 1968. 39 pp.

The purpose of range of motion exercises is to prevent further disability and help maintain existing function. Ideally, this is the function of a physiotherapist, but often one is not available in nursing homes or other smaller institutions and the nurse is most involved in the patient's care. This manual is meant to aid her in this purpose, but may be useful to all health care personnel and even the layperson who is involved in home care. The manual includes information on planning a range of motion exercise program, as well as describing the exercises themselves. Extensive illustrations are accompanied by explanatory text. A definition of terms is also included. Recommended for medical libraries and larger public libraries.

Food, Nutrition and the Disabled; An Annotated Bibliography. Compiled by Alison Furse and Elyse Levine. Toronto: Nutrition Information Service, Ryerson Polytechnical Institute Library, 1981. 82 pp.

This useful bibliography was developed because of a lack of basic information in these areas and covers primarily material published since 1970. In compiling this bibliography the term "disabled" was defined as those unable to shop or prepare food for themselves, or eat normally, or who suffered from a nutrition imbalance due to their disability. Cardiovascular, renal, and gastrointestinal disabilities were excluded because of the availability of other materials on those subjects. Both print and audiovisual materials are covered in separate sections. These sections are further divided by subject, organized into areas such as general, mealtime skills, child care, home management, aids and devices, and cookbooks. A list of organizations in the United States and Canada during this project is included, as is a selective list of suppliers of equipment for the disabled. Because of a lack of other materials on the subject this bibliography is recommended for all medical libraries.

Friedmann, Lawrence W. The Psychological Rehabilitation of the Amputee. Springfield, Ill.: Charles C. Thomas, 1978. 157 pp.

For an evaluation of this work, see Chapter 1.

Friedmann, Lawrence W. The Surgical Rehabilitation of the Amputee. Springfield, Ill.: Charles C. Thomas, 1978. 553 pp.

MEDICAL ASPECTS 223

This monograph is intended for the entire health care team who will operate and rehabilitate the amputee. It advocates "treating the patient as a whole," when amputation is involved. The most workable and logical approach to rehabilitation is advocated and various surgical procedures are presented. A bibliography, glossary, name and subject indices, and many instructive photographs are included. Intended more for research and teaching than utilized by patients or laypersons. Recommended for medical school libraries.

Garcia, Rebecca M. Rehabilitation After Myocardial Infarction. New York: Appleton-Century-Crofts, 1978. 83 pp.

This text is based on the author's experience with myocardial infarction as well as a review of the literature. It discusses the need for rehabilitation, the importance of patient instruction in rehabilitation, and the physical reconditioning of the patient. Meant as a self-study guide for the nurse, each chapter lists objectives and study questions, and ends with a self-examination. A post-test and answers are included. This text is more theoretical than practical, and is useful primarily for the nurse or nursing student to update her knowledge in the area covered. Recommended for hospital and medical school libraries.

Greif, Elaine, and Matarazzo, Ruth G. Behavioral Approaches to Rehabilitation: Coping with Change. (Springer series on Rehabilitation, v. 3) New York: Springer, 1982. 158 pp.

Written by two physicians specializing in clinical psychology and based on their experiences with patients, this text gives an overview of the common patterns of behavior of patients in the rehabilitation setting and recommends ways the professional can help. Subjects discussed include rehabilitation in general, principles of learning, common feelings among the disabled such as depression, anxiety and confusion, and coping skills needed by caretakers, including family members and health professionals. An epilogue includes a detailed case history illustrating principles discussed in the text. Appendices on charting progress, examples of reward and praise, scheduling a routine, relaxation training, and resources are included. Bibliographies and an index are also included. Useful to all health care professionals who work with patients and their families. Recommended for all medical libraries.

Hardy, Alan G., and Elson, Reginald. Practical Management of Spinal Injuries: A Manual for Nurses. 2d ed. Edinburgh: Churchill Livingstone, 1976. 162 pp.

A specialized text on the management of spinal injuries for nurses. The causes and treatment of vertebral injuries are discussed first, then the complications that might result from that treatment. Among the complications discussed are pressure sores, spasms, urinary complications, and psychological distress. The importance of physiotherapy and occupational therapy is also stressed. The text is well-illustrated and includes an index. Although written especially for nurses it might also be of interest to doctors, physiotherapists, and other health professionals. Recommended for larger hospital and medical school libraries.

Hardy, Richard E., ed. Counseling and Rehabilitating the Cancer Patient. Springfield, Ill.: Charles C. Thomas, 1975. 147 pp.

This publication is #946 of the American Lecture Series, and is not intended as a research or medical textbook, but rather as a psychological approach to cancer. Aimed at the layperson, the psychologist, rehabilitation counselor, social worker and occupational therapist, this text is concerned with educating those who do rehabilitation work with cancer patients. Good clear definitions and explanations are included as well as case studies and an index. Recommended for medical school and hospital libraries.

Haynes, William O. Understanding Aphasia: A Guide for Medical and Paramedical Professionals. Danville, Ill.: The Interstate Printers and Publishers, 1976. 63 pp.

Intended for nurses and allied health personnel as an aid in helping them extend their knowledge of aphasia. The following information is included: 1) a semi-technical description of aphasia disturbances, 2) a description of the procedures followed by speech clinicians in evaluating and treating this disorder, and 3) a description of the behavior changes in aphasic patients. Examples are given throughout the text in order to give the reader a better understanding of the situation discussed. A bibliography is provided with each chapter and a glossary of terms is also included. The reading is not too technical, so the text may also be useful to the family of the aphasic patient, to help them better understand the disorder. Recommended for medical and large public libraries.

Humm, W. Rehabilitation of the Lower Limb Amputee: For Nurses and Therapists. 3rd ed. London: Bailliere Tindall, 1977. 142 pp.

This text discusses the rehabilitation of those who have lost one or two legs. The text is arranged in the order of treatment: part one discusses early and intermediate phases (pre-prosthetic) and part two deals with prosthetic and late phases of treatment. Among the topics covered are psychological problems of the amputee, exercise, stump care, prosthetic training techniques, and types of functions of prostheses. The text is illustrated and includes an index. Although written for nurses and therapists it would be useful to all health care professionals. Recommended for larger hospital and medical school libraries.

Ingenito, Rosalie, and Priestley, Lorraine. Hemiplegia, Current Approaches to Patient Positioning: An Instructional Manual. Washington, D.C.: George Washington University Medical Center, 1979. 38 pp.

This text emphasizes the importance of proper positioning to prevent secondary disabilities, pain, or deformity. The problem involved is described, then the proper techniques of positioning to aid the problem. Problems include the spastic hand, flaccid hand, edema control, whole body positioning on involved and non-involved sides and stomach, sitting in bed, and use of wheelchairs. The text is illustrated and very basic, so it can be used by family members as well as nursing staff and students in health related professions. Appendices include a glossary, references, and a ready reference sheet of bedside instructions. Recommended for medical and large public libraries.

James, John I. P. Scoliosis, 2d ed. Edinburgh: Churchill Livingstone, 1976. 348 pp.

Written primarily to update the first edition published in 1967, it contains new information for those involved with scoliosis. Rehabilitation chapters include: instrumentation and other surgical procedures, correction and fusion, and conservative methods and treatment. A bibliography appears at the conclusion of each chapter. Could be utilized as an auxillary textbook in a subject specialty and is recommended for medical school libraries.

Johnstone, Margaret. Restoration of Motor Function in the Stroke Patient: A Physiotherapist's Approach. Edinburgh: Churchill Livingstone, 1978. 187 pp.

A follow-up to The Stroke Patient: Principles of Rehabilitation, this text discusses controlled movement, positioning, sensory loss, treatment plans, and assessment. It includes a glossary, index, and reading lists for further information. Straightforward style and good illustrations, as in the author's previous work. The information is given in a practical rather than a theoretical approach. Although written primarily for physiotherapists, this text would be of interest to all who handle stroke patients, including the layperson. Recommended for medical libraries.

Johnstone, Margaret. The Stroke Patient: Principles of Rehabilitation. Edinburgh: Churchill Livingstone, 1976. 84 pp.

In this text the author advocates a simple approach based on her own work with hemiplegic patients. The emphasis is on the technique of handling patients, with accompanying illustrations. The author emphasizes the team approach to stroke rehabilitation, with the nurse as the most important member of the team, due to having the most contact with the patient. Individual chapters were written for the nurse, the physiotherapist, the occupational therapist, and the speech therapist. Index and glossary are included. A well-written, straightforward book for the stroke care team. Recommended for medical libraries.

Kaplan, Paul E., and Materson, Richard S., eds. The Practice of Rehabilitation Medicine. Springfield, Ill.: Charles C. Thomas, 1982. 558 pp.

Written primarily by physicians, this text is intended as an introduction to the field for nonphysiatristsis; that is, residents in other fields of medicine. It is organized by diagnosis and includes chapters on arthritis, oncologic rehabilitation, cardiovascular disease, orthotics, spinal cord injury, stroke, and other disorders. This text deals primarily with common problems of inpatient care; another text is planned to discuss issues in outpatient care. Illustrations, bibliographies, and an index are all included. This text is very technical and for that reason is useful primarily to physicians. Recommended for larger medical school and hospital libraries.

Keith, Robert L., and Darley, Frederic L., eds. Laryngectomee Rehabilitation. Houston, Tex.: College-Hill Press, 1979. 533 pp.

Proceedings of the 5th Laryngectomee Rehabilitation Seminar, held June 10-15, 1979 at the Mayo Clinic. Papers include historical reviews on various aspects of laryngectomee rehabilitation, as well as descriptions of current techniques and research. Emphasis is on speech rehabilitation, but many other topics are also covered, including physical therapy, occupational therapy, nursing care, and the patient's viewpoint. Many papers are technical; others are less so. Each paper includes a bibliography -- many are illustrated. Because the papers cover a diversity of topics from so many viewpoints, this book could be of interest to anyone involved with laryngectomee rehabilitation, including the patient. Recommended for medical and large public libraries.

Kenedi, R. M.; Paul, J. P.; and Hughes, J., eds. Disability. Baltimore, Md.: University Park Press, 1979. 524 pp.

Two hundred fifty-two international participants contributed to this volume which is a "proceedings of a seminar on rehabilitation of the disabled in relation to clinical and biomechanical aspects, costs of effectiveness," held in August 1978 at the University of Strathclyde, Glasgow. The papers presented on worldwide rehabilitation, clinical and laboratory methodology and techniques, orthopedic implants, prosthetics and orthotics comprise this international "state-of-the-art" publication. Practicing clinicians as well as research physicians will be interested in this symposium. Recommended for large medical research libraries.

Kostuik, John P., ed. Amputation Surgery and Rehabilitation: The Toronto Experience. Edinburgh: Churchill Livingstone, 1981. 448 pp.

This text was written by orthopedic surgeons and allied health professionals and is directed toward students in relevant disciplines such as surgery, rehabilitation medicine, physical and occupational therapy, nursing, social work and bioengineering.

Introductory chapters cover the history of epidemiology of amputation surgery and are followed by chapters on specific types of amputations. Up-to-date topics such as the replantation of extremities through neurosurgery and the use of externally powered prostheses are included. The final chapter is comprised of questions and answers on the material covered in the text. Illustrated, with bibliographical references, and an index, this is a good introductory text. Recommended for hospital and medical school libraries.

Kottke, Frederic J; Stillwell, G. Keith; and Lehmann, Justus F., eds. Krusen's Handbook of Physical Medicine and Rehabilitation. 3rd ed. Philadelphia: Saunders, 1982. 1023 pp.

This is the latest edition of a comprehensive text originally edited by a pioneer in the field of physical medicine and rehabilitation, Frank Hammond Krusen. It is meant as a text for medical students, residents and therapists as well as a reference for practicing physicians and is composed of three general sections on the evaluation, therapy, and rehabilitation of major disabling conditions. The section on evaluation covers such topics as gait analysis, psychological assessment, and vocational assessment; the section on therapeutics includes heat and cold therapy, electrotherapy, massage, exercise, positioning, and orthotics; the third section covers specific conditions such as stroke, arthritis, fractures, spinal cord injuries. The text is illustrated and includes an index and bibliographic references. As the classic text in its field it is recommended for all medical libraries.

Krenzel, Judith, R., and Rohrer, Lois M. Paraplegic and Quadriplegic Individuals. 4th ed. Chicago: The National Paraplegia Foundation, 1977. 69 pp.

This text is divided into two sections: the first, on initial care, cover skin care, positioning, diet, urinary and bladder problems, and emotional adjustment; the second, on readmission and wheelchair living, covers hygiene, organizations, and nurse patient relations. The final chapter on organizations describes the National Paraplegia Foundation and the Paralyzed Veterans of America. Each chapter includes references and is well-illustrated. An index is also included. Written especially for nurses and nursing students, but the information could also be useful to other health care personnel and even the interested layperson. Recommended for all medical libraries.

Lehman, Wallace B. The Clubfoot. Philadelphia: Lippincott, 1980. 109 pp.

Intended for surgeons, this report covers a surgeon's experiences in the desert of the Negeu concerning the surgical treatment of the clubfoot. Contents cover the definition, a brief history, soft and hard tissue surgery, tendon transfer surgery and surgical treatment of the clubfoot. References and good illustrations are included. This is the only monograph in its field which was recent enough for inclusion in this chapter. Recommended for medical school libraries for the purpose of research and further study by medical students and future orthopedic surgeons.

Licht, Sidney, ed. Stroke and Its Rehabilitation. (Physical Medicine Library; v. 12) Baltimore, Md.: Waverly Press, 1975. 562 pp.

Paints a rather grim future for the stroke patient and covers the full range of stroke explanation, treatment, and rehabilitation. A very comprehensive text and the only source found which discusses electrical devices for the stroke patient. In the preface the author touts the book as the most updated source of stroke rehabilitation information and probably is the most updated source of 1975. Appendix of electrical aids of hemiplegia, glossary of terms, and index are included. Recommended for medical school library as a research tool.

Logigian, Martha K., ed. Adult Rehabilitation: A Team Approach for Therapists. Boston: Little, Brown and Company, 1982. 354 pp.

This text provides an overview of rehabilitation programs for entry level allied health professionals. The function of the interdisciplinary rehabilitation team is emphasized. Individual chapters cover a variety of topics including aging, oncology, orthopedic disorders, rheumatic diseases, cardiac and pulmonary rehabilitation, burns, stroke, brain trauma, and spinal cord injuries. Each chapter discusses the disease process and rehabilitation problems related to that disorder, and evaluates suggested treatments. Each chapter has an extensive bibliography, and the text is illustrated and has an index. A good basic introductory text for all health professionals. Recommended for hospital and medical school libraries.

Longacre, J. J. Rehabilitation of the Facially Disfigured: Prevention of Irreversible Psychic Trauma and Early Reconstruction. Springfield, Ill.: Charles C. Thomas, 1973. 124 pp.

Primarily intended for physicians, this monograph discusses the psychological and socioeconomic effects of facial disfigurement. It covers observations of cases over thirty years and points out the long range results of early care as opposed to later care on the "body image" of the facially disfigured. No more current title covering this subject was discovered for evaluation. Has many fine photographs for teaching visual aids and includes name and subject indices. A teaching and reference tool not recommended for the layperson. Recommended for medical school libraries.

Lower-Limb Orthotics: A Manual. Philadelphia: Rehabilitation Engineering Center, Moss Rehabilitation Hospital, 1978. 132 pp.

This text discusses efforts to produce functional orthoses with minimal restrictions using thermoplastics and explains the philosophy and details of the new designs. General principles of patient/orthosis matching are discussed first, then specific orthoses and their fabrication techniques are described. Only those orthoses that the staff at the Rehabilitation Engineering Center is familiar with are discussed. Subsequent editions are intended to update the information. The text is well-illustrated, especially the section on fabrication techniques. Meant especially for clinical personnel--orthotists, therapists, and physicians--this text contains useful information for experienced health care personnel working with thermoplastic orthoses or interested in learning more about them. Recommended for larger medical libraries with specialized collections in orthotics.

Malick, Maude H., and Meyer, Christa M. H. Manual on Management of the Quadriplegic Upper Extremity: Using Available Modular Splint and Arm Support Systems. Pittsburgh: Harmarville Rehabilitation Center, 1978. 216 pp.

As indicated from the title, the emphasis of this text is on the application of orthoses to the upper extremity. The text describes the different types of orthoses available, the criteria for selecting the appropriate device, training methods in the use of orthoses, and types of control systems available. Helpful features include a glossary, bibliography, list of sources of supply, index, and extensive illustrations. The text is intended for "all people concerned with the rehabilitation of quadriplegics" although a statement on the cover reads "for physicians, occupational therapists, physical therapists, orthotists." Recommended for all medical libraries.

Martin, Nancy; Holt, Nancy B.; and Hicks, Dorothy. Comprehensive Rehabilitation Nursing. New York: McGraw-Hill. 1981. 792 pp.

A collection of articles written by authors from different health care disciplines, this text is divided into four parts: 1) conceptual and theoretical considerations. Includes articles on such topics as attitudes toward the handicapped, coping, and stress; 2) assessment and modalities for management. Covers urinary and bowel management, speech and language therapy, physical therapy; 3) nursing management of selected physical impairments. Includes stroke, multiple sclerosis, spinal cord injuries, amputations, burns, cancer, and heart disorders; and 4) the world out there. Deals with topics such as discharge planning and vocational rehabilitation. This is a comprehensive text covering both theoretical and practical considerations in rehabilitation nursing. Illustrated, includes a bibliography and index. Although directed toward nurses it might also be useful to the layperson working in the field of rehabilitation and to other health care personnel. Recommended for all medical libraries.

Mastro, Brian A., and Mastro, Robert T., eds. Selected Reading: A Review of Orthotics and Prosthetics. Washington, D.C.: American Orthotic and Prosthetic Association, 1980. 406 pp.

A selection of articles intended to be useful to the practitioner for reviewing procedures currently being used in the field. Described by the editors as "the most clinically significant articles appearing in Orthotics and Prosthetics -- a journal of the American Orthotic and Prosthetic Association." The articles selected cover a variety of topics -- types of amputations, various prosthetic and orthotic devices, and the use and fabrication of these devices. Each article includes a bibliography and is well-illustrated. An index is also included. A useful review of current developments in the field of orthotics and prosthetics especially to the practitioner. Recommended for hospital and medical libraries.

Menelaus, Malcolm B. The Orthopaedic Management of Spina Bifida Cystica. 2d ed. Edinburgh: Churchill Livingstone, 1980. 217 pp.

The main objective of this new edition is to convince orthopedic surgeons that "not all deformities should be corrected, but rather, simple surgery should be performed to prevent recurrent deformity and ensure maximum functional capability." for the patient. It also updates new developments and procedures in the orthopedic management of spina bifida cystica. New sections on embryology, genetics, antenatal diagnosis, and detailed management of pressure sores and anesthetics are also included. References and index are included as well as many good tables and photographs. All these combined make this text invaluable for the future orthopedic surgeon and is recommended for all medical school libraries.

Miller, T. Rothrock. Evaluating Orthopedic Disability: A Common-Sense Approach. Oradell, N.J.: Medical Economics Co., 1979. 114 pp.

A very good quick reference book to help physicians in an area that the author admits is not covered in the medical school curriculum. Included are chapters on essential steps in evaluating disability, preparation of the medical report, and giving legal testimony. A handy self-help reference tool for all general physicans and specialists alike. Recommended for hospital, personal, and medical school libraries.

Moberg, Erik. The Upper Limb in Tetraplegia: A New Approach to Surgical Rehabilitation. Stuttgart: Thieme, 1978. 104 pp.

A very small but worthwhile specialized book for surgeons and those who work to rehabilitate the upper limb disabled. It is an international state of the art publication on upper limb surgical procedures and treatment which contains many good illustrations, references, and a subject index. Would be best utilized as a teaching and research text for specialists and not intended for laypersons or nonsurgeons. Recommended for medical libraries within teaching institutions.

Monteiro, Lois A. Cardiac Patient Rehabilitation: Social Aspects of Recovery. New York: Springer Publishing Co., 1979. 178 pp.

Based on case studies of patients enrolled in a research project at Harvard University, this excellent reference book could be used on a daily basis by clinicians and nurses. Although it is intended for Cardiac Care Unit nurses, it can be used as a text for nursing research, medical-surgical nursing, and rehabilitation nursing. Could even be given to recovering patients. Contains excellent chapters on alternative cardiac patient careers and the wife's role in rehabilitation. Recommended for medical and hospital libraries.

Morrison, Andrew W. <u>Management of Sensorineural Deafness</u>. Boston: Butterworth, 1975. 294 pp.

Diagnosis is the emphasis in this collection of essays on adult sensorineural deafness. Intended primarily for postgraduate students of otolaryngology who will specialize as clinicians this text has many fine illustrations, charts, and references. Its chapters on acoustic neuroma, differential diagnosis of neuroma, late syphilis, endolymphatic hydrops, sudden deafness, diseases of the otic capsule and post-operative sensorineural problems make this an excellent supplementary text and research monograph. This is the only title in its field which could be located for examination. Recommended for specialized and large medical school libraries.

Mossman, Philip L. <u>A Problem-Oriented Approach to Stroke Rehabilitation</u>. Springfield, Ill.: Charles C. Thomas, 1976. 456 pp.

This good "how-to" problem-oriented approach to the treatment of stroke and its rehabilitation is intended for all allied health professionals. It is very comprehensive with good references and bibliography at the conclusion of each chapter as well as fine illustrations, graphs, charts, and line drawings. A good teaching tool for medical students, occupational therapists, and physical therapists alike. Recommended for medical school libraries.

Mulder, Donald W., ed. <u>The Diagnosis and Treatment of Amyotrophic Lateral Sclerosis</u>. Boston: Houghton Mifflin, Medical Division, 1980. 397 pp.

This contributed monograph is a result of "The Care and Treatment of Amyotrophic Lateral Sclerosis" symposium held in February 1979 in Tucson, Arizona by the Amyotrophic Lateral Sclerosis Society of America (ALSSOA). Written by specialists for physicians and paramedical personnel, it stresses the role of neurologic physician in patient care. Includes chapters on diagnosis and treatment and research strategies and outstanding chapters on rehabilitation and the role of exercises. Many photographs of assistive devices, references, illustrations, and an index make this a very useful supplemental and research monograph. Recommended for large medical libraries and private libraries of specialists.

Murray, Rosemary, and Kijek, Jean C. <u>Current Perspectives in Rehabilitation Nursing</u>. St. Louis, Mo.: C. V. Mosby, 1979. 232 pp.

Intended as a continuing series to update the nurse's knowledge of rehabilitation; however, only volume one has been published to date. The text is organized into three sections. The first emphasizes the role of the nurse and covers topics such as the organization of nursing care, the role of clinical nurse specialists, nursing education, and leadership. The second section is on patient care, and covers various disabilities and techniques--spinal cord injuries, cardiovascular diseases, intensive care, and biofeedback. The third section covers the psychology of rehabilitation--the role of the team, physical therapy, sex therapy, and communication. The text is oriented toward nurses, but could be useful to other members of the health care team who wish to increase their knowledge in the field of rehabilitation. Recommended for hospital and medical school libraries.

Musselwhite, Caroline R., and St. Louis, Karen W. Communication Programming for the Severely Handicapped Vocal and Non-Vocal Strategies. Houston, Tex.: College-Hill Press, 1982. 325 pp.

This text, intended for the communication professional, is divided into four parts. Part 1 covers general principles of communication programming and preliminary training strategies. Part 2 provides an overview of 24 selected vocal language programs. Part 3 discusses non-vocal communication systems, including both gestural and symbolic modes. Part 4 consists of four useful appendices, including a lengthy annotated bibliography, a review of selected communication programs, a list of relevant organizations, agencies and publications, and a discussion of assessment procedures and tools. Although most useful to the speech pathologist, this text could also be used by occupational and physical therapists, psychologists, and social workers. It is quite technical thus it would be most useful to professionals in those fields. Recommended for larger medical libraries.

Nichols, P. J. R., ed. Rehabilitation Medicine, 2d ed. Boston: Butterworth, 1980. 353 pp.

The 1976 edition of this title was a classic in the field. This much needed update will prove to be the same. Divided by type of injury to be rehabilitated this text deals with rehabilitation of the total patient and all his injuries. Occupational and physical therapists, as well as clinicians and general practitioners will utilize this title as a ready reference tool and a text. Some instructors may be discouraged from using this title as a main text because of its lack of illustrations, however its current chapters on head injury, spinal paralysis, and sexual problems of the physically disabled may more than compensate for the shortcoming. Recommended for hosptial, nursing and clinical medicine libraries.

O'Brien, Mary T., and Pallett, Phyllis J. Total Care of the Stroke Patient. Boston: Little, Brown, and Company, 1978. 379 pp.

This text is based on a study carried out at Peter Bent Brigham Hospital, Boston, on the effectiveness of nursing measures in the prevention and control of complications in the acute state of stroke which inhibit effective rehabilitation. The physiological basis of stroke and its pathological manifestations are viewed as a standard for nursing care. Topics discussed include the anatomy and physiology of the brain, standards of care, patient assessment, language disorders, perceptual disorders, respiratory care, fluid and electrolyte balance, nutrition, bowel and bladder function, and skin care. The text is illustrated, with an index and references for each chapter. The theory rather than the practice of patient care is emphasized. The text is directed primarily to hospital nurses, but would also be helpful to other health care professionals dealing with the stroke patient. Recommended for larger hospital and medical school libraries.

Pearman, John W., and England, Ernest J. The Urological Management of the Patient Following Spinal Cord Injury. Springfield, Ill.: Charles C. Thomas, 1973. 280 pp.

A joint work by a clinical microbiologist and a urologist summarizing the present knowledge of the physiology, pathology and anatomy of the urinary tract of persons suffering from spinal paralysis. Based on actual case studies of urological management at the spinal unit of the rehabilitation branch of the Royal Perth Hospital, Western Australia. An excellent reference book for all those who deal with spinal cord injury victims because it stresses the great attention to detail needed to produce successful results in rehabilitation of the spinal cord injured patient. It is included in this chapter because it is the only book in its field on the subject. A good supplementary teaching and reference text for medical students. Recommended for medical school libraries.

Pierce, Donald, and Nickel, Vernon H. The Total Care of Spinal Cord Injuries. Boston: Little, Brown, and Company, 1977. 340 pp.

A contributed work by "paraplegists" to present the most current material on surgical and medical management of the spinal cord injured patient and is intended for those who deal with his treatment and rehabilitation. It contains many good photographs and more surgical information than other titles examined. References are provided at the conclusion of chapters, as well as an index. Good supplementary text for occupational and physical therapists and surgeons interested in the spinal cord injured patient. Recommended for medical school libraries for student and research purposes.

Pollack, Michael L., and Schmidt, Donald H., eds. Heart Disease and Rehabilitation. Boston: Houghton Mifflin, 1979. 725 pp.

A "state of the art" book written to provide the most current and comprehensive information on heart disease and its rehabilitation. Primarily aimed at cardiologists, internists, generalists, physicians-in-training, medical students, physiologists, physical educators, exercise therapists, nurse supervisors, and postgraduate students in medical sciences. Based on the "Heart Disease and Rehabilitation State of the Art" symposium held at Mount Sinai Medical Center in Milwaukee, Wisconsin in 1972. Because it is a contributed work as well as symposium publication, it might be suitable as a main basic text. Includes references at end of chapters, good index, and many graphs. Recommended for medical and nursing school libraries.

Preston, Ronald Philip. The Dilemmas of Care: Social and Nursing Adaptations to the Deformed, the Disabled, and the Aged. New York: Elsevier, 1979. 220 pp.

This text discusses what the author calls the Gregor effect (so named from the character who changes into a cockroach in Kafka's The Metamorphosis, that is, the influence of human abnormality on people. The author first discusses theoretically the nature of man as related to human frailty and mortality--this is based on the ideas of Ernest Becker as developed in his books, The Denial of Death and Escape from Evil. In the second section, the author relates these ideas to nursing--this is based on the author's experiences as a sociologist working in a hospital setting. Useful to nurses and all others dealing with abnormalities as an aid in helping them understand themselves and their reactions better. A philosophical rather than a practical approach to disability. Recommended for larger hospital and medical school libraries.

Providing Early Mobility. Horsham, Pa.: Intermed Communications, 1980. 160 pp.

Written by nurses and physical therapists, this text discusses the physical and emotional preparation of the patient for early mobility. It includes step-by-step procedures and photographs of turning and positioning, range of motion exercises, isometrics, and transfer techniques. An especially useful section gives instructions on the use of transfer and positioning equipment, with very good illustrations. The extensive illustrations make this text very useful for self-teaching, especially for nurses and physical therapists, but also for other health care personnel. The text includes a bibliography, index, and a list of agencies for further information. Recommended for all medical libraries.

Rantz, Marilyn Fresen, and Courtial, Donald. Lifting, Moving and Transferring Patients: A Manual. 2d ed. St. Louis, Mo.: Mosby, 1981. 182 pp.

"This text is to be used to teach health care personnel who perform bedside patient care the safest and easiest methods of patient handling and transfers." General transfer techniques are discussed first, then specific techniques for different types of disabilities. Included are specific directions for lifting, moving, and transferring patients. The text is well-illustrated, with step-by-step procedures. Information on specific types of equipment is also given. A glossary and index are included. Useful for all health care personnel involved in direct patient care and to laypersons involved in home care. A good text for training new employees because of its simplified instructions. Recommended for all medical and larger public libraries.

Redford, John B., ed. Orthotics Etcetera. 2d ed. Baltimore, Md.: William and Wilkins, 1980. 776 pp.

Written primarily by and for clinicians in the field of rehabilitation medicine. Preliminary chapters discuss in a general sense the mechanics of orthotics. The term orthotics is used liberally, as the book also discusses such topics as beds, housing, automobile modification, and self-help aids for the disabled. Well-illustrated, with extensive references given for each chapter. Also, includes an index. Several chapters include an appendix discussing the terminology used in that chapter. Because it is very comprehensive and clearly written, it is a useful reference for health care professionals, laypersons working with the disabled, and even the patients. Recommended for all medical and larger public libraries.

Rehabilitation Nursing. The Nursing Clinics of North America. vol. 15, 1980. Philadelphia: Saunders. 210 pp.

This issue of "Nursing Clinics of North America" deals specifically with the "rehabilitation of individuals with neurologic conditions leading to a significant degree of disability." Disability is defined as partial or complete inability to function physically, mentally, socially, or economically. It consists of a series of articles by contributors with expertise in rehabilitation nursing. The first four articles deal with specific conditions--spinal cord disorders, multiple sclerosis, Guillain-Barre syndrome, and stroke. The next two articles discuss rehabilitation in general, rather than discuss specific disorders, and the final article deals with psychosocial changes. Each article has a bibliography and is illustrated. This text is useful to update and complement the working nurse's knowledge, rather than to provide basic information. It could also be of interest to other health care personnel involved in rehabilitation. Recommended for medical libraries.

Rehabilitation Nurses and Related Readings: A Bibliography. Compiled by Boucher, Rita J., and Dittmar, Sharon S. Evanston, Ill.: Rehabilitation Nursing Institute, 1980. 63 pp.

This bibliography was compiled while the authors were working in a graduate program in rehabilitation nursing at State University of New York at Buffalo. It includes books and journal articles arranged by 50 specific subject areas. Articles included are not limited to those discussing rehabilitation but emphasize nursing issues as well. Some of the subject categories used include specific disorders such as cancer and stroke, geriatrics, nursing administration, the team approach, professional issues, bowel and bladder training, human sexuality, the handicapped child, and many more.

Unfortunately, such a publication is out of date as soon as it is published and must be supplemented by other sources. However, it is still a useful bibliography covering a diversity of topics. A good starting point to begin reading in a particular area of rehabilitation. Recommended for all medical libraries.

Riffle, Kathryn L., ed. Rehabilitative Nursing, Case Studies. Garden City, N.Y.: Medical Examination Publishing Co., 1979. 380 pp.

A collection of 30 case studies, intended as a study tool for baccalaureate and graduate nursing students. Each case covers a different problem, among them leukemia, alcoholism, mastectomy, systemic lupus erythematosis, and multiple sclerosis. A variety of age groups and both sexes are included in the cases discussed. A case is presented, followed by review questions and answers, and then references for further study. This format makes the text useful primarily for review and self-study. Strongly oriented toward nurses, but may be helpful to other health care personnel. Recommended for medical libraries.

Rosenstein, Solomon N. Dentistry in Cerebral Palsy and Related Handicapping Conditions. Springfield, Ill.: Charles C. Thomas, 1978. 167 pp.

In the past, some cerebral palsied and other handicapped individuals have been denied dental care because dentists did not have adequate understanding and knowledge of the mental and physical capabilities of the cerebral palsied patient. This book aims to rectify this situation by educating the general dentist and specialist. It contains principles, procedures, observations and findings of clinical practice, and studies developed during 25 years of the Cerebral Palsy Dental Program, initiated in 1951. A major section is devoted to neurological factors in cerebral palsy and related conditions, preoperative sedation and use of general anesthesia for dental treatment. Author and subject indices and many illustrations are included in this very excellent monograph. It is a much needed addition in a rarely explored field and a valuable teaching and research monograph. Recommended for dental and medical libraries.

Ross, Deborah, and Spencer, Sara. Aphasia Rehabilitation: An Auditory and Verbal Task Hierarchy. Springfield, Ill.: Charles C. Thomas, 1980. 237 pp.

Intended for use by clinicians in the treatment of the aphasic adult, this text is divided into two major sections: auditory and verbal. Each section contains activities presented in a task hierarchy, and arranged in order of increasing difficulty. Each "task" gives information on materials needed for that activity, task instructions, clinician instructions, and suggested criteria for mastery of the task, as well as descriptions of the activities or sample exercises. Includes a bibliography and an appendix with sample score sheets and pictures for exercises. The exercises could also be used by involved family members, since all instructions are included. Recommended for medical libraries.

Rossi, Paolo, ed. Functional Evaluation and Rehabilitation of Cardiac Patients. Chicago: Year Book Medical Publishers, 1979. 384 pp.

A contributed work primarily for cardiologists and physicians derived from the International Symposium in Functional Evaluation and Rehabilitation of Cardiac Patients, held in Stresa, Italy. Major sections of interest are rehabilitation of cardiac patients, drugs and rehabilitation, and psychological aspects of rehabilitation. Sections on drugs in habilitation were not found in other books evaluated. Charts, tables, and a subject index are included. Recommended for medical and special libraries.

Russell, W. Ritchie. Multiple Sclerosis: Control of the Disease. New York: Pergamon Press, 1976. 77 pp.

In the introduction of his work, Mr. Russell expresses his hope that other MS sufferers will read this monograph and "plan their own programs for a better and more healthy life." This title includes case studies of MS sufferers who have studied the factors which influence their disease and have modified their lifestyles accordingly. The study covers 15 years of progressive disease and is intended for all health care professionals who deal with multiple sclerosis. Recommended for hospital libraries for the purpose of patient education in MS.

Sahs, Adolph L.; Hartman, E. C.; and Aronson, S. M. Stroke: Cause, Prevention, Treatment, and Rehabilitation. London: Castle House Publications, 1979. 282 pp.

This contributed work tries to present the best and most current facts about stroke. It serves as a handbook of ready reference for general physicians, nurses, neurologists, therapists, and geriatric physicians. It includes chapters on manpower organization and community health services for stroke and medical and surgical treatment of stroke in children which are subjects seldom dealt with in other books. A very fine concise book and the best and most updated of all books evaluated on stroke rehabilitation. Recommended for medical school and nursing school libraries.

Shedd, Donald P., and Weinberg, Bernd . Surgical and Prosthetic Approaches to Speech Rehabilitation. Boston: G. K. Hall, 1980. 321 pp.

Papers presented at a workshop held in Buffalo in May 1978. The purpose of the workshop was to define the state of the art in the development of surgical and prosthetic approaches to speech following removal of the larynx. The papers discuss a variety of techniques used in speech rehabilitation. Each paper is illustrated and lists references for further information. A summary article at the end of the text discusses and evaluates the previous papers. Participants in the workshop included speech specialists, biomedical engineers, and surgeons, and the papers should be of interest to these same professionals. Recommended for larger medical school and research libraries.

Stolov, Walter C., and Clowers, Michael A., eds. Handbook of Severe Disability: A Text for Rehabilitation Counselors, Other Vocational Practitioners and Allied Health Professionals. Washington, D.C.: U.S. Department of Education, Rehabilitation Services Administration, 1981. 445 pp.

This text is oriented toward the vocational rehabilitation counselor. It was developed as a course for the first year graduate student in rehabilitation counseling and as a reference for the worker in the field. General introductory chapters on rehabilitation, psychosocial adjustment, and descriptions of significant body systems are followed by chapters on specific disabilities. The disabilities covered include many not usually covered in rehabilitation literature, including alcoholism and drug abuse, mental retardation, sickle cell disease, and epilepsy as well as the more commonly discussed problems such as stroke, cerebral palsy, cardiovascular and pulmonary disorders, blindness, and hearing disorders. Many illustrations are included and an annotated bibliography is given for each chapter. A glossary and index are also included. A useful introductory text especially for those with less technical background. Recommended for all medical libraries.

Stryker, Ruth. Rehabilitative Aspects of Acute and Chronic Nursing Care. 2d ed. Philadelphia: Saunders, 1977. 272 pp.

A basic nursing text, intended to be used in dealing with patients with neuromuscular problems, primarily adult and elderly patients. It covers physical rehabilitation in a general fashion, rather than dealing with specific disabilities. The text is divided into four basic sections: 1) introduction--includes the history of rehabilitation and basic concepts; 2) nursing care--includes the information on planning patient care, nutrition, bowel and bladder problems, and patient education; 3) nursing skills--covers positioning, transfer techniques, range of motion exercises; and 4) after rehabilitation--deals with the disabled in the community. Each chapter contains a list of references for further information. Many sample forms are included in the text. The sections on techniques are very detailed and well-illustrated, and include information on sources for the supplies mentioned. An index is also included. A useful text for the nursing student or the nurse just entering the field of rehabilitation as well as other health care personnel. Recommended for hospital and medical libraries.

Stryker, Stephanie. Speech After Stroke: A Manual for the Speech Pathologist and the Family Member. 2d ed. Springfield, Ill.: Charles C. Thomas, 1981. 427 pp.

MEDICAL ASPECTS   239

   Written by a speech pathologist with eleven years experience, and meant to be used by the speech pathologist, with learning reinforced by a family member. Each section includes instructions to the therapist, followed by exercises. The exercises are printed in large type so as to be easily read, and are arranged in order of increasing difficulty, so the patient can progress at his own pace. Words and pictures used are appropriate for adults and relevant to everyday needs and activities. Materials are arranged in five sections: 1) comprehension of the spoken word, 2) imitative abilty and articulation drills, 3) vocal recall, grammar, and syntax, 4) reading development skills, and 5) writing development skills. Includes a bibliography and index. An especially useful collection of materials, because it can be used as is or adapted to fit an individual situation. The exercises are simple, but not childish, and adapted to practical situations. Explanations are clear enough for the family member to understand and apply. Recommended for all medical libraries.

Symposium on "Dental Management of the Handicapped Child," Iowa City, 1973. Iowa City: University of Iowa, 1974. 94 pp.

   This collection of papers presented at the Symposium on Dental Management of the Handicapped Child held May 23 and 24, 1973 at the University of Iowa, is one of the few titles written addressing the subject of dentistry for the disabled individual. It is intended to be utilized as a continuing education tool for practicing dentists as well as dentistry students. It is unfortunate that a more current title dealing with this subject could not be located for examination. Recommended for medical school and dentistry libraries.

Total Hip Prosthesis. Baltimore, Md.: Williams and Wilkins, 1976. 328 pp.

   This text presents findings of a study on the effects of artificial joint replacements, with emphasis on the complications that may result. Over 2500 cases were studied and evaluated by use of a computer. This study would be of interest to the orthopedist and the general surgeon, the rheumatologist, and the doctor of internal medicine, for advising patients in need of artificial joint replacement. The study would be of interest to the engineer and the technician dealing with the construction of artificial joints. Illustrated, and includes references and an index. Recommended for larger medical school and research libraries.

Trieschmann, Roberta B. Spinal Cord Injuries: Psychological, Social, and Vocational Adjustment. New York: Pergamon Press, 1980. 234 pp.

   For an evaluation of this work, see Chapter I.

Vash, Carolyn L. The Psychology of Disability. (Springer series on Rehabilitation. v. 1) New York: Springer, 1981. 268 pp.

Written by a rehabilitation psychologist who is herself disabled, this text is useful reading for disabled people as well as for professionals dealing with the disabled. It is also interesting reading as it includes many cases, examples, and individual experiences. The text is divided into two parts. The first part covers the disability, relationships of the disabled with others, sex, employment, and recreation. Part 2 on interventions discusses how the disabled can be helped by legislation, counseling, and psychotherapeutics. A bibliography and an index are included. Recommended for all medical and larger public libraries.

Vitali, Miroslaw; Robinson, Kingsley P.; Andrews, Brian G.; and Harris, Edward. Amputations and Prostheses. London: Baillierc Tindall, 1978. 241 pp.

The author discusses the various types of amputation operations and the impact the operation has on choosing a suitable prosthesis. The advantages and disadvantages of prostheses suitable for various amputation levels are discussed, as are the types of complications that may result from using a certain prosthesis. Each prosthesis is described in detail, with illustrations. This text was written as an aid in prescribing the most suitable prosthesis for a given condition. An appendix gives a list of amputation and artificial limb centres in the United Kingdom. Includes a bibliography and an index. Especially written for the surgeon but useful to the non-specialist clinician or to those just starting out in the field who need basic, rather than intensive, information on the relationship between amputations and prosthesis. Its British influence does not limit the usefulness of the work. Recommended for hospital and medical libraries.

Walker, Frank C., ed. Modern Stoma Care. Edinburgh: Churchill Livingstone, 1976. 193 pp.

This book deals specifically with ileostomy, colostomy, and ileal conduit. The book is divided into five sections. A preliminary section contains general information about stoma and the organization of a stoma clinic; three chapters each dealing specifically with a type of stoma mentioned above; and a final section covers equipment. Written for the doctor, the nurse, and/or the stomatist, but with a minimum of technicality, which makes it useful to patients as well as health care professionals. Includes illustrations, references, and index. A useful appendix includes manufacturers' descriptions of various appliances used by stoma patients. Recommended for hospital and medical school libraries.

Wallace, Roberta; Heiss, Marie L.; and Bautch, Judith C. Staff Manual for Teaching Patients About Rheumatoid Arthritis. Chicago: American Hospital Association, 1982. 408 pp. (looseleaf)

This manual was designed for use by health care professionals in educating patients and their families about rheumatoid arthritis. As a result, it contains many sample forms and patient handouts. Topics covered include what patients should know about their disease, psychosocial issues affecting patients, medications, therapy, exercises and nutrition. Examples are geared toward the hospital setting, but the manual could be used in outpatient settings as well. The publication is looseleaf, so as to permit the inclusions of local material. It could be used for groups or for individual self-study, as each chapter begins with learning objectives and ends with study questions. The text is easy to understand, illustrated, and contains many references scattered throughout. Especially useful for patient education programs in the hospital or community. Recommended especially for hospital libraries and other medical libraries involved in patient education.

Walsh, Angela, ed. The Expanded Role of the Rehabilitation Nurse. Thorofare, N.J.: Charles B. Slack, 1980. 92 pp.

Proceedings of a three day symposium held in the spring of 1978 on the "Changing Role and Future Direction of Rehabilitation Nursing." The primary objectives of the conference were: 1) to define the expanded role and responsibilities of the rehabilitation nurse, 2) to identify specific educational preparation in rehabilitation nursing, and 3) to identfy the means of contributing nursing expertise in the care of the disabled on a local, state, regional, and national level. Papers included cover such diverse topics as the California Department of Rehabilitation, the Center for Independent Living (Berkeley), educational preparation in rehabilitation nursing, home health care, and the role of rehabilitation nursing in the insurance industry. Each chapter includes a list of references. Especially useful to nurses currently active in the field of rehabilitation nursing who are interested in any changes in their role. Recommended for medical libraries.

Wannstedt, Gunilla, and Craik, Rebecca. Evaluation of the Limb--Load Monitor. Philadelphia: Rehabilitation Engineering Center, Moss Rehabilitation Hospital, 1977. 75 pp.

The limb-load monitor is a clinical tool used to enhance the relearning of posture and locomotor skills in patients. It provides an auditory signal which correlates with the amount of weight placed on the limb. This study discusses the effect of the device on patient performance, the utilization of the device, and practical methods of introducing the device to the clinician. Includes a bibliography. Appendices include sample questionnaires and information on trial sites used in the study. For specialists in the field of orthotics and prosthetics who are interested in new developments from either the research or the clinical point of view. Recommended for larger medical school and research libraries.

Weinberg, Bernd. Readings in Speech Following Total Laryngectomy. Baltimore, Md.: University Park Press, 1980. 588 pp.

This text is meant to be a representative set of readings of important journal articles in the field. Both research and clinical articles are included. A variety of techniques are covered, including esophageal speech, the artificial larynx, and surgical-prosthesis methods of speech rehabilitation. Intended especially for speech and medical specialists, such as speech pathologists and head and neck surgeons. It is useful for extending the knowledge of those working in the field, but too technical to be useful to nonspecialists or the layperson. Includes bibliographies, illustrations, and an index. Recommended for larger hospital and medical libraries.

Weiss, Marian, ed. Early Therapeutic, Social, and Vocational Problems in the Rehabilitation of Persons with Spinal Cord Injuries. New York: Plenum Press, 1977. 378 pp.

This title is intended for the physician who cares for the spinal cord injured patient. Chapter 3 discusses experiences with treatment and rehabilitation of patients with spinal cord injury, pathology of spinal cord lesions in the light of dynamic alloplasty, biomedical studies in dynamic alloplasty of the spine, clinical results and the general evaluation of clinical material. It is intended for the professional and should not be used in patient education as the language is too complicated for the layperson. Recommended for medical school libraries.

Wenger, Nanette K., and Hellerstein, Herman K., eds. Rehabilitation of the Coronary Patient. New York: Wiley, 1978. 323 pp.

Designed to provide basic information about the medical, physiologic, and social problems of myocardial infarction, and intended to give realistic programs of rehabilitation. Contributors are specialists in the fields of medicine and psychiatry. It is particularly useful for "primary care physicians," mainly the chief individual responsible for continuing care of patient and entire health care team. Intended for medical students as a supplementary text and a research monograph. It is not a patient education tool because the terminology is too complicated for laypersons. Recommended for medical school libraries.

Wilson, A. Bennett, Jr. Limb Prosthetics, 5th ed. Huntington, N.Y.: Robert E. Krieger, 1976. 95 pp.

A description of current practices in limb prosthetics, intended for nontechnical personnel. Contents include the reasons for amputations, a description of the different types of amputation operations, a discussion of prostheses suitable for various types of amputations, and special considerations needed for children and the elderly. Also discussed are care of the stump and methods of training in using prostheses. Good illustrations of the different types of prostheses available are included as is an extensive bibliography. Fairly technical, but could be understood with a minimum of effort and therefore would be useful to patients and their families as well as to health care personnel. Recommended for all medical libraries.

Wilson, A. Bennett, Jr.; Boblitz, Michael H.; and Meece, A. Roger. Limb Prosthetics for Vocational Rehabilitation Workers. Philadelphia: Moss Rehabilitation Hospital, Texas University, 1978. 63 pp.

Similar in context to his book, Limb Prosthetics, but intended specifically for the rehabilitation counselor. This text gives basic information on amputees, the various types of amputations, the types of prostheses used, prosthetic training, and the functional capabilities of different types of amputees. It includes two tables of functional capabilities of upper and lower limb amputees, detailing which activities of daily living can be done and how they can be done for various levels of amputation. It also includes a bibliography and an appendix on specific body movements. Emphasis is on what the amputee can do so as to aid the vocational rehabilitation counselor in advising and placing his client. For this reason it could also be of value to prospective employers and to the patient himself. Recommended for medical and larger public libraries.

Wilson, A. Bennett, Jr.; Pritham, Charles; and Stills, Melvin. Manual for an Ultralight Below-Knee Prosthesis. 2d ed. Philadelphia: Drexel University, Temple University, Moss Rehabilitation Hospital, 1979. 68 pp.

This booklet is essentially a how-to manual. It discusses the development and evaluation of an ultralight below-knee level prosthesis. The fabrication of the device is described in great detail and with the use of many illustrations. This text should be of interest primarily to specialists in the field of prosthetics who are interested in keeping up with new developments. Recommended for larger medical school and research libraries, especially those with specialized collections in prosthetics.

8 LEGAL RIGHTS: ADVOCACY, LEGISLATION, LITIGATION, AND PROGRAMS

NANCY P. JOHNSON/Reference Librarian, Georgia State University,
Law Library, Atlanta, Georgia

INTRODUCTION

In the early 1970s civil rights for America's handicapped became a pressing issue. Large numbers of disabled individuals demonstrated in Washington, D.C. demanding new laws and regulations to end discrimination in key areas of employment, education, transportation, and accommodation. Fortunately, several public laws were enacted and regulations were issued that set forth the principles necessary to ensure that all disabled persons are guaranteed their civil rights.

These laws which had the resultant goal of equality for the disabled are discussed, some in greater detail than others, in the literature set forth in this bibliography. Public Law 94-142, the Education for All Handicapped Children Act, is a comprehensive law guaranteeing the availability of free appropriate public education to disabled children. Another important law, Section 504 of the Rehabilitation Act of 1973, P.L. 93-112, is the basic civil rights provision with respect to terminating discrimination against handicapped citizens under any program or activity receiving federal financial assistance. The Architectural Barriers Act, P.L. 90-480, requires that buildings constructed, altered, leased, or financed by the U.S. Government be accessible to physically handicapped persons. In 1974, the U.S. Congress substantially altered the federal government's assistance to states in providing social services with Title XX of the Social Security Act, P.L. 93-64. The regulations implementing these laws are also extremely important in the areas of education, employment practices, and accessibility.

The titles listed in this bibliography grew out of the need for professionals, parents, and disabled individuals to understand the laws and regulations which guarantee certain civil rights. Many of the titles focus on individual laws, whereas, other titles present an overview of the topic.

A major act which is discussed in much of the legal literature is Public Law 94-142, the Education for All Handicapped Children Act. Under this Act, each child must be provided with non-discriminatory evaluation and full rights of due process of law in all placement decisions. Additionally, the act requires that each child be educated in a "least restrictive environment."

Many of the books annotated in this bibliography explain the significance of P.L. 94-142. An important book which answers questions on P.L. 94-142 raised by parents of handicapped children is Schmidt and Williams' Law and the Handicapped Child: A Primer for Illinois Parents published by the Illinois Regional Resources Center, Northern Illinois University. Another title, A Primer on Due Process: Education Decisions for Handicapped Children is one of the several titles published by The Council for Exceptional Children and written for educators to understand and implement the federal law. Two excellent compilations on the topic are published by Research Press, Educating Handicapped Children: The Legal Mandate and Workshop Materials: The Impact of Current Legal Action of Educating Handicapped Children. These books, written by an attorney, Reed Martin, cover individualized education programs, procedural safeguards, record keeping, and cases. An important source for information on higher education and physically disabled students is the Proceedings of the Supreme Court Davis Decision. For an historical look at laws affecting the education of handicapped children, refer to State Law and Education of Handicapped Children: Issues and Recommendations. Legal Rights Primer for the Handicapped: In and Out of the Classroom is designed to act as a primer to the interaction between the law and the handicapped child. An expensive, but comprehensive reporter, Education For the Handicapped Law Report, is extremely important for keeping on top of major legal developments in the field.

Another landmark act, The Rehabilitation Act of 1973, Public Law 93-112, contains four important sections. Section 501 requires that all government agencies establish affirmative action programs to employ handicapped individuals. Section 502 created the Architectural and Transportation Barriers Compliance Board to oversee enforcement of federal laws mandating access to buildings constructed or operated with federal funds. Section 503 mandates affirmative action in the employment of qualified disabled persons on the part of all employers holding federal contracts totalling at least $2500. Section 504, possibly the most familiar section, is the basic civil rights provision with respect to terminating discrimination against handicapped citizens under any program or activity receiving federal financial assistance.

Several of the publications listed in this bibliography summarize the requirements and implementation of the laws and regulations on educational process and employment rights under the Rehabilitation Act of 1973. The most comprehensive work on Section 504 is published by the Federal Programs Advisory Service titled Handicapped Requirements Handbook. The Handbook has compiled in one easy-to-use binder all essential information and requirements relating to Section 504 and amendments. Other notable titles on the topic include Clellan's Section 504: Civil Rights for the Handicapped. Biehl's Guide to the Section 504 Self-Evaluation for Colleges and Universities, and Hermann's Handbook of

Employment Rights of the Handicapped: Section 503 and 504 of the Rehabilitation Act of 1973.

The Architectural Barriers Act of 1968, P.L. 90-380, requires that buildings constructed, altered, leased, or financed by the U.S. Government be accessible to physically handicapped persons. An excellent, two-volume work which covers the state statutes and regulations of four Eastern states is Barrier Free Design: The Law.

In 1974, the U.S. Congress substantially altered the federal government's assistance to states in providing social services with Title XX of the Social Security Act, P.L. 93-64. One work devoted to assisting blind individuals in understanding Title XX is Duncan's A Guide to Expanding Social Services to the Blind Under Title XX of the Social Security Act.

Judicial efforts to protect and advance the rights of handicapped Americans are presently evolving; therefore, the judicial field of legal rights for disabled persons is in its embryonic stage. Few discrimination cases have been tried because of the expense of such suits. This lack of judicial precedent and the complexity of the laws and regulations discourages attorneys from accepting cases on behalf of disabled people. Fortunately, this situation is changing and these cases will soon be appearing in the literature. There is a need for looseleaf reporting services that will cover legal developments in a timely manner. An unpolished, but valuable, reporter is the Case Reporter published by the University of Maryland Law School Developmental Disabilities Law Project. This service provides, on a quarterly basis, summaries of court decisions dealing with P.L. 94-142 and Section 504. Abeson's Legal Change for the Handicapped Through Litigation was written for persons unfamiliar with the judicial process who may be considering filing a complaint, lawsuit, or appeal.

The lack of training in law schools concerning issues basic to the civil rights of disabled individuals may be remedied by the comprehensive casebook, The Legal Rights of Handicapped

Persons, edited by Robert L. Burgdorf, Jr. As stated in the preface, Burgdorf's intent for the book is to facilitate the training of attorneys and other professionals who will be vigorous and knowledgeable advocates for the legal rights of their handicapped clients. This volume is exceptionally comprehensive in the coverage of the legal rights of the disabled in the following areas: employment, accessibility, guardianship, confinement, housing, medical services, marriage, contract, and voting.

Within the last ten years, advocacy groups have improved the quality of life for disabled persons. These groups have been effective in getting legislation passed and requesting better services from public and private agencies. Two detailed books directed towards the parents of handicapped children, How to Organize an Effective Parent/Advocacy Group and Move Bureaucracies and Let Our Children Go are tools for teaching parent advocacy skills. The American Coalition of Citizens With Disabilities published another practical guide appropriately titled Planning Effective Advocacy Programs by Bowe. The United Cerebral Palsy Association presents a very complete guide on advocacy, Thinking/Learning/Doing by Dickman.

Fortunately, in this age of legal rights for the disabled, there are several books directed at disabled individuals and/or the parents of disabled children. One guide, Hull's The Rights of Physically Handicapped People, part of the ACLU handbook series, sets forth the rights of the handicapped and offers suggestions on how these rights can be protected. There are also a few texts available on the legal rights of persons with specific disabilities. Works dealing with specific disabilities include The Legal Rights of Persons with Epilepsy by the Epilepsy Foundation, The Rights of Hearing-Impaired Children by Nix, and the 1956 and 1966 editions of Epilepsy and the Law by Barrow and Fabing.

Two sources have been devoted to disabled individuals as consumers. Bruck's Access: The Guide to a Better Life for Disabled Americans is the most comprehensive, action-oriented guide for disabled consumers. Many areas of concern to the disabled consumer--attitudinal problems, advances in technology, laws and regulations--are highlighted. Another consumer guide, Bean and Schapiro's Consumer Warranty Law: Your Rights and How to Enforce Them, explains warranties on medical devices and equipment.

Resource manuals and directories of programs or services for disabled persons have been published within the last few years. Information about state and federal organizations and attorneys specializing in the field are provided in such reference aids. These directories, such as Walker's A Guide to Organizations, Agencies, and Federal Programs for Handicapped Americans and National Center for Law and the Handicapped's A Selective Listing of Legal Resources for the Handicapped help meet the need for information by caseworkers, attorneys, and other persons concerned with the legal rights of the disabled.

Recently, several excellent books have been published and deserve special notice because of their comprehensive nature. These books should be models for future publications on legal aspects of rehabilitation. One source, already mentioned previously, Handicapped Requirements Handbook, combines all essential information and requirements related to Section 504 of the Rehabilitation Act. An excellent state manual, published by the Illinois Developmental Disabilities Advocacy Authority, entitled Manual on Legal Rights and Responsibilities of Developmentally Disabled Persons in Illinois by Kerns' et al, surveys various areas of Illinois and Federal law of importance to the disabled. An exceptional compilation of materials presented at a National Public Law Training Center workshop, Advocacy For/With the Mentally Ill and Handicapped, presents current information on advocacy roles, employment, housing, education, and health care.

More research is greatly needed by legal scholars in the general area of legal rights for the disabled and in the specific areas of problems faced by handicapped persons in the criminal justice system. There is also a definite need for more reporters, such as the University of Maryland Law School, Developmental Disabilities Law Project, Case Reporter, that cover case law, legislation, and regulatory developments. There is also the need for periodicals, such as the discontinued periodical, Amicus; the current National Center for Law and the Deaf Newsletter; and the current In the Mainstream; to act as awareness tools for legal rights advocates. The monographic series published by the National Center for Law and the Handicapped helps fulfill the need for brief papers on specific topics affecting the rights of the handicapped.

There are a number of legal citations and documents that are used in the literature and may need a very brief explanation. For example, P.L. 94-142 means that Public Law 142 was enacted during the 94th Congress. Laws in force are codified in the United States Code, which is divided into titles and sections. For example, 42 U.S.C. Sec. 6001 refers to Title 42 and Section 6001. The citation 34 C.F.R. 5.63 means section 5.63 of Title 34 of the Code of Federal Regulations. The C.F.R. is a codification of general and permanent regulations.

Special legal language exists that permits professionals to communicate easily with others. Therefore, some legal phrases, such as due process, warranty law, reasonable accommodation, may need to be defined. Some of the sources include a glossary of terms, or reference should be made to Black's law dictionary (St. Paul, Minn.: West, 1979).

ANNOTATED BIBLIOGRAPHY

Abeson, Alan, ed. A Continuing Summary of Pending and Completed Litigation Regarding the Education of Handicapped Children. Arlington, Va.: Council for Exceptional Children, 1973. 50 pp.

The Council for Exceptional Children's State-Federal Information Clearinghouse for Exceptional Children (SFICEC), a project supported by the U.S. Bureau of Education for the Handicapped, collected and organized this summary of litigation. Federal and State cases on education of handicapped children are summarized. Unfortunately, the cases are not cited correctly so it would be difficult to find the full decision in a law library. It contains a detailed table of contents, but no index. Each new edition updates and supercedes earlier editions. This material will be valuable only if updated on a regular basis.

Abeson, Alan, ed. Legal Change for the Handicapped Through Litigation. Reston, Va.: Council for Exceptional Children, 1975. 35 pp.

This book was written for persons unfamiliar with the litigation process who may be considering instigating a lawsuit. Topics covered include: preparation for the trial, and litigation expenses. This pamphlet is unique in that it explains very common legal terms, e.g., complaint, deposition, appeal, in a very concise and non-technical manner. The information could be applied to any type of legal action.

Abeson, Alan; Bolick, Nancy; and Hass, Jayne. A Primer on Due Process: Education Decisions for Handicapped Children. Reston, Va.: Council for Exceptional Children, 1976. 57 pp.

Discusses the requirements of due process in the identification, evaluation, and educational placement of handicapped children. Attention is devoted to the steps needed to meet the requirements and the sequence in which these steps could be implemented. Written for educators to comply with the due process requirements. The information is concise and clear. The legal forms, covering due process, evaluation, and educational placement could be very useful to school administrators.

Amicus. South Bend, Ind.: National Center for Law and the Handicapped, 1975-79. Bimonthly (Replaced Newsline, former NCLH newsletter).

For an evaluation of this work, see Chapter XIV.

Ballard, Joseph. Public Law 94-142 and Section 504: Understanding What They are and Are Not. Reston, Va.: Council for Exceptional Children, 1978. 13 pp.

Written in a question and answer format, this pamphlet would serve as a quick reference guide for school administrators in understanding and implementing the two federal laws. Recommended for school officials. References are scattered among the pages.

Barrow, Roscoe, L., and Fabing, Howard D. Epilepsy and the Law. 2d ed. New York: Harper and Row, 1966. 174 pp.

The first edition of Epilepsy and the Law, published in 1956, exposed the archaic laws relating to epilepsy and proposed reform of these laws. To describe the great change in the epilepsy laws since 1956, the second edition had to be completely rewritten. The following topics are covered in this volume: eugenic marriage laws, sterilization laws, and driver's license laws. The authors, a law professor and a doctor, clearly and ably report on the legal reform of laws in the light of medical progress in treating epilepsy. This is the classic work in understanding the legal rights of epileptics.

Bean, Belinda, and Schapiro, Susan. Consumer Warranty Law: Your Rights and How to Enforce Them: A Guide for Users of Medical Devices. Washington, D.C.: Disability Rights Center Inc. 1977. 22 pp.

A practical guide written to provide consumers of medical devices and equipment with information about their legal rights. Includes sample complaints and solutions, explanation of warranties, small claims court, and steps to follow if a problem arises. This slim pamphlet would be helpful to disabled individuals in acquainting them with their consumer rights. Although it focuses only on one aspect of consumer rights, it adequately covers consumer warranty law. Includes a few addresses for further help.

Berkowitz, Edward D., ed. Disability Policies and Government Programs. New York: Praeger, 1979. 185 pp.

Seven essays, complete with tables and figures, describe the state of the art and need for change in disability policies. Intended for scholars and researchers.

Berkowitz, Monroe,; Johnson, William G.; and Murphy, Edward H. Public Policy Toward Disability. New York: Praeger, 1976. 150 pp.

This work brings together the legal and institutional background of the disability system and statistical models which seek to explain the limitations in role functions that have been labeled as disability. Selective topics cover worker's disability income system, disability insurance program, and an applied model of the disability process. Tables, figures, references, and an index complement the text. The authors are Ph.D.'s in Economics and publish on the topic of disability. Highly scholarly; recommended for researchers in the field.

Biehl, G. Richard. Guide to the Section 504 Self-Evaluation for Colleges and Universities. Washington, D.C.: National Association of College and University Business Officers, 1978. 127 pp.

The self-evaluation under Section 504 of the Rehabilitation Act of 1973 is the principal process through which compliance with the statute is assessed. This guide is aimed at assisting college and university officials in the completion of their self-evaluation. The HEW Regulations are summarized and pertinent parts of the regulations are published. Written in a clear and informative manner. The appendix, "Sources of Additional Information and Technical Assistance" includes a listing of organizations and agencies that represent handicapped persons. Includes a bibliography. This guide would be very helpful to higher education administrators.

Biklen, Douglas. Let Our Children Go: An Organizing Manual for Advocates and Parents. Syracuse, N.Y.: Human Policy Press, 1974. 144 pp.

This book describes how parents of children with disabilities, and their allies, can fight for their rights. Provides very helpful chapters on self-evaluation; identifying community needs; action (lobbying, letter writing), and legal action. The author explains the basic steps to successful organizing. The information is well-organized, specific, and includes sensitive photos. The bibliography includes books, articles, and films. Highly recommended for parents and advocates.

Bolick, Nancy. Digest of State and Federal Laws: Education of Handicapped Children. 3rd ed. Reston, Va.: Council for Exceptional Children, 1974. Looseleaf.

Part I presents, in digest form, the laws of the 50 states. Each state's laws have been organized along 11 subject categories. Citations are provided for those who may wish to refer to the original text of the laws and update the laws if necessary. Part II is a digest of federal laws which have relevance to education of handicapped children. A compilation of this type is very valuable for attorneys, educators, and advocates. The information aids in understanding, evaluating, and comparing the education of handicapped children in each state.

Bowe, Frank. Coalition Building. Washington, D.C.: American Coalition of Citizens with Disabilities, 1978. 66 pp.

The American Coalition of Citizens with Disabilities (ACCD) found in their research project that cooperation among people with diverse disabilities and their organizations enhances the capacity of rehabilitation program officials to ascertain the needs of the disabled, design approaches to meet these needs, and evaluate the impact of these efforts. Coalition Building describes the efforts to construct and refine a model for structuring cooperation and communication across disability. Presents interesting reading and an annotated bibliography on rehabilitation consumerism and political coalitions.

Bowe, Frank, and Williams, John. Planning Effective Advocacy Programs. Washington, D.C.: American Coalition of Citizens with Disabilities, 1979. 61 pp.

Offers guidelines for enhancing the capabilities of existing self-help organizations for disabled people and ensuring the effectiveness of new ones. The ACCD is a nationwide association of 84 national, state, and local organizations of and for disabled people. Chapters cover: consumer participation, leadership programs, support, and workshops. Presents a practical guide for effective advocacy programs. Offers additional sources of information. A unique and helpful book that focuses on advocacy programs for a specific audience.

Bruck, Lilly. Access: The Guide to a Better Life for Disabled Americans. New York: David Obst Books, 1978. 251 pp.

Written with an activist slant, this book explains to disabled individuals how they can better make use of their resources to obtain needed goods and services in the marketplace. Discusses consumerism, civil rights, purchase of goods and services, recreation, and barrier-free travel. A unique and comprehensive book on disabled individuals as consumers. The author has been active in New York and on the national level with the education of disabled consumers. Written in an easy-to-read format and style. Just about every page offers suggestions for additional information: organizations and their addresses and publications with complete bibliographic information. Indexed. Highly recommended.

Burgdorf, Robert L., Jr., ed. The Legal Rights of Handicapped Persons: Cases, Materials, and Text. Baltimore: Paul H. Brookes Publishers, 1980. 1127 pp.

An excellent volume covering cases and legislation dealing with the rights of handicapped individuals. The scope is focused on those areas in which disabled persons have traditionally been denied some right, e.g., employment, education, housing, medical services, and marriage. It is designed for use in law school courses or clinical education. The author, an attorney, is the Director of the Developmental Disabilities Law Project, University of Maryland School of Law. It is the only casebook available on the topic. Extremely comprehensive in coverage. Contains an index and table of contents. This well-written landmark book is definitely a valuable acquisition for law libraries.

Clellan, Richard. Section 504: Civil Rights for the Handicapped. Arlington, Va.: American Association of School Administrators, 1978. 128 pp.

The purpose of this handbook is to: 1) examine the statutory and regulatory requirements of Section 504, and 2) delineate the various dimensions of local educational agency administrative responsibilities relative to the successful implementation of various Section 504 subparts. The four chapters, introduction, employment practices, program accessibility, comparison of P.L. 94-142 and Section 504, are heavily footnoted and include charts. References are included. Dr. Richard Clellan, Ed.D., attempts to describe, analyze, and identify critical issues and problems relative to Section 504. Recommended for school administrators.

Crosson, Anita; Browing, Philip; and Krambs, Robert E. Advancing Your Citizenship. Eugene, Ore.: Center on Human Development, University of Oregon, 1979. 78 pp.

The first section introduces the reader to the three major pieces of federal legislation pertaining to handicapped individuals: P.L. 94-142, P.L. 93-112, and P.L. 94-103. The second section overviews specific mechanisms which can be used in implementing these rights, while the third section is a demonstration of the application of these rights and mechanisms. The format is easy to read. The references to additional information are complete and could be very helpful. This manual would be useful to handicapped persons in interpreting and implementing the laws.

DeJong, Gerben. Disability, Home Care, and Relative Responsibility: A Legal Perspective. Boston, Mass.: Research and Training Center No. 7 Medical Rehabilitation Institute, Tufts-New England Medical Center, 1978. 41 pp.

DeJong presents a thorough study of the role of relatives in providing in-home assistance to disabled persons. He explores in detail the legal traditions, cases, and statutes, which explain the issue of relative responsibility and home care. The state law and policies of Massachusetts are explained in-depth. Citations to cases and statutes are provided, as well as a complete bibliography. Because this topic is not covered in other sources, this paper is recommended for attorneys and others involved in shaping public policy towards the role of relatives in providing in-home assistance to the disabled.

Des Jardins, Charlotte. How to Organize an Effective Parent/Advocacy Group and Move Bureaucracies. Chicago: Coordinating Council for Handicapped Children, 1980. 131 pp.

CCHC is a very strong group which continues to be in the forefront of the movement to implement P.L. 94-142 and train hundreds of parents to advocate for the rights of their handicapped children in individualized education programs. This "how-to" guidebook is an excellent resource for planning advocacy groups. The detailed explanation on every topic is extremely valuable. Highly recommended for parents of handicapped children and other advocacy groups.

Dickman, Irving R. Thinking/Learning/Doing. New York: United Cerebral Palsy Association, 1975. 128 pp.

The National Advocacy Project of United Cerebral Palsy Associations presents a very complete and compassionate guide on advocacy. All aspects of advocacy projects for the rights of disabled persons are discussed: Project Model Sites; Replication Sites; and Advocacy and UCPA. Recommended reading for families of the disabled and others committed to the rights of the disabled.

DuBow, Sy. <u>National Center for Law and the Deaf: Final Report</u>. Washington, D.C.: National Center for Law and the Deaf, 1978. 8 pp.

This brief final report describes how the National Center for Law and the Deaf (NCLD) between 1975 and 1977 provided legal services, legal education, and legal advocacy for hearing-impaired individuals. The information presented would be helpful to organizations and law groups interested in providing legal assistance to the deaf.

Duncan, John L. <u>A Guide to Expanding Social Services to the Blind Under Title XX of the Social Security Act</u>. New York: American Foundation for the Blind, 1976. 113 pp.

The purpose of this guide is to enable blind individuals, advocates for the blind, and those who provide services to the blind to better understand Title XX and to have a larger share in the decision-making processes which determine whether or not programs are responsive to the blind. The appendices include a state by state account of special services for the blind, agency addresses, fees, eligibility determination, etc. This guide would be greatly enhanced by more complete bibliographic information, especially citations to the "Comprehensive Annual Services Program" which is the source of most of the statistical information.

<u>Education for the Handicapped Law Report</u>. Washington, D.C.: CRR Publishing, 1979- . Biweekly.

The biweekly looseleaf reporter is a thorough compilation of the basic documents-interpretations, administrative rulings, statutes, regulations, and federal and state court decisions. This service alerts users to all important legal developments affecting education of the handicapped. Comprehensive indexes by topic, statute and regulation permits fast location of specific documents. Because education for handicapped children is a rapidly changing area, this service is valuable for keeping school administrators, education agencies, and attorneys informed. Unfortunately the cost ($400) may limit the number of organizations and libraries that can subscribe to it.

Epilepsy Foundation of America. <u>Education for Children with Epilepsy: The Education for All Handicapped Children Act</u>. Washington, D.C.: Epilepsy Foundation of America, n.d. 22 pp.

Presents a basic explanation of the significance of P.L. 94-142 for epileptic children. Also provides sources for more information. This brief document would be useful to parents of epileptic children.

Epilepsy Foundation of America. <u>The Legal Rights of Persons with Epilepsy</u>. Washington, D.C.: The Foundation, 1976. 154 pp.

This work is the fourth edition of a study conducted by the Epilepsy Foundation of America. It briefly summarizes current state statutes and administrative policies relating to epilepsy. Also contains a special section on model legislation. Published in 1976, but still is valuable. The survey of state statutes and regulations is extremely useful for a researcher wishing to efficiently compare various state laws.

Goltz, Diane L., and Behrmann, Michael M. Getting the Buck to Stop Here: A Guide to Federal Resources for Special Needs. Reston, Va.: The Council for Exceptional Children, 1979. 225 pp.

This manual was developed to help individuals identify and access relevant sources of federal funding. Section I of the manual consists of a series of matrices divided into seven areas of interest. Information in the matrices is provided to facilitate the selection of federal programs which may be appropriate funding sources. Section II of the manual, Program Descriptions, presents more than 100 individual federal programs relating to the provision of education and services for exceptional individuals. The information is complete and accurate. Once the information is obtained from this manual, it could be updated by consulting the latest Catalog of Federal Domestic Assistance. Washington, D.C.: Government Printing Office.

Handicapped Requirements Handbook. Washington, D.C.: Federal Programs Advisory Service, 1979. Looseleaf.

This handbook consists of two sections: the Basic 504 Compliance Guide and Agency Requirements that analyze the requirements. Appendices include a glossary, annotated bibliography, text of regulations, set of ANSI standards, discussion of relevant court cases, and complete index. This book adequately meets the needs of different groups that must understand all essential information and requirements related to Section 504. The coverage is comprehensive and the index is very easy to use. Since it is in a looseleaf format, the material could be updated. The advisory service is also available to serve subscribers in an individual capacity by phone or letter. Definitely highly recommended for purchase for those individuals complying with the law and implementing programs.

Hermann, Anne Marie C., and Walker, Lucinda. Handbook of Employment Rights of the Handicapped: Section 503 and 504 of the Rehabilitation Act of 1973. Washington, D.C.: George Washington University. Regional Rehabilitation Research Institute of Attitudinal, Legal and Leisure Barriers, 1978. 87 pp.

Discusses hiring practices by providing a detailed explanation of Sections 503 and 504 of the Rehabilitation Act, and Post-hiring Practices, e.g., benefits, pay, and promotion. This book is written for the mentally or physically handicapped person who is looking for a job or already has one. It's descriptive format is clear and helpful. Contains a thorough bibliography of statutes, regulations, and cases. Complete index and glossary of legal terms. Both authors are attorneys involved in legal issues affecting the handicapped.

Howards, Irving; Brehm, Henry P.; and Nagi, Saad Z. Disability, from Social Problem to Federal Program. New York: Praeger, 1980. 171 pp.

The in-depth data and discussion presented in this volume provide the basis for conclusions and assumptions about disability and the Social Security Disability Insurance program. The background and developmental history to the present legislation authorizing the SSDI program is reviewed and the social problem toward which the underlying policy was aimed is described. The bibliography is comprehensive. The three authors are academicians and leaders in the field of research on disability. This analytical study would be of great interest to sociologists, policy formulators, and researchers.

Hull, Kent. The Rights of Physically Handicapped People. New York: Avon Books, 1979. 235 pp.

This guide, part of the American Civil Liberties Union handbook series, sets forth rights of the handicapped under the present law and offers suggestions on how these rights can be protected. The following topics are covered: architectural barriers, transportation, education, and employment. Contains extensive, well-cited footnotes. Written from an activist viewpoint, this guide not only explains the legal rights of handicapped people, but outlines the avenues of legal recourse when those rights are violated. Highly recommended; paperback edition makes it very affordable.

In the Mainstream. Washington, D.C.: Mainstream, Inc., 1976-   . Bimonthly.

This bimonthly newsletter on affirmative action for disabled persons includes articles on compliance, regulations, legislation, and litigation. The articles and columns would be of great interest to employers, educators, and handicapped individuals. This type of newsletter is greatly needed to keep professionals informed of the law as it relates to the disabled.

Institute on Rehabilitation Issues. Report from the Study Group on Legal Concerns of the Rehabilitation Counselor. Menomonie, Wis.: Research and Training Center, University of Wisconsin - Stout, 1976. 143 pp.

This document was prepared by a Committee of the Institute on Rehabilitation Issues, which is a cooperative endeavor of representatives from the state, federal, and private sectors of vocational rehabilitations. Developed specifically for the rehabilitation counselor. Contents include: client rights affecting the counselor, confidentiality, and liability. Comprehensive coverage of laws and the sources are footnoted. Glossary of legal terms. No index, but detailed table of contents. This is a valuable text since it is a working document developed for the practitioner.

Kerns, Elizabeth; Kiley, Ann; and Siedar, Greig. Manual on Legal Rights and Responsibilities of Developmentally Disabled Persons in Illinois. Springfield: Illinois Developmental Disabilities Advocacy Authority, 1980. 317 pp.

This well-written manual provides a survey of various areas of the law - confidentiality, consent, criminal law, education, housing, marriage, sexual activity, and voting - having importance to physically and mentally disabled persons. Excerpts are taken from Federal and Illinois law. Cases are excerpted and cited throughout this work. Very comprehensive in scope; covers topics not in other manuals, e.g., estate planning, insurance, and voting. Extremely valuable since it states the Illinois requirements that enforce the federal laws. The authors intend periodically to up-date this manual, therefore, it should always contain current information. Many attorneys and advocates are responsible for compiling the material. Indexed. Appendices include: resources, legal terms, and acronyms. Very highly recommended for all Illinois libraries.

Lobbying for the Rights of Disabled People: Views from the Hill and from the Grass Roots. Falls Church, Va.: Institute for Information Studies, 1980. 50 pp.

The authors have written this brief document to inform disabled people and their families, friends, and advocates on how to influence legislators and policy makers. Presents specific information on communicating with representatives and testifying before official bodies. It would be very useful to advocates of the disabled.

Martin, Reed. Educating Handicapped Children: The Legal Mandate. Champaign, Ill.: Research Press Co., 1979. 181 pp.

Examines in-depth laws, regulations, and court cases affecting the education of handicapped children. Covers public education, individualized education programs, procedural safeguards, and record-keeping. Although legal citations abound in this book, all of the references are cited correctly and the laws and cases could be located in a law library. Written by an attorney for administrators and others who work with the legal requirements governing educational services to handicapped children. Unfortunately, it is not indexed. Appears to be one of the better publications available for school administrators on the topic.

Martin, Reed, ed. Workshop Materials: The Impact of Current Legal Action on Educating Handicapped Children. Champaign, Ill.: Research Press Co., 1980. 309 pp.

This compilation of workshop materials consists of two basic parts. Part one details the legislative and judicial history of the federal acts governing special education, along with complaints and defenses, evaluation, and IEP. Part two, an appendix, contains recent cases applying the act to current special education services. The information is presented in a clear format. Highly recommended for administrators and attorneys.

McGarry, Barbara D. Federal Assistance for Programs Serving the Visually Handicapped. 5th ed. New York: American Foundation for the Blind, 1979. 56 pp.

This compilation is based on the Catalog of Federal Domestic Assistance (1979) published by the U.S. Government. From this Catalog, the author selected 136 federal programs with potential for specific assistance for the visually handicapped. The subject index cross references the listed programs by type of services offered. This directory, if updated yearly, is a very useful tool for directors seeking federal funds.

Meade, James G. The Rights of Parents and The Responsibilities of Schools. Cambridge, Mass.: Educators Publishing Service, 1978. 186 pp.

The first part of this work is devoted to the texts of P.L. 94-142 and P.L. 93-112 and the HEW regulations interpreting the two acts. The second part of the text is devoted to questions and answers about the laws. Information centers, books, and directories are also listed. Because the text of the laws and regulations appear in so many other sources, this book would be useful to libraries that have limited access to legal materials.

Mental Health Law Project. Combatting Exclusionary Zoning: The Right of Handicapped People to Live in the Community. Washington, D.C.: Mental Health Law Project, 1976. 113 pp.

While the materials explore case law, state statutes, and articles which deal with zoning barriers to the developmentally disabled, the legal principles found in these materials can be applied to the physically disabled. Recommended for attorneys and city planners.

Moakley, Terence J. Barrier Free Design: The Law. New York: Eastern Paralyzed Veterans Association, 1976. 2 vols.

Provides explanation and illustration of building laws and construction code provisions for the physically handicapped under P.L. 90-480, within the city of New York, and in the states of New York, New Jersey, Connecticut, and Pennsylvania. This two volume publication is directed toward architects, engineers, and building officials involved with building design, code implementation, and enforcement. State statutes, regulations, and code provisions are set forth followed by concise explanation of the law. Includes tables and illustrations. Excellent, simplified version of building laws for one city and four states that should set an example for other states' publications. Highly recommended for building officials in states covered.

National Association of State Directors of Special Education. The Education for all Handicapped Children. Washington, D.C.: The National Association of State Directors of Special Education, Inc., 1975. 26 pp.

Presented in tabular form, this brief document is a section-by-section analysis of the law and a general comparison of P.L. 94-142 with previous law. This booklet would provide educators with quick reference to provisions of the law.

National Center for Law and the Handicapped. A Comprehensive Guide to Employment Discrimination of the Handicapped. South Bend, Ind.: National Center for Law and the Handicapped, 1980. 64 pp.

This document is designed to explain laws relating to employment of the handicapped to non-lawyers. The laws which protect the handicapped against employment discrimination are identified and discussed. The last chapter explains how an individual can use the laws. Citations to cases and statutes are provided for those who wish to go directly to the sources. This guide is highly recommended for handicapped employees and all employers.

National Center for Law and the Handicapped. The Rights of Special Education and Handicapped Students in School Disciplinary Procedures. South Bend, Ind.: National Center for Law and the Handicapped, n.d. 18 pp.

This brief document examines, in detail, the topic of disciplinary procedures and handicapped children. Cases, statutes, and regulations which relate to the topic are discussed. The information is clear and concise. This topic is not covered in other sources, therefore, this paper is highly recommended for educators and advocates for the disabled.

National Center for Law and the Handicapped. Selected Litigation and Legislation Affecting the Handicapped: Employment. South Bend, Ind.: National Center for Law and the Handicapped, 1978. 45 pp.

As stated in the title, this document is a compilation of cases and statutes affecting the handicapped in the area of employment. The cases and statutes are abstracted. Provides easy access for legal materials in the field of employment and the handicapped.

National Center for the Law and the Deaf. Newsletter. Washington, D.C.: National Center for the Law and the Deaf, 1976-

This NCLD Newsletter, issued irregularly, is designed to inform deaf and hearing-impaired individuals about the Center's plans, programs, activities, and achievements. In addition, the Newsletter, reports on legislation, litigation, and legal clinics affecting the legal rights of the hearing-impaired. This current awareness resource is valuable for lawyers and advocates working with the hearing-impaired community.

National Federation of the Blind. The Blind and Physically Handicapped in Competitive Employment: A Guide to Compliance. Washington, D.C.: National Federation of the Blind, 1975. 43 pp.

Includes background information on Title V of the Rehabilitation Act of 1973 and compliance procedures. Also includes an address delivered by Kenneth Jernigan, "Blindness: Is the Public Against Us?" Written for persons who must comply with Section 504 of the Rehabilitation Act. The information presented is fairly general. The lack of an index and bibliography limits its usefulness.

National Federation of the Blind. Section 504 and Blind Employees: A Guide to Reasonable Accommodation and An Illustrative List of Job Opportunities. Baltimore, Md.: National Federation of the Blind, 1979. 60 pp.

This publication provides insight into the kinds of accommodations that can be made for blind employees to enable them to be productive individuals as employees of a company. Includes a discussion of reasonable accommodations, list of job opportunities, resource guides, and an address delivered by Kenneth Jernigan (a common inclusion in other National Federation of the Blind publications). The information provided is general and very basic.

National Federation of the Blind. Why Section 504: Discrimination Against the Blind in Employment: A Case Review. Baltimore, Md.: National Federation of the Blind, 1979. 109 pp.

A collection of articles reprinted from The Braille Monitor. These articles, which appeared in the Monitor from 1976-79, present background for the understanding of Section 504 of the Rehabilitation Act. The articles cover: blind teachers discrimination cases, discrimination by the U.S. State Department, and the Sheltered Shop System. Similar to other compilations of reprints, this book presents the information in one convenient place. If the library already receives The Blind Monitor, this title is not needed.

National Public Law Training Center. Advocacy For/With the Mentally Ill and Handicapped: Legal Concerns for Persons with

Disabilities. Washington, D.C.: National Public Law Training Center, 1981. 762 pp. in various pagings.

This thick volume is a compilation of materials presented at a workshop on the legal rights of the mentally ill and handicapped held April, 1981 at the National Public Law Training Center. The following topics are included: Advocacy Roles; Legal System; Employment; Housing; Education; Health Care; and Community Organizations. The material is clear, complete, and very well presented. Cases, laws, and regulations are accurately cited. The regulations and other legal materials are up-to-date and even include proposed revisions. This volume is extremely valuable to all who are involved in maintaining and expanding the rights of all disadvantaged people. Highly recommended.

Nix, Gary W., ed. The Rights of Hearing-Impaired Children. Washington, D.C.: Alexander Graham Bell Association for the Deaf, 1977. 92 pp.

A collection of essays covering various aspects of rights of hearing-impaired children, i.e., educational options, case history, challenge to parents. The essays are well-written with references. The editor is involved nationally with education of the hearing-impaired. Valuable for parents of hearing-impaired children.

Overdue Process: Providing Legal Services to Disabled Clients. Washington, D.C.: Regional Rehabilitation Research Institute on Attitudinal, Legal, and Leisure Barriers, 1979. 24 pp.

A unique booklet designed for attorneys who may encounter disabled people as clients. This pamphlet was prepared by the School of Education and Human Development, George Washington University. The purpose of this booklet is to show some of the common myths, stereotypes, and attitudinal barriers faced by disabled persons and how these attitudes apply to the legal profession.

Parks, A. Lee, and Rousseau, Marilyn, K. The Public Law Supporting Mainstreaming: A Guide for Teachers and Parents. Austin, Tex.: Learning Concepts, 1977. 92 pp.

Written in a cartoon format, this book is divided into three chapters: purpose and definition of the law, assessment of handicapped children, and serving handicapped children. Intended to help teachers work more effectively with exceptional children. The illustrated format allows for easy, light reading. Both authors are professors in education. This text provides very basic information on mainstreaming and would be useless to those already acquainted with the law.

Phillips, William R. F., and Rosenberg, Janet. Changing Patterns of Law: the Courts and the Handicapped. New York: Arno Press, 1980. 324 pp. in various pagings.

This hardbound book is a compilation of eight law review articles on the topic of the legal rights of the handicapped. Because this book lacks an introduction, it is difficult to ascertain why these articles were selected. Not recommended.

Proceedings of the Supreme Court Davis Decision: Implications for Higher Education and Physically Disabled Students, November 14-15, 1979. Detroit: Wayne State University, 1979, 153 pp.

Southeastern Community College vs. Davis, decided by the U.S. Supreme Court on June 11, 1979, was the first case concerning the rights of disabled persons under Section 504 of the Rehabilitation Act of 1973. It dealt with the refusal of the Southeastern Community College to admit Francis B. Davis to an associate degree nursing program, based on the presence of her hearing impairment. In addressing the impact of the decision, the symposium offers insights regarding the process of integrating disabled students into higher education along with issues relating to admitting physically impaired individuals to nursing and the implications of the Davis decision. The proceedings are very informative and recommended reading for administrators, educators, and attorneys.

Redden, Martha Ross; Levering, Cricket; and DiQuizio, Diane. Recruitment, Admissions, and Handicapped Students. Washington, D.C.: The American Association of Collegiate Registrars and Admissions Officers and the American Council on Education, 1978. 36 pp.

Written for college and university administrators, this document is a guide for compliance with Section 504 of the Rehabilitation Act of 1973. Topics covered include recruitment, admissions, financial aid, orientation, registration, and grievance procedures. Appendices include organizations supporting handicapped persons. No index, but complete table of contents. Provides basic information for compliance of the law.

Rice, B. Douglas. Consumer Involvement/Policy Development Consultation: A Resource Manual for Staff Development Personnel and Rehabilitation Trainers. Hot Springs: University of Arkansas, Arkansas Rehabilitation Research and Training Center, 1979. 40 pp.

Written in outline form, this manual is designed to serve as a basic resource document for staff development personnel, rehabilitation trainers, and others who conduct training programs in the areas of consumer involvement for the severely handicapped. Includes: definition of terms, legislation and regulations, consumer rights and responsibilities, and staff training. The outline format is effective for some of the chapters (legislation), but lacks clarity for the others. Information presented is sketchy.

Roberts, Joseph and Hawk, Bonnie. Legal Rights Primer for the Handicapped: In and Out of the Classroom. Novato, Calif.: Academic Therapy Publications, 1980. 141 pp.

This book is designed to act as a primer to the interaction between the law and the handicapped child. The authors are educators who use clear, concise, non-legal jargon to explain the legal rights of the handicapped. The laws and cases are adequately explained, but without complete citations, it would be difficult to read the texts of these materials in the original sources. In addition to the following "In the Classroom" topics: appropriate assessment and individualized education plan, the following "Out of the Classroom" topics are also discussed: parenthood, work, and access. Recommended for educators, administrators, and parents of disabled children.

Schmidt, Carl, and Williams, Mary Claire. Law and The Handicapped Child: A Primer for Illinois Parents. DeKalb: Illinois Regional Resources Center, Northern Illinois University, 1978. 51 pp.

The purpose of this manual is to provide answers to questions on P.L. 94-142 which may be raised by the parents of handicapped children. Divided into four sections: 1) answers to questions, e.g., due process; 2) a sample case which follows a child and her parent from the time the child's problems are first detected through the writing of the actual individualized education plan; 3) a glossary of mostly educational terms; and 4) a list of service providers (particularly useful list). This well-written manual will definitely help parents of handicapped children better understand their rights and responsibilities, as well as the rights of the local school district and the child. Legal documents are summarized and source of information is clearly stated. This work along with the manual by Kerns, are highly recommended for all Illinois libraries.

A Selective Listing of Legal Resources for the Handicapped. South Bend, Ind.: The National Center for Law and the Handicapped, 1979. 55 pp.

NCLH has compiled a selective listing of attorneys and advocacy groups plus their addresses, telephone numbers, and areas of specialization. The resources are arranged alphabetically by state. NCLH plans to update this directory periodically. The directory in no way presumes to be an exhaustive listing of all attorneys or groups working for the rights of the handicapped, but was compiled from a list of resources which the Center has called on in the past and relies on regularly to give legal assistance to the handicapped.

Smith, Fran Tupper, Jr., and Smith, Jill. Annotated Bibliography: The Exceptional Child and the Law. N.P. 1975. 18 pp.

Exceptional child encompasses the mentally and physically handicapped. Materials included in this bibliography are book, pamphlets, audiovisuals, and periodical articles. The items are divided into four major subject areas. Availability statements are given for most items, but the items are not annotated. The materials listed dated from 1970-74, therefore, one would have to update their search. Good, unannotated, bibliography for years covered.

A Summary of Selected Legislation Relating to the Handicapped: 1975-76. Washington, D.C.: Clearinghouse on the Handicapped, 1976. 42 pp.

This booklet is the sixth in a series first published in 1967. The booklet includes tables tracing the development of each law through the legislation process, and cross references to laws described in earlier editions.

Switzer, Lucigrace, ed. Understanding the Rights of the Handicapped: A Guide for Government Contractors and Grantees. Washington, D.C.: McGraw-Hill, 1977. 109 pp.

Review of the requirements under the federal law on the rights of the handicapped. The regulations issued by HEW and the Labor Department are analyzed. The text follows the regulations section-by-section. Written for government contractors and grantees who need an analysis of the federal regulations which implement Section 504 of the Rehabilitation Act. The review of the regulations is only 88 pages (more white space than typing), and without an index, it is difficult to believe that this publication cost $75.00. Definitely not recommended for libraries.

University of Maryland Law School, Developmental Disabilities Law Project. Case Reporter. Baltimore, Md.: Developmental Disabilities Law Project, University of Maryland Law School, v. 1, 1980- Quarterly.

This slim, mimeographed Reporter is prepared as a research tool for attorneys and other advocates who are engaged in asserting the rights of handicapped people. It provides a summary of court decisions dealing with P.L. 94-142 and Section 504. Divided into three segments: 1) alphabetical list of the cases with a descriptive summary of each; 2) list of the categories into which the cases have been indexed with a descriptive summary of each category; and 3) list of cases under the appropriate category. Published by a law project at the University of Maryland Law School, it is designed to keep interested people informed of current cases. It is the only case reporter on developmental disabilities. Law libraries should purchase this serial and support this type of greatly needed publication.

Walker, Janet M., ed. A Guide to Organizations, Agencies, and Federal Programs for Handicapped Americans: Report I. Washington, D.C.: Plus Publications, Handicapped American Reports, 1979. 72 pp.

Intended as a handy desk guide, this work contains addresses and telephone numbers of national offices and organizations that serve handicapped people - federal offices, federal programs, congressional committees, associations and foundations. Although the information is brief, it appears complete and accurate. The introduction states that it will be out-of-date within a few years. Because of the narrow margins, the print is rather difficult, but not impossible, to read. Refer to A Selective Listing of Legal Resources for the Handicapped for attorneys' addresses. It should be an asset to persons working in this area.

Weintraub, Frederick J.; Abeson, Alan R.; and Braddock, David L. State Law and Education of Handicapped Children: Issues and Recommendations. Arlington, Va.: The Council for Exceptional Children, 1971. 142 pp.

This book is the result of five years of research on the part of The Council for Exceptional Children. It presents issues relating to the education of handicapped children. State laws and cases are excerpted throughout this text. It offers to those seeking legal change of direction, a rationale, and in the final chapter, a model. It is an important book for researching the historical beginnings of the legal rights movement for the disabled.

Yohalem, Daniel, and Dinsmore, Janet. 94-142 and 504: Numbers that Add Up to Educational Rights for Handicapped Children. Washington, D.C.: Children's Defense Fund, 1978. 47 pp.

This slim guide for parents and advocates is extremely informative. It is published by the Children's Defense Fund which is a national nonprofit public charity created to provide long-range and systematic advocacy on behalf of the nation's children. The following areas are concisely, but adequately, covered: legislation, school district's responsibilities, evaluation process, and resources. The question and answer format should help parents understand their child's educational rights.

Zimmer, Arno B. Employing the Handicapped: A Practical Compliance Manual. New York: AMACOM, 1981. 374 pp.

This book addresses and interprets the employment rights of America's disabled citizens. It covers the following topics: federal and state laws affecting employers, the Office of Federal Contract Compliance Programs, accessibility and mainstreaming, financial incentives for employers, and development of an affirmative action plan. The Appendices include lists of organizations, federal agencies, and a bibliography of publications helpful to employers. The index is detailed and complete. This book provides extremely practical information for employers on bringing handicapped workers into the mainstream of our society's worklife. It is a well-researched and easy to read source -- highly recommended.

9 HEALTH EDUCATION

FRANCESCA ALLEGRI/Assistant Health Sciences Librarian,
University of Illinois, Urbana, Illinois

INTRODUCTION

There are many variations on the theme of health education, now popular in the current literature, which also appear in the rehabilitation literature. Some of these variations are evident in the terms used to describe them: patient education, patient teaching, and health promotion. The aspect of health education which emphasizes the patient care setting has been defined as

"...both the formal and informal teaching you (the health professional) do each time you explain to patients or clients what is wrong with them, how to avoid certain conditions, what is to be done to them (for their own information or for informed consent), what medications they are being given, why, and how to take them, or what they need to know while at home or once they go home in order to get well, stay well, strengthen themselves, avoid relapses, etc."(1)

The health education literature of rehabilitation reviewed in this chapter covers the above aspects of patient education, and also health education in a broad sense: literature designed to facilitate voluntary changes in behavior which will promote the health of the disabled individual. These changes in behavior may be effected by parents or families of disabled persons as well as by disabled persons themselves, and thus the literature addresses both audiences.

Norris describes the self-care movement which has prompted publication in the area of health education. She breaks self-care into seven areas of activity, three of which are stressed by materials in this chapter: "...supporting life processes," "...therapeutic and corrective self-care," "...and auditing and controlling the treatment program."(2) The current interest in self-care centers around the concept labeled "wellness," or a desire to prevent illness or complications of illness. The prevention of complications is the motivating factor for self-care in the disabled, as further illness as a result of a disabling condition is often a likely possibility. This desire to avoid complications is exemplified in Rosenberg's Living with Your Arthritis: A Home Program for Arthritis Management and Fallon's So You're Paralysed... .

The recent emphasis on health education is due to several interrelated factors. Some of these are 1) the "crip lib" movement for rights of the disabled, 2) increased consumerism in the area of health care resulting in "A Patient's Bill of Rights,"(3) 3) the Joint Commission on Accreditation of Hospitals' statement of a patient's right "...to obtain from the practitioner responsible for coordinating his care, complete and current information concerning his diagnosis (to the degree known), treatment, and any known prognosis. This information should be communicated in terms the patient can reasonably be expected to understand...," (4) 4) hospitals' responsibilities in the area of informed consent, 5) increasing incidence of malpractice suits against health professionals, 6) evidence that patient education has positive effects on treatment outcomes, and 7) supporting statements from health profession organizations on the subject of patient education. Other factors have also contributed to the emphasis on health education in a less direct way. One of these is the technological advances in the communications field, e.g., mass use of photocopying and use of closed circuit television in educational and health care settings.

Along with the emphasis on health education, then, has come the literature designed to inform patients, in this case the disabled, about their varied disabling conditions. This chapter provides a selected list of health education materials, covering psychological as well as physical aspects of disability. The psychological aspects cover emotional self-help and coping strategies from the disabled individual's perspective. These differ from materials in the Chapter IV, "The Social and Psychological Contexts of Physical Disability," which discusses psychological and attitudinal concerns and barriers that the disabled experience from others. The physical aspects covered in this chapter are descriptions of the disability, effects on the individual's function, medical treatment, and personal care techniques. A broad range of materials was examined in this chapter to show the variety of formats, subjects, and sources of health education items.

The materials reviewed fall into three broad categories. General works discuss living as a disabled person and cover the coping strategies described above as well as sociopsychological implications for disabled individuals themselves. A second category covers specific disabilities or groups of disabilities and the concerns and medical or self-care procedures specific to them. The third category deals with specific adaptive techniques such as attendant care, education and career opportunities for the physically disabled. These differ from the "Independent Living" chapter in that they are broader concerns of disabled individuals. Some examples are Katz's et al. The Deaf Child in the Public Schools and Your Future: A Guide for the Handicapped Teenager by Feingold and Miller.

In the first group, several of the books attempt to persuade the disabled to have a positive attitude toward their disability. Two of these, directed toward adolescents, are particularly good: Living Fully: A Guide for Young People with a Handicap, Their

Parents, Their Teachers and Professionals by Gordon and What Can I Do About the Part of Me I Don't Like? by Belgum. Another of this type describes a Christian response to disability: Coping with Physical Disability by Cox-Gedmark. The author leads the reader through various discussions and situations of disabled individuals in an attempt to help the reader discover how God fits into the picture and to think creatively about coping with the disability. Several others in this group emphasize the psychological impact on the parents. Parents of a disabled child often undergo a grief process similar to that of the person experiencing a disabling injury or illness; they must work through feelings of shock, anger, guilt, and grief. This is also similar to the process described by Elisabeth Kubler-Ross in her book, On Death and Dying.(5) Some parents may also suffer the additional stresses of rejecting the child or having false or unrealistic hopes about treatments or cures. One of the better books dealing with these concerns is Helping Your Handicapped Child by Paterson. Another excellent general work, The Special Child Handbook by McNamara and McNamara, emphasizes the practical concerns parents have, examples of which are detecting problems at birth, preparing the child for the diagnostic process, locating parent groups, and managing financial concerns.

The majority of health education materials which deal with specific disabling conditions cover arthritis, blindness, deafness, epilepsy, multiple sclerosis, ostomies, spina bifida, and spinal cord injuries. It appears to be more difficult to locate materials in the areas of multiple physical handicaps, cleft lip/palate, congenital amputees, and muscular dystrophy. In general, the coverage is better for disabilities of adults rather than children, for example, in the area of spinal cord injury. Two sources of information in laypersons' terminology for some of the lesser known disabilities are Physically Handicapped Children: A Medical Atlas for Teachers,(6) and the chapter, "Defining Disabilities," in Serving Physically Disabled People: An Information

Handbook for All Libraries.(7) The intended purposes of these materials varies widely. Some, like A Resource Guide for Parents and Educators of Blind Children by Willoughby, are fairly comprehensive discussions of a disabling condition and cover a variety of aspects, both physical and psychological. Some, like The Ostomy Handbook, are intended as a simple introduction to the topic or a description of only one aspect of the disability. This treatment is most typical of those health education materials dealing with ostomies. These works primarily discuss appliances used and related topics such as surgical procedures, skin care, and product manufacturers. Many of the materials in this group deal with the techniques for managing physical problems associated with a particular disability. A good example, because of its comprehensiveness, is The Arthritis Book: A Guide for Patients and Their Families by Engleman and Silverman. It contains such information as recent data on the costs of treatment and lists questions the physician may ask the patient.

In the third category are specific adaptive techniques or strategies such as mainstreaming, attendant care, consumerism, and career planning. As explained previously, these are broad adaptive skills applicable to a variety of disabilities. They are generally not living skills pertaining to health or medical care. Examples of these are Attendees and Attendants: A Guidebook of Helpful Hints by DeGraff and Access: The Guide to a Better Life for Disabled Americans by Bruck. Other titles on attendant care are annotated in Chapter V, "Independent Living."

Although the area of special education was determined to be out of the scope of this literature guide, there is some overlap among the materials annotated in this chapter and special education materials, particularly those for parents of mentally retarded children. Several of these materials were reviewed, as they would be valuable to parents of children with physical disabilities and this has been indicated in the annotation. Naturally, the materials would be of use for children with multiple disabilities.

Due to the recent emphasis on and importance of sexuality and sex education, these materials appear in a separate chapter, "Sexuality and Disability." The importance of this topic to physically disabled persons, their families, spouses, and rehabilitation professionals has been heavily stressed in the literature. The number of titles available warranted dividing the chapter into materials for the professional and materials for the general audience, thus, the health education materials on sexuality are easily identified. Other chapters which are related to health education are "Independent Living" and "Disabled Children."

In general, health education materials are aimed at the patient or health educator. As would be expected, the distinguishing feature of these materials -- the language level -- varies to a great degree from title to title. Some terms treated as "technical" by one author, are not considered such by another author. The manner in which technical terminology or jargon is handled by the authors differs as well. In addition to no explanation at all, some include explanations within the text, while others include glossaries. Very few of those reviewed use the technique of footnoting the terms. Generally, the most effective technique is that of including an explanation directly within the text. Another distinguishing feature of health education materials is their illustrations. These need not be as detailed as in medical texts, but need to be easily understood. Because of their importance, illustrations were examined for their effectiveness. As most of the texts were well-illustrated, the exceptions are noted in the annotations. Where illustrations would have been helpful but were lacking was also noted.

Many of the health education materials reviewed were prepared or sponsored by various associations in the field of rehabilitation, for example, the National Easter Seal Society and the United Ostomy Association. It is well known that such associations are excellent sources of health education materials and several of these associations produce a list of their publications, e.g., The Ostomy Library by the United Ostomy Association.

The tremendous expansion of health education literature necessitated that the following be a selective list. The literature has grown so rapidly in recent years that any "comprehensive" list would be outdated immediately. Thus, this is a representative sample of what materials have been published.

NOTES

1. Carol R. Freedman, Teaching Patients: A Practical Handbook for the Health Care Professional (San Diego: Courseware, Inc., 1978), p. v.
2. Catherine M. Norris, "Self-Care," American Journal of Nursing (March 1979), pp. 486-9.
3. American Hospital Association, A Patient's Bill of Rights (Chicago: American Hospital Association, 1975).
4. Joint Commission on Accreditation of Hospitals, Accreditation Manual for Hospitals, 1983 Edition (Chicago: Joint Commission on Accreditation of Hospitals, 1982), p. xiv.
5. Elisabeth Kubler-Ross, On Death and Dying (New York: Macmillan, 1969).
6. Eugene E. Bleck and Donald A. Nagel, eds., Physically Handicapped Children: A Medical Atlas for Teachers, 2nd ed. (New York: Grune & Stratton, 1982).
7. Ruth A. Velleman, "Defining Disabilities," in Serving Physically Disabled People: An Information Handbook for All Libraries (New York: R. R. Bowker Company, 1979), pp. 25-50.

ANNOTATED BIBLIOGRAPHY

Adams, John M. Multiple Sclerosis, Scars of Childhood: New Horizons and Hope. Springfield, Ill.: Charles C. Thomas, 1977. 78 pp.

Reports history, etiology, epidemiology, treatment and recent research on multiple sclerosis. Describes other related diseases, and includes selected reading list, glossary and index. Provides a great deal of information but the language level is more technical than the author claims. Glossary is very helpful but this appears to be geared to more sophisticated readers.

Atkinson, Jean. Multiple Sclerosis: A Concise Summary for Nurses and Patients. Bristol: John Wright and Sons, Ltd., 1974. 60 pp.

Written by a nurse who is also a nineteen year victim of multiple sclerosis. Although written in a more technical vein than most, this provides a unique perspective on the disease: a view from the professional and patient as one person. Includes fairly thorough description of disease but needs updating in areas of etiology and treatment. Contains a pretty extensive glossary to assist the layperson. Information on social services is on British services. Due to the nature of its authorship, this is a particularly interesting and personal description of multiple sclerosis.

Baer, William P. The Aphasic Patient: A Program for Auditory Comprehension and Language Training: Patient's Edition. Springfield, Ill.: Charles C. Thomas, 1976. 211 pp.

Consists of the visual cues to be used with the Clinician's Edition of the same title. No accompanying text therefore not useful to patient or professional without instructions and auditory cues for the clinician. Includes thirty vocabulary pages and thirty pages showing a sequential activity. Also includes additional pages showing rearrangements of the vocabulary and sequence pages in order to discourage patients from responding to the location of an image rather than its content. Portrays the same patient, a middle aged white male, in all the sequences. Would have limited use due to its focus on portrayal of male patient only and daily activities of hospital setting.

Belgum, David R. What Can I Do about the Part of Me I Don't Like? Minneapolis: Augsburg Publishing House, 1974. 102 pp.

Psychological self-help book for those with various "stigmas", particularly physical disabilities. Confronts the reader with thought provoking questions regarding living with a disability. Has fairly extensive bibliography of autobiographies and biographies of disabled persons. Also includes list of pamphlets and articles on various disabilities. Lists organizations and self-help groups. This is one of the most extensive patient education monographs coming from a psychological/attitudinal viewpoint about disabilities.

Bland, John H. Arthritis: Medical Treatment and Home Care. London: Collier Macmillan, 1960. 221 pp.

Although published over twenty years ago, much of the information presented is still applicable. The emphasis given to home care and family involvement in treatment is surprising, considering the age of this publication. Has useful glossaries on self-help devices and lists major organizations and clinics specializing in arthritis treatment. Includes glossary and index. Major drawback is need for updating, especially in areas of ultrasonic therapy, drug therapy and current research and status of the disease.

Blumenfeld, Jane; Thompson, Pearl E.; and Vogel, Beverly S. *Help Them Grow! A Pictorial Handbook for Parents of Handicapped Children.* New York: Abingdon Press, 1971. 64 pp.

   Primarily aimed at parents of educable or trainable mentally retarded. Would be of help to professionals working with disabled on daily living skills. Illustrated throughout. Contains list of information sources: agencies and associations. Includes extensive book list, not limited to special education. May be helpful for parents of physically disabled children. Emphasizes the positive things parents can do for or with their children but also points out some "don'ts". Very straightforward language. Would aid in giving parents some sense of control or helpfulness in teaching their child daily living skills.

Bruck, Lilly. *Access: The Guide to a Better Life for Disabled Americans.* New York: David Obst Books, 1978. 252 pp.

   Extensive review of consumer information for the disabled person. Ties in information about civil rights for disabled consumers. Advocates "consumerism" on the part of disabled individuals and offers suggestions on how to become involved. Index and in-depth table of contents make the information available in a handbook-type style. Unique contribution to the literature. Author, who developed the New York City Division of Consumer Education, is well-qualified. Lists many sources for additional information throughout. Highly recommended for disabled persons or anyone else interested in consumer rights for the disabled.

Cooper, I. S. *Living with Chronic Neurologic Disease: A Handbook for Patient and Family.* New York: W. W. Norton and Company, 1976. 318 pp.

   Presents the idea of the "fourth world," or world of chronic illness. Discusses parkinsonism, dystonia, chorea, and amyotrophic lateral sclerosis, among others. Authored by leading brain surgeon. Includes sections on diagnostic tests, chronic pain, neurosurgical procedures, questions most frequently asked, and separate sections for relatives and for patients. Covers how to select a physician and other self-help topics. Appendix lists agencies to contact for further help. Has index. Authoritative guidelines presented to assist patient and family in making decisions regarding life with this particular type of disability. Gives examples of actual cases throughout. Unique information from a professional's perspective.

Cox-Gedmark, Jan. *Coping with Physical Disability.* Philadelphia: The Westminster Press, 1980. 119 pp.

   Discusses emotional and psychological adjustment to physical disability. Describes stages of grief and adjustment and Christian response to a disabling condition. Written by a chaplain at a rehabilitation institute. Book includes many quotes and stories of actual patients. Includes list of resources.

Davis, Judy A., and Spillman, Shirley J. Cardiac Rehabilitation for the Patient and Family. Reston, Va.: Reston Publishing Company, Inc., 1980. 162 pp.

Excellent introduction to coronary artery disease and rehabilitation. Clearly written and illustrated (includes list of illustrations) in a format adaptable to any institution's patient education efforts. Includes review questions and answers, pages for notes and questions, and diagrams for physician's illustrations and remarks. Rather than a glossary, appropriate chapters list definitions after their individual introductions. Provides individual charts for commonly used medication. Charts state purpose of drug, symptoms indicating adverse reactions, and provide space for physician's instructions. Blank charts are included for other medications prescribed.

DeGraff, Alfred H. Attendees and Attendants: A Guidebook of Helpful Hints. Washington, D.C.: College and University Personnel Association, 1979. 38 pp.

Concise guide discusses the "how-to's" of attendant care. Most of the text is aimed at the disabled person (attendee) and is useful to give insight to persons employed or volunteering as attendants. Covers all aspects from responsibilities to tax deductions. Does not deal with specific duties which may be performed but rather with recruiting, instructing, employing, and terminating an attendant. Primarily refers to short-term care. See Eldridge's Caring for the Disabled Patient-An Illustrated Guide, annotated in Chapter VII.

Dorros, Sidney. Parkinson's: A Patient's View. Washington, D.C.: Seven Locks Press, 1981. 220 pp.

Autobiographical account of living twenty years with Parkinson's disease, twelve of which were as an experimental research patient. Author underwent cryosurgery and L-Dopa and bromocriptine treatment in attempting to alleviate symptoms. Summarizes with ten tips for coping with Parkinsonism. Appendices cover a description of the disease, past and current treatment, and current research as well as what it feels like to be Parkinsonian. Also lists books about the disease and national and local information sources and self-help groups. The book is sensitively written and extremely valuable and informative for patients or family members desiring an understanding of the effects of the disease on the individual, family and friends.

Doyle, Phyllis B.; Goodman, John F.; Grotsky, Jeffery N.; and Mann, Lester. Helping the Severely Handicapped Child: A Guide for Parents and Teachers. New York: Thomas Y. Crowell, 1979. 150 pp.

Aimed primarily at parents of children with severe physical impairments who are also mentally retarded. Takes into consideration current social developments affecting child care, e.g., both parents working and legislation requiring equal education. Includes reading lists after most sections. Sections on "Special Services and Agencies," "Special Equipment" and "Transportation" provide a great deal of information. Addresses the questions of what the public school can do to help the severely handicapped and retarded child, what parents can do at home and where special help can be obtained. Discusses legal aspects of the child's education. Contains fairly detailed table of contents and index. Good introduction to a broad range of concerns, from improving communication skills to income tax deductions. Highly recommended.

Engleman, Ephraim P., and Silverman, Milton. The Arthritis Book: A Guide for Patients and Their Families. Sausalito, Calif.: Painter Hopkins Publishers, 1979. 199 pp.

Discusses various myths about arthritic diseases. Unique features of this book include 1) table of monthly retail costs of oral arthritis drugs, 2) discussion of cost of surgery, 3) discussion of role of individual members of the patient care team, and 4) extensive list of questions physician might ask patient. Authoritative yet easy to read. Statistics are recent. Contains separate chapters on some forms of arthritis, e.g., gout, but also discusses rarer manifestations, e.g., bursitis, sjögren's syndrome, systemic lupus erythematosus. Contains good illustrations. Has index and short list of references. Recommended.

Evans, Joyce. Working with Parents of Handicapped Children. Reston, Va.: The Council for Exceptional Children, 1976. 45 pp.

A guide for teachers working with parents of disabled children. Each chapter is introduced with a brief summary of purpose and content. Suggests many questions that teachers should ask themselves for certain situations, e.g., preparing for meetings with parents. This guide would also be helpful for parents although they are not intended as the primary audience. Appendices list specific organizations, an annotated bibliography and suggested parent interview forms and home visit records.

Fallon, Bernadette. So You're Paralysed... . London: Spinal Injuries Association, 1975. 116 pp.

Concise introduction to spinal injury. Contains good illustrated description of spinal cord and spinal injury. Also contains detailed discussion of pressure sores as well as less common problems: frostbite and sweating. Brief discussion of sex and possible problems. Especially useful items are description of immediate effects of spinal injury and checklist of warning signals of problems, what they could be and what to do. This is one of the better books describing spinal injury. Appears to be well-researched.

Feingold, S. Norman, and Miller, Norma R. <u>Your Future: A Guide for the Handicapped Teenager</u>. New York: Richards Rosen Press, Inc., 1981. 177 pp.

    Thorough and informative career/life planning handbook for high school age disabled persons. Covers planning, research, finding the right school, financing education, life-style and leisure activities. Each chapter contains conclusion, helpful aids and selected resources for further information. Contains pictures and comments throughout from disabled persons on each of the topics discussed. Does not "talk down" to the reader. An excellent handbook.

Fraser, Beverly A., and Hensinger, Robert N. <u>Managing Physical Handicaps: A Practical Guide for Parents, Care Providers, and Educators</u>. Baltimore: Paul H. Brookes, 1983. 246 pp.

    Describes a team management approach for health professionals, educators, and parents for care of the severely impaired (multiply impaired) child or young adult. Emphasizes the roles of physical therapists and orthopedists in this care, particularly the role of physical therapists in the school setting. Gives a brief history of care of the severely disabled; describes specific disabilities and the implications for care providers and educators; and discusses communicating, handling, positioning, and transporting the disabled person. One chapter gives questions and answers most often asked by persons meeting the severely impaired for the first time. Another chapter describes normal movement and movement terminology with succeeding chapters explaining how various disabilities affect movement. Ends with a chapter describing new trends in treatment and management. Terms in glossary are identified in bold face type the first time they are used. Has a list of manufacturers and distributors of equipment mentioned in the text. References accompany each chapter. The text is heavily illustrated, including many photographs, and well-organized. This is an excellent introduction to neuromuscular disabilities and the terminology, adaptive equipment, and surgical management involved.

Fries, James F. <u>Arthritis, A Comprehensive Guide</u>. Menlo Park, Calif.: Addison-Wesley Publishing Company, 1979. 258 pp.

    Emphasizes management of the disease. Written in conversational style and a basic question/answer format. Self-help guide to arthritis treatment includes diagnostic decision charts followed up with chapters devoted to the particular type of arthritis. Discusses medications, tests, prevention and saving money, among others. Includes arthritis status test, reading list of recommended and not recommended titles, Arthritis Foundation chapters, and index. Good discussion of treatment of arthritis for layperson.

Goldfinger, Glenn H., and Hanak, Marcia A., eds. <u>Spinal Cord Injury: A Guide for Care. Revised Primer for Spinal Cord Injured</u>.

New York: New York Regional Spinal Cord Injury Center, New York University Medical Center Institute of Rehabilitation Medicine, 1979. 91 pp.

Produced for a particular rehabilitation program but useful for any recently spinal cord injured person. Provides detailed explanation of a comprehensive rehabilitation program from admittance to discharge planning. Well-organized by categories such as medications, nutrition, and vocational services. Has eight appendices, including a glossary of medical terms and a personal medical·record. Valuable to the disabled individual for its descriptions of common procedures and therapies in a rehabilitation center. Unique in its detail and slant. One appendix describes attendant care agencies in New York area and rates charged.

Gordon, Sol, ed. Living Fully: A Guide for Young People with a Handicap, Their Parents, Their Teachers and Professionals. Toronto: The John Day Company, 1975. 296 pp.

Written in second person and in nontechnical terms. Provides a great deal of practical information to the reader. Directed primarily towards young disabled persons who would like to be part of the "mainstream of life" but are not. Addresses specific audiences: the disabled, their parents and families, and professionals. Would be valuable to anyone interested in integration of disabled persons into society. Includes a chapter devoted to various resources for the disabled, e.g., media, work opportunities, leisure reading. Also includes an index and a glossary of rehabilitation terms. Recommended especially for young adults.

Griffith, Valerie Eaton. A Stroke in the Family. London: Wildwood House, 1970. 122 pp.

Aimed at the family and friends of stroke victims. Describes the beginnings of what is now known as the Volunteer Stroke Scheme in Britain. The preface and three forewards explain how this scheme of using volunteers to teach stroke victims evolved. The majority of the book consists of sample lesson plans used at different stages of progress of two stroke victims. Emphasizes that these volunteer teachers are all nonprofessionals. Also discusses some general observations the author has made concerning stroke victims and methods of teaching them. Has a very practical orientation and would provide family some sense of helpfulness and control in the rehabilitation of stroke victims. Should probably be used in consultation with the speech therapist in order to maximize results.

Gross, Linda. Ileostomy: A Guide. Los Angeles: United Ostomy Association, 1974. 48 pp.

Illustrated throughout. Contains detailed table of contents. Refers throughout to other related United Ostomy Association publications. Contains many photographs of persons with ileostomies. Appendix lists 48 manufacturers and their products, but is probably out-of-date. Contains brief glossary and index. Describes appliances, problems the ostomate may have, and detailed instructions for using appliances and skin care products. Contains some unique information: 1) section for parents of children with ileostomies, 2) unique self-help aids such as stoma measuring card, 3) cost of equipment, insurance, and tax deductions. Unfortunately, this information needs updating.

Heisler, Verda. A Handicapped Child in the Family: A Guide for Parents. New York: Grune & Stratton, 1972. 160 pp.

Emphasizes psychological aspects of parenting a disabled child. Tries to create empathy between the reader and parents described in the book. Does this through descriptions of group therapy sessions with parents of cerebral palsied children. These sessions took place over a two year period with the author, who is a psychologist and disabled by poliomyelitis. Author tends to bring in psychotherapeutic techniques and her own responses and successes more than is warranted by the purpose of this book. Would be more useful if information were synthesized, although personal quotations help to solicit empathy.

Hess, George H. Living at Your Best with Multiple Sclerosis: A Handbook for Patients. Springfield, Ill.: Charles C. Thomas, 1962. 111 pp.

Written in a clear manner. Provides extensive information about multiple sclerosis. Table of contents shows clear organization of this handbook. The latter, with the book's thorough indexing, make it easy to read and refer to. Appendices provide 1) lists of daily exercises for balance, coordination, dizziness, 2) allergic substances and related foods, and 3) an allergy treatment dosage chart. Good tool to assist the professional in patient education but should be checked for dated material.

INA Mend Institute. General Information to Help the Recently Disabled. Albertson, L.I., N.Y.: Insurance Company of North America and Human Resources Center, 1974. 24 pp.

Much of the information provided is included in other sources. References several publications, agencies, and sources of information on a variety of topics, e.g., motels, sports, financial assistance, and bathroom aids. This latter feature is somewhat useful but more informational and up-to-date publications are available. This is first in a series.

Jayson, Malcolm, and Dixon, Allan. Understanding Arthritis and Rheumatism: A Complete Guide to the Problems and Treatment. New York: Pantheon Books, 1974. 228 pp.

Clearly written explanations of numerous aspects of arthritis and rheumatism. Covers straightforward description of the "slipped disk" to discussion of how arthritis affects family life. Includes section on "Facts on Arthritis" (as of January, 1974), and resource directory consisting of lists of agencies, homebound services and self-help devices. Has illustrations throughout and an index. Emphasizes physiological aspects of the disease. A very comprehensive introduction to this topic.

Jeter, Katherine F. These Special Children: The Ostomy Book for Parents of Children with Colostomies, Ileostomies, and Urostomies. Palo Alto, Calif.: Bull Publishing Co., 1982. 192 pp.

Introduces parents to the world of ostomies: the various types; preceding conditions; vocabulary involved; and resources such as associations, financial aid, books for children and parents, and appliances and manufacturers. Suggests ways to discuss ostomies with family, friends, and others and contains an alphabetical list of questions most frequently asked. Discussions of ostomy care include examples of several parents' techniques for handling a particular aspect. Unique information is presented in the review of child development and how this relates to ostomies, hospitalization, previous illness, and surgery. Introduces ways to alleviate stress on marital and family relationships as well as with teachers and in classrooms. Includes a glossary and a bibliography. Appendices cover diet, nutrition, and intermittent catheterization. Also has a coloring section for children and drawings to use to illustrate locations of a stoma, etc. Very good tool for patient educators in counseling parents before and after surgery but also excellent for parents to use on their own.

Jeter, Katherine F. Urinary Ostomies - A Guidebook for Patients. Los Angeles: United Ostomy Association, Inc., 1972. 36 pp.

One of the more detailed guides for ostomates. Covers topics not covered elsewhere: preparation for surgery, treatment of various skin irritations, advantages and disadvantages of various appliances and skin care products. In addition, includes many pictures of ostomates of various ages in everyday activities. Gives brand names of appliances and other products. Includes glossary with fairly detailed definitions and list of equipment manufacturers. This edition was revised in 1978. Most comprehensive guide reviewed to date.

Katz, Lee; Mathis, Steve L.; and Merrill, Edward C. The Deaf Child in the Public Schools. Danville, Ill.: Interstate Printers & Publishers, Inc., 1978. 149 pp.

Handbook written in question/answer format with nontechnical language. Answers many general questions parents of deaf children may have and specifically answers questions regarding education of the child in the local public school. Includes index plus several appendices; questions to ask about a child's educational program; list of organizations and government agencies; bibliography of supplemental reading. Is well-organized and has self-explanatory chapter headings.

Lagos, Jorge C. Seizures, Epilepsy, and Your Child: A Handbook for Parents, Teachers, and Epileptics of All Ages. New York: Harper & Rowe, Pub., 1974. 239 pp.

Written in question/answer format and directed toward the adult lay person. Although the author has attempted to explain in the text many of the terms used, some of the information provided may still be beyond the average reader's level of comprehension. Provides very detailed discussion of many aspects of epilepsy: causes, conditions that resemble epilepsy, genetic aspects and diagnosis. Unique aspects covered are liability in case of car accidents or acts of violence, voluntary and involuntary sterilization, and policies of insurance companies in regard to epileptics. Contains appendices of drugs used in treatment, "milestones of psychomotor development" to age six, and risk of epilepsy of centrencephalic origin with family history of epilepsy. Includes index.

Larson, Darlene. Living Comfortably with Your Ileostomy. Minneapolis: Sister Kenny Institute, 1973. 37 pp.

A guide to self-care techniques. Covers skin care, diet and appliances used. Also provides general information on the surgical procedure and physiological responses to the surgery. Uses step-by-step explanations, including photographs, to illustrate the various techniques. Helpful feature is diet guideline for the period immediately following surgery. Includes information sheet for ordering supplies, list of manufacturers of ileostomy equipment, and an index. Photographs and illustrations are clear. Good basic guide to self-care.

Lenneberg, Edith, and Mendelssohn, Alan N. Colostomies: A Guide. Los Angeles: United Ostomy Association, 1971. 32 pp.

Discusses physical aspects of colostomies and how they affect daily living. Describes intestinal tract, how it works, and types of colostomies in some detail. Includes brief section on practical aids and suppliers of equipment. Provides straightforward descriptions and illustrations but "talks over" some points - summarizes too much. Good for its description of intestinal tract and description of various colostomies.

McDonald, Eugene T. Understand Those Feelings. Pittsburgh: Stanwix House, 1962. 196 pp.

Written for parents of handicapped children. Discusses the emotions and reactions parents of handicapped children experience and how parents and professionals working with them can manage those feelings. Table of contents contains a brief synopsis of each chapter. Although primarily written for parents, a secondary audience is the professional dealing with the family of the disabled child. Uses many quotes from actual situations. Lack of index is not a drawback. Appears to be fairly thorough and helpful. Discusses emotional impact of having disabled children and effects on the family. Author has much experience dealing with parents.

McDonald, Eugene T., and Berlin, Asa J. <u>Bright Promise for Your Child with Cleft Lip and Cleft Palate</u>. Chicago, Ill.: The National Easter Seal Society for Crippled Children and Adults, 1979. 46 pp.

Discusses all aspects of cleft lip and palate from etiology to effects on personality. Has no table of contents but topics are divided by headings. Language is much easier to understand than <u>Advice to Parents of a Cleft Palate Child</u> by Wicka and Falk, which summarizes scientific studies on the topic. Actual comments of parents are presented throughout. Includes several illustrations and photographs and has glossary. Lists four agencies to contact for further information. Better introduction for parents than previously mentioned book.

McNamara, Joan, and McNamara, Bernard. <u>The Special Child Handbook</u>. New York: Hawthorn Books, Inc., 1977. 330 pp.

An excellent resource book for parents of children with physical, mental, developmental or learning disabilities. Covers topics from genetic counseling and other measures used to prevent disabilities to tips for the disabled interviewing for a job. Provides chart of routine childhood immunizations, advice on preparing a child for diagnostic testing, list of diagnostic clinics, advice on how to start programs for disabled children where none exist, and financial problems and solutions, among others. Some valuable aspects of this handbook are its comprehensiveness and detail, lists of resources after each chapter, and the use of specific examples of parents and their children throughout. In addition, it contains a selected, annotated bibliography and an index.

Miller, Alfred L. <u>Hearing Loss, Hearing Aids and Your Child: A Guide for Parents</u>. Springfield, Ill.: Charles C. Thomas, 1980. 97 pp.

Contains forms describing hearing responses of infants and young children and forms used to observe reactions to auditory stimuli. Explains how to prepare a child for a hearing evaluation, what tests are commonly done, how hearing loss is described, hearing aid training, and problems and therapy for children in the regular classroom. Includes "testimonials" of hearing impaired children. Has index. Author tends to "talk down" to the reader, particularly in initial chapter.

Norris, Carol. All About Jimmy and His Friend: An Ostomy Coloring Book. Los Angeles: United Ostomy Association, 1973. 24 pp.

Coloring book story about how a boy overcomes his embarrassment in being an ostomate. Simple language is inconsistent, using words like "bladder" and "birth defect". Makes no attempt to explain the surgery or appliances used. Recommendation is qualified unless used with a parent or health educator.

The Ostomy Handbook. Los Angeles: United Ostomy Association, n.d. 28 pp.

This is a general information work on ostomies directed towards the lay public and/or ostomate. Introduces the reader to the nature of abdominal stomas and how they affect peoples' lives. Lists types of service organizations which may be of assistance but no specific names or addresses are given. Includes a pictorial glossary of ostomy-related terms. Contains a dated (1973) reference bibliography. Indexed and written in a clear concise manner. This type of information would be available in more comprehensive texts; however, it could be useful to the patient educator.

The Ostomy Library. Los Angeles: United Ostomy Association, n.d. 6 pp.

Annotated bibliography produced by the United Ostomy Association. Lists ostomy and related publications. Covers colostomy, urostomy, ileostomy and combined ostomies. Gives bibliographic and ordering information for subject-related print and nonprint materials. Lists materials intended for the ostomate. Published in 1978, many of the items listed may no longer be available. It is not indexed and contains no illustrations. However, may still be a useful acquisition tool for the patient educator.

Ostomy Review II. Los Angeles: United Ostomy Association, n.d. 76 pp.

A review of articles from five years (1968 to 1973) of the Ostomy Quarterly. Covers helpful articles for the ostomate. Directed to the lay ostomate, these dated articles still contain helpful information. Contains only an advertisers' index. Would be useful for collections not subscribing to the Ostomy Quarterly; however, much of the information can be found elsewhere. Contains glossary of ostomy-related terms.

Paterson, George W. Helping Your Handicapped Child. Minneapolis: Augsburg Publishing House, 1975. 104 pp.

Using the examples of three children with different disabilities (deafness, mongolism, and cerebral palsy), the author describes the parents' responses to the birth of a disabled child, grief and adjustment stages and the part religion might play in these responses. Discusses various views of suffering and how parents can respond to family, community, and religious community. Includes annotated list of references and list of organizations and agencies. Well-written and organized.

Perlmutter, Alan D., and Crowell, William M. Your Child and Ileal Conduit Surgery: A Guidebook for Parents. Springfield, Ill.: Charles C. Thomas, 1970. 99 pp.

Introduction to ileal conduit surgery for parents of children undergoing this surgery. Is organized into useful chapters aiding the parent from the time of diagnosis to life with the conduit. Unique features of this book are actual photographs of the procedure of attaching an appliance to the stoma and two brief, illustrated stories for children about ileal conduit surgery, "Judy's new bladder" and "Jeff's new bladder". Has index. Includes chapter with suggested sources of help. Introduction was written by person other than authors and the language used is not as straightforward as the rest. Introduction also includes an explanation of ileal conduit surgery which seems out of place and confusing. Despite these flaws, this book is recommended as a useful guide for parents, especially of young children in need of this surgery.

Pieper, Betty. By, For and With ... Young Adults with Spina Bifida: A Discussion for Young People. Chicago: Spina Bifida Association of America, 1979. 74 pp.

Written for teenagers, this book emphasizes learning to be independent and making decisions affecting one's lifestyle. Discusses this in several contexts: relationships with other people, personal health care, work and lifestyle, nature of disability and how it affects others. Language level is appropriate and it includes quotes from others with spina bifida which would be very helpful for young adults. Reference pamphlets and other sources of information within each section as well as having an appendix of sources on such topics as architectural accessibility, assertiveness, college, housing, sports and travel, among others.

Pieper, Elizabeth. Sticks and Stones: The Story of Loving a Child. Syracuse, N.Y.: Human Policy Press, 1970. 88 pp.

Autobiographical account of mother of a child with spina bifida. Unfortunately realistic account of one woman's experiences with societal discrimination against persons with disabilities. Describes the learning experiences the author goes through as she moves from knowing little about disabilities to being an advocate for her child and others. Describes the shocking insensitivity and ignorance of professionals encountered by her. Recommended for professionals dealing with the disabled and families of the disabled.

Pilling, Doria. The Child with Spina Bifida: Social, Emotional and Educational Adjustment: An Annotated Bibliography. Upton

Park, Slough, Bucks, NFER Publishing Company Ltd. Great Britain, 1973. 46 pp.

Introduction contains concise description of spina bifida and its treatment history. Refers to other publications which are part of this series summarizing research literature on physically disabled children. Not evaluative. Has general section which contains references to materials for parents and family; otherwise this is directed towards the professional. Includes author index. Each section on adjustment of the child and his family and educational status begins with a summary of the literature.

Prensky, Arthur L., and Palkes, Helen Stein. Care of the Neurologically Handicapped Child: A Book for Parents and Professionals. New York: Oxford University Press, 1982. 331 pp.

For an evaluation of this work, see Chapter 12.

Rogers, Michael A. Paraplegia: A Handbook of Practical Care and Advice. London: Faber & Faber, 1978. 166 pp.

Written by a quadriplegic for paraplegics or quadriplegics and their families. Contains practical information on wide range of topics: anatomical aspects of spinal cord injury, home treatment of minor pressure sores, lifting with and without an assistant, physiotherapy, sexuality, and management of the urinary system, among others. Although many references to legislation, the health care system and manufacturers are British, the reader would be able to find comparable information for this country. Discusses psychological adjustment of the disabled and the family and suggests ways the family can aid this adjustment. Contains glossary and several appendices of addresses and references useful to the disabled. This is a very thorough description of paraplegia and resources available to the disabled; contains excellent advice for the family of a disabled person.

Rosenberg, Alan L., ed. Living with Your Arthritis: A Home Program for Arthritis Management. New York: ARCO Publishing Co., 1979. 226 pp.

Table of contents lists fourteen topics related to arthritis. Includes a discussion of medications used. Lists generic and brand names in most cases. A chapter on exercises includes illustrations. One chapter describes self-help aids. Includes a glossary and index. Also contains a brief appendix covering distributors and manufacturers of aids and equipment, addresses for clothing, recreation and arthritis information. Language is easy to understand. Technical terms used are explained in the text or in the glossary. Some illustrations are not as clear as they could be but generally this is a good guide for anyone afflicted with rheumatoid arthritis, osteoarthritis or gout.

Silverstein, Alvin, and Silverstein, Virginia B. Epilepsy. New York: J. B. Lippincott Company, 1975. 64 pp.

Includes brief discussion of how epilepsy has been perceived in history, its etiology, symptoms, and treatment. Also discusses research at the time of publication (1975). Contains good illustrations including photographs of famous epileptics. Describes what to do if a person has a seizure. Includes index and scientific terms are explained within the text. Very good introduction to epilepsy for young readers.

Splaver, Sarah. Your Handicap - Don't Let It Handicap You, 2d ed. New York: Julian Messner, 1974. 224 pp.

Difficult to judge what age range this is geared toward even though directed to young people; has simplistic explanation of feelings in first chapter, but later chapters are geared to older audience. Overwhelms the reader with its positive approach. Author has written other books in the area of psychology and career counseling. Includes a list in one chapter of state departments of special education and exceptional children. Includes extensive list of sources of further information in each state divided by type of source. Might have been more useful if organized by state. Includes list of further reading. Has index. This is not best of its type.

Swinyard, Chester A. The Child with Spina Bifida. Chicago: Spina Bifida Association, 1977. 54 pp.

An introduction for parents of children with spina bifida. Uses question/answer format with no index or table of contents but the information is clear and authoritative. Diagrams and tables are very clear. Is well-written, would be an excellent resource for parents. Covers a broad range of questions on the topic. Highly recommended.

Volle, Frank O., and Heron, Patricia A. Epilepsy and You. Springfield, Ill.: Charles C. Thomas, 1978. 72 pp.

Primarily concerned with social and psychological aspects of epilepsy rather than medical. Written in lay terminology for parents of older children or adolescents or for adults who have epilepsy. Uses a lot of stories from the authors' clinical experiences, which might be helpful but other texts are more informative and better organized.

Wicka, Donna Konkel, and Falk, Mervyn L. Advice to Parents of a Cleft Palate Child. Springfield, Ill.: Charles C. Thomas, 1970. 57 pp.

Reviews older literature on cleft lip and palate and presents summaries on topics ranging from speech characteristics to dental management. Language level is sometimes difficult; a glossary would have been helpful. Has no index. Lists sixty-two items, most of which are from period 1950-1969. Comprehensive in scope and one of few reviewed on this topic for layperson. Contains few illustrations.

Willoughby, Doris M. A Resource Guide for Parents and Educators of Blind Children. Baltimore, Md.: National Center for the Blind, 1979. 142 pp.

Directed primarily at parents of blind children from infancy through high school. Would also be helpful for anyone concerned about blind children. Answers many questions which parents of blind children and others have about blindness and the capabilities of blind persons. Discusses attitudinal aspect throughout. Relates actual situations as examples of "what to do" and "what not to do". Includes many practical suggestions such as how blind children can be taught to play various games, what to tell a child about his/her blindness, and how to teach orientation and travel techniques. Chapters are divided into broad categories. No index is provided. Contains brief bibliography and list of addresses at the end. Author's preface gives description of author's qualifications and experiences with the blind, (she is the wife of a blind electrical engineer, a classroom teacher and teacher of blind children). Recommended as a good orientation to blindness - provides a philosophical approach as well as many practical applications and techniques.

10 SEXUALITY AND DISABILITY

FRANCESCA ALLEGRI/Assistant Health Sciences Librarian,
University of Illinois, Urbana, Illinois

INTRODUCTION

Like other areas of rehabilitation, the literature on sexuality is experiencing a phenomenal period of growth. This growth is due, in part, to two factors: the emphasis on a holistic approach throughout the field of rehabilitation and the consumer's movement among disabled individuals.

The holistic approach of rehabilitation professionals toward sexuality reflects what Daniels describes as the establishment of sexuality as part of the health system: "Today sexual health and sexual health care are recognized as a major component of a total health-care system."(1) Because this emphasis on sexuality is causing a new push for sexuality in health professionals' education, we see a steady flow of these materials from publishers. In the past five years this has been particularly noticeable, and a large number of materials on sexuality have been published for both the professional and the disabled person.

The holistic movement goes hand in hand with what Rabin discusses regarding trends in treatment.(2) As medical care for the disabled improved, sustaining life was no longer the primary concern of health professionals, but rather improving the quality of life for these individuals. This new concern required an interdisciplinary approach and thus interest in the sexual readjustment of the disabled came forward to take a place beside vocational and psychological counseling. The interrelationship of the sexual, psychological, and social aspects of rehabilitation is gaining acceptance by professionals in this field. One author states that there is also considerable support for the idea that a satisfactory sexual life is related to productivity, thus pulling vocational concerns closer to these other areas of interest to the disabled.(3)

The women's movement, in conjunction with consumerism, has definitely been a contributing factor to the growth of literature on sexuality. Sha'ked describes this influence in the context of spinal cord injuries:

> "Interest in the effects of spinal cord injury on sexual functioning of women has increased markedly in the last decade and can be linked in several ways to the women's movement. With the increased involvement of women in work and other activities outside the home, the incidence of spinal cord injury among women has increased. The evolving belief in the right of women to enjoy and engage in sexual activity has generated interest in the special concerns of spinal cord injured women as well."(4)

Traditionally, there has been a lack of information for and about disabled females, even in the area of spinal cord injury, which is the single most prevalent disability in the literature. A larger percentage (three-fourths) of the spinal cord injured population has been male, and thus a lack of literature on women followed as a result.(5) As Cornelius states, "Although a wealth of literature is available on sexuality and the male spinal cord injured, little information is written concerning sexuality and the disabled woman, beyond mention of fertility and passive sexual participation."(6) Examples of this treatment are in the Handbook of Spinal Cord Medicine(7) and Gregory's Sexual Adjustment: A Guide for the Spinal Cord Injured. In the Handbook, just a little over four pages is devoted to the topic of sexual function, of which one page pertains to female concerns, almost exclusively pregnancy. In addition, the treatment of the subject often has a strong sexist bias. In Sexual Adjustment the author states, "... The female paraplegic is usually better able to satisfy the normal partner, because of the passive role she can play during sexual relations."(8) Fortunately, this situation is being corrected by the publication of several valuable books including Becker's Female Sexuality Following Spinal Cord Injury and Duffy's ... All Things are Possible.

Not only was the earlier literature on sexuality and disability concentrated in the area of spinal cord injury, but most authors emphasized the male and female reproductive capacities following injury and the possibility of medical complications. There also tended to be an excessive emphasis on the male's virility and erectile capabilities. The recent literature, however, tends to put these topics in the context of a broader picture of sexuality, which includes femininity, masculinity, intimacy, and emotional and physical relationships not limited to sexual intercourse.

In reviewing the literature there appears to be few materials for the following disabilities: deafness, amputation, cerebral palsy, multiple sclerosis, epilepsy, spina bifida, and other neurological or neuromuscular impairments. These are sometimes mentioned in the general texts, however, along with those which appear more frequently: ostomies and spinal cord injuries. Examples of general texts are Stewart's The Sexual Side of Handicap: A Guide for the Caring Professions and Bullard and Knight's Sexuality and Physical Disability: Personal Perspectives.

Although the general materials tend to cover topics such as attitudes of society and the disabled, sexual physiology, and dysfunction and emotional/psychological aspects, there are some books devoted solely to a single one of these topics, for example, Personal Relationships, the Handicapped and the Community by Lancaster-Gaye. This book concentrates on the role of institutionalization and independent living facilities in the life of disabled persons, particularly as they relate to sexuality.

Physiological aspects of sexuality and sexual dysfunction, however, are still more prominent in the literature than counseling of psychological concerns.

In addition to a lack of literature on sexuality for particular disabilities, there appears to be gaps in information on particular aspects of sexuality. Materials relating to child and adolescent sexuality are scant and those that do exist are generally in the context of a sex education curriculum; few publications are directed toward young disabled persons. There is also a lack of research or information for laypersons from the perspective of marital relationships. One of the few is Peterson's Marital Adjustment in Couples of Which One Spouse is Physically Handicapped. Another title, Handicapped Married Couples was not annotated because of its overwhelming emphasis on mental disability.(9) However, it does contain a literature review divided by topic and subdivided by mental and physical disability. Homosexuality, transsexualism, and transvestism are other topics rarely discussed. One of the few titles which contains any reference to these is the Task Force on Concerns of Physically Disabled Women's Toward Intimacy: Family Planning and Sexuality Concerns of Physically Disabled Women. There is a chapter in Califia's Sapphistry: The Book of Lesbian Sexuality entitled, "Disabled Lesbian," but no similar information was discovered for male homosexuals.(10) "Disabled Lesbians" discusses the problems of discrimination for lesbians compounded by a disability as well as concerns of body image, finding partners, sexual techniques for particular disabilities, and sex in institutional settings.

As mentioned earlier, the expansion of the literature on sexuality and disability is a recent phenomenon, considering that the field of human sexuality research has been developing since World War II.(11) This recent proliferation is borne out by an examination of the publication dates of items which were identified for inclusion in this chapter. Of 73 titles (two had no publication date listed) ranging from 1942 to 1982, 68% were published in 1975 or later and 95% were published in 1970 or later. Several of the 75 items which were identified for this chapter were unavailable for review and a list of those not annotated is included at the end of this introduction.

Despite particular gaps in the literature, one author has stated that, "A comprehensive review of the literature on sexuality and disability would require an extensive effort producing several volumes."(12) Therefore, the coverage of this chapter has been defined as follows. The annotations are of published monographs solely or primarily devoted to the topic of sexuality and disability. The journal literature in this area is extensive, but several bibliographies exist which cover it fairly comprehensively and these have been annotated. Examples are Eisenberg's <u>Sex and Disability: A Selected Bibliography</u>, <u>Sex and the Handicapped: A Selected Bibliography (1927-1975)</u> by the Veterans Administration Hospital, and Lassen's <u>Sex and the Spinal Cord Injured: A Selected Bibliography</u>. In addition, three serial publications which provide many of the articles on sexuality and disability are <u>Rehabilitation Literature</u>, <u>SEICUS Report</u>, and <u>Sexuality and Disability</u>. Proceedings and sex education curriculum guides are only selectively included. As in other chapters, mental retardation and other developmental disabilities have been considered out of the scope of this reference text. Areas such as aging and chronic diseases have been included selectively if the primary emphasis is on orthopedic, genetic, traumatic, or similar physical disability. An example of materials available on sexuality in disabling illness is Stoklosa's <u>Sexuality and Cancer</u>.

As was mentioned earlier, the social and psychological impact of physical disability relates closely to the whole area of sexuality. Such concepts as body image, self concept, and attitudes of others toward the physically disabled are intertwined with concepts of femininity, masculinity, and sexual expression. Chapter 4 in this book, "Social and Psychological Contexts of Physical Disability," attempts to pull together references which deal with the emotional, social, and psychological effects of disability without particular emphasis on sexuality. Examples of related titles in Chapter 4 which have not been included here are McDaniel's <u>Physical Disability and Human Behavior</u> and De Loach and Greer's <u>Adjustment to Severe Physical Disability: A Metamorphosis</u>. The De Loach and Greer text has a fine chapter, "The Third Disabling Myth: The Asexuality of the Disabled," which includes information on little-discussed topics such as disability-related expenses and pace-of-life differences as sources of stress in marriage. Because of the close relationship of psychological aspects of disability with sexuality, these two chapters should be used together.

The annotations have been divided into two sections: those that have professionals as their primary audience and those primarily for the general lay public or disabled persons themselves. Bibliographies are included with the professional literature. The separation of the annotations by audience was thought to be valuable due to the small number available for the nonprofessional and the need librarians have for selecting materials appropriate for their clientele, particularly in a sensitive subject area such as sexuality. As can be seen by this division of the chapter, a need is demonstrated for more materials for the nonprofessional, particularly materials covering the less well-known disabilities. However, although the majority of titles were aimed at professionals working with the disabled, several of these titles would be helpful to the layperson as well. This has been indicated in the annotation.

In examining the literature, two broad statements can be made regarding both the professional and lay literature. In the professional literature, most of the research on sexuality and disability is reported in journals with the exception of a few titles such as Janz's <u>Epilepsy, Pregnancy, and the Child</u>; the monographic literature tends to concentrate on general physiology, pathology, management, and psychological concerns. The nonprofessional literature concentrates on educating the disabled to the universality of their concerns among disabled and able-bodied alike and suggests techniques for accomodating various physical impairments during sexual activities. There is little for the layperson on the less well-known disabilities.

In summary, the topic of sexuality and disability is a newly expanding one receiving a great deal of attention from professionals and nonprofessionals. The fact that sexuality is just as vital a concern to the disabled as it is to able-bodied individuals is emphasized again and again in the literature. The inclusion of sexual concerns in health care, influenced by a holistic approach in treatment, is just now being reflected in the literature. Several gaps, primarily in information for the deaf and neurologically or neuromuscularly impaired, need to be filled in order to satisfy the needs of a varied disabled population.

NOTES

1. Susan Daniels, "Sexual Health Care Services for the Disabled" in Sexuality Article Packet (Washington, D.C.: Regional Rehabilitation Research Institute on Attitudinal, Legal and Leisure Barriers, George Washington University, 1977), p. 1.

2. Barry J. Rabin, The Sensuous Wheeler: Sexual Adjustment for the Spinal Cord Injured (San Francisco: Multi-Media Resource Center, 1980), p. v.

3. Roberta B. Trieschmann, ed., Spinal Cord Injuries: Psychological, Social and Vocational Adjustment (New York: Pergamon Press, 1980), p. 127.

4. Ami Sha'ked, ed., Human Sexuality and Rehabilitation Medicine: Sexual Functioning Following Spinal Cord Injury (Baltimore: Williams and Wilkins, 1981), pp. 3-4.

5. Robert M. Goldenson, ed., Disability and Rehabilitation Handbook (New York: McGraw-Hill, 1978), p. 566.

6. Debra Cornelius, "A Brief Consumer's Guide to Sexuality and the Disabled Woman" in Sexuality Article Packet, p. 1.

7. David C. Burke, and D. Duncan Murray, Handbook of Spinal Cord Medicine (New York: Raven Press, 1975).

8. Martha Ferguson Gregory, Sexual Adjustment: A Guide for the Spinal Cord Injured (Bloomington, Ill.: Accent on Living, 1974), p. 68.
9. Ann Craft and Michael Craft, Handicapped Married Couples: A Welsh Study of Couples Handicapped from Birth by Mental, Physical or Personality Disorder (London: Routledge and Kegan Paul, 1979).
10. Pat Califia, Sapphistry: The Book of Lesbian Sexuality (Tallahassee, Fla.: Naiad Press, 1980), pp. 97-105.
11. Paul H. Gebhard, "Human Sex Behavior Research" in Perspectives in Reproduction and Sexual Behavior, ed. Milton Diamond, (Bloomington, Ind.: Indiana University Press, 1968), pp. 391-394.
12. Daniels, "Sexual Health Care", p. 1.

MATERIALS UNAVAILABLE FOR REVIEW

Cole, T. M. and Cole, S. S. A Guide for Trainers: Sexuality and Physical Disability. Minneapolis: University of Minnesota Medical School, Multi-Resource Center, Inc. 1976.

Cole, T. M., and Cole, S. S. A Guide for Trainers: Sexuality and Physical Disability. Minneapolis: University of Minnesota Medical School, Multi-Resource Center, Inc., 1976.

Cole, T. M., and Cole, S. S. Sexuality and Physical Disability: Resources for Rehabilitation Practitioners. Minneapolis: University of Minnesota Medical School, Multi-Resource Center, Inc., 1975.

Committee on Sexual Problems of the Disabled. Sex and the Physically Handicapped. Horsham, Sussex, England: National Fund for Research into Crippling Diseases, 1975.

Gordon, Sol. Facts about Sex. East Orange, N.J.: New Jersey Association for Brain-Injured Children, 1969.

Gordon, Sol. Facts about Sex for Exceptional Youth. Plainview, N.J.: Charles Brown (New Jersey Association for Brain-Injured Children), 1969.

Illinois School for the Deaf. The Development of a Sex Education Curriculum for a State Residential School for the Deaf and Social Hygiene Guides. Jacksonville, Ill.

Lassen, Peter L. Sex and the Spinal Cord Injured: A Selected Bibliography. Washington, D.C.: Paralyzed Veterans of America, Inc., 1973. 15 pp.

Monograph on Sexual Function and Paraplegia. Handicapped Forum, vol. 1, 12 July, 1972. Reprinted by the Massachusetts Association of Paraplegics, Bedford, Mass.

National Paraplegia Foundation. Paraplegics Discuss Their Sexual Problems. The Foundation, 1973. 12 pp.

Poling, Daniel A. Socio-Sexual Distance: The Emotional, Social and Sexual Obstacles the Disabled Encounter When Interacting with the Able-Bodied (Monograph 1). New York: United Cerebral Palsy of New York City, 1974.

Shearer, Ann. A Right to Love? A Report on Public and Professional Attitudes toward the Sexual and Emotional Needs of Handicapped People. London: The Spastics Society and the National Association for Mental Health, 1972. 13 pp.

Spastics Society and SPOD. Love Matters. London: Spastics Society and the Committee on the Sexual and Personal Relationships of the Disabled, 1976. (leaflet)

Stewart, W. F. R. Sex and Spina Bifida. London: Association for Spina Bifida and Hydrocephalus, 1978. (pamphlet)

Wilson, D. Counseling the Person with Spinal Cord Injury on Sex and Sexuality. Vancouver, British Columbia, Canada: Canadian Paraplegic Association, 1973.

ANNOTATED BIBLIOGRAPHY:
Materials for Professionals

Anderson, Frances; Bardach, Joan; and Goodgold, Joseph. Sexuality and Neuromuscular Disease. New York: The Institute of Rehabilitation Medicine and The Muscular Dystrophy Association, 1979. 52 pp.

Reports results of interviews with 40 patients at the Neuromuscular Disease Center at the Institute of Rehabilitation Medicine. Discusses particular problems of early onset neuromuscular disease vs those affected later in life. Includes quotes from interviewees, illustrations of possible sexual positions, and guidelines for sexual counseling. Recommendations for the professional accompany each topic. References section includes materials for the adolescent, awareness of sexual options and organizations providing information on sexual functioning. Bibliography is good and these references are also cited in the text. Excellent guide for the professional. Well-organized. Recommended for health science libraries.

Bass, Medora S., and Lang, Joyce. Sex Education for the Handicapped and an Annotated Bibliography of Selected Resources. Eugene, Ore.: E. C. Brown Center for Family Studies, 1972. 37 pp.

Begins with reprint of article by first author which is a review of sex education and family life programs available in the fifties and sixties. Contains quotes of responses from researchers and educators in the field when few programs existed. Includes programs for blind, culturally disadvantaged, and parents.

Covers such areas as family life, sexual relations, genetic counseling, health and safety, sterilization, and marriage. Summarizes fourteen points as implications for further study. Annotated bibliography is selective and contains some materials not specifically for disabled. Divides items by format. Includes audiovisuals and curriculum guides. Has list of publishers and agencies in this area. Emphasizes mentally retarded heavily in the bibliography. Despite age of materials and emphasis on mental retardation, this work is excellent for historical perspective and description of early programs and philosophies of program personnel. Recommended for education, health science and research libraries.

Beasley, Mary Catherine; Burns, Dorothy; and Weiss, Janis M. Human Sexuality: The Handicapped, The Aging (A Resource Guide to Printed Materials). University, Ala.: Division of Continuing Education, University of Alabama, 1978. 53 pp.

Excellent bibliography covering developmental disabilities, mental retardation, aging, and physical disabilities. Monographic coverage is particularly good; includes papers, proceedings, other unpublished items, and government documents in addition to periodical articles. Not annotated but bibliographic and availability information is more complete than in other bibliographies examined. Recommended for a reference collection.

Blum, Gloria J., and Blum, Barry. Feeling Good about Yourself: A Human Sexuality and Social Learning Resource Guide. Mill Valley, Calif.: Gloria J. Blum, 1975. 40 pp.

Interim edition of bound edition to have been published by Academic Therapy Publications in 1977. Aimed at teachers of a course on sexuality. Discusses particular concerns of disabled and parents of disabled children. Lists activities and techniques for discussion. Each section lists objectives: covers veneral disease, homosexuality, nonverbal communication, sex roles, and so on. Has list of resources and bibliography. Good as a guide for teachers in developiong a program as it contains many suggestions for topics of discussion and statements with which to react. Recommended for education libraries.

Boller, Francois, and Frank, Ellen. Sexual Dysfunction in Neurological Disorders: Diagnosis, Management, and Rehabilitation. New York: Raven Press, 1982. 94 pp.

Written by two professors, one of neurology and psychiatry and one of psychiatry and psychology. Provides an overview for the professional of effects on sexual behavior of neurologic syndromes, spinal cord and cerebral lesions, among others. Discusses anatomy and physiology of the central nervous system, particularly those structures which relate to sexual behavior. Majority of book however, discusses clinical treatment of sexual disorders including a section on drugs affecting sexual behavior through action on the central nervous system. Unique contribution to the field for its review of the literature on sexuality and neurological disorders other than spinal cord injury. Recommended for health sciences libraries.

Bullard, David G., and Knight, Susan E., eds. Sexuality and Physical Disability: Personal Perspectives. St. Louis: C. V. Mosby Company, 1981. 318 pp.

Excellent as a broad overview of the professional as well as personal issues in this area. Covers the spectrum of physical disability and includes several seldom seen in other texts: head injury, mastectomy, hysterectomy, penile prosthesis, and hereditary physical disability. Divided by sections covering individual, family and professional perspectives. Includes sections on social skills, sex education, counseling, therapy, and family planning. Has brief paragraphs describing the authors after each chapter. Recommended for special and public libraries.

Comfort, Alex, ed. Sexual Consequences of Disability. Philadelphia: George F. Stickley Co., 1978. 296 pp.

Covers sexual effects of common disorders as well as the question of sex and disability. Emphasizes male problems, however, female problems are discussed. Little attention given to the sexual problems of the institutionalized patient. Directed towards the physician. Refers to materials published as late as 1978. Contains extensive index and some illustrations. Covers only common disorders. The information may be located elsewhere but difficult to find. Each chapter contains a bibliography of references. Recommended for medical libraries.

Cornelius, Debra A.; Chipouras, Sophia; Makas, Elaine; and Daniels, Susan, M. Who Cares? A Handbook on Sex Education and Counseling Services for Disabled People. 2d ed. Baltimore: University Park Press, 1982. 260 pp.

The first edition of this handbook was a result of a grant project to do a needs assessment, describe the state of the art and develop models for sexual adjustment counseling services. The second edition updates the section for consumers and the various resource lists provided. Would be helpful to any professional setting up or evaluating such services. Many resources and references are listed throughout. Includes lists of sexuality-related and disability-related journals, audiovisuals and audiovisual producers, consultants and organizations, among others. Excellent resource. Recommended for special or public libraries.

Cornelius, Debra; Makas, Elaine; and Chipouras, Sophia. Sexuality and Disability: A Selected Annotated Bibliography. Washington, D.C.: Regional Rehabilitation Research Institute on Attitudinal, Legal and Leisure Barriers, 1979. 78 pp.

Lists 412 articles, books and pamphlets divided into two large categories: those dealing with specific disabilities and those discussing sex education, counseling, attitudes, programs or functioning. There are twenty-eight subheadings under these two large headings. Majority of items have nonevaluative content note. Does not include cross referencing. Contains list of organizations from which some of the materials are available. Useful reference tool for professionals primarily but also for laypersons. Unique features are inclusion of elderly, mastectomy, and renal disease. Recommended for special and public libraries.

Daniels, Susan M. Sexual Health Care Services for the Disabled. Washington, D.C.: Regional Rehabilitation Research Institute on Attitudinal, Legal and Leisure Barriers, (between 1977 and 1979). 17 pp.

Includes three articles. Describes status of sexuality in total health and reviews literature regarding the role sexual health plays in the rehabilitation process. Discusses developmentally disabled as well as physically disabled. 45 references listed. Comprises a brief introduction to the topic for professionals. Summarizes research findings. The article, "Brief Consumer's Guide to Sexuality and the Disabled Woman," reviews Toward Intimacy and Within Reach. Recommended for special libraries.

Dickman, Irving R. Sex Education and Family Life for Visually Handicapped Children and Youth: A Resource Guide. New York: Sex Information and Education Council of the American Foundation for the Blind, 1975. 86 pp.

Title is somewhat misleading. Resource guide itself is one of three parts of this text and lists print, braille, recorded, audiovisual, and large-type materials on the topic for both teachers and students. Lists publishers' addresses and organizations in the area of family life and sex education. Lists sources of anatomical models as well. Unique and valuable contributions of this publication are the first two sections which provide guidelines in setting up a program, training staff, and involving parents. Covers background and philosophy of teaching blind children in this area, and provides concepts and appropriate learning activities and students' common questions in each of five areas which should be covered in sex education. Aimed at the professionals or parents working with visually disabled youth and useful as an orientation or starting point for a program. Recommended for education and public libraries.

Eisenberg, M. G. Sex and Disability: A Selected Bibliography. Tempe, Ariz.: Rehabilitation Psychology, 1978. 113 pp.

Covers primarily journal literature from 1942 to 1978. All references are English language or English abstracts. References appear only once in bibliography despite overlap in subject and are not annotated. However, the preface contains a brief eleven-point analysis of the literature. Lists films and audiocassettes with brief description of content. Includes references on topics not found easily in monographic literature, for example, amputation, poliomyelitis, and arthritic and orthopedic impairments. Includes other disabling conditions such as cancer, head injuries, cardiovascular disorders, and renal transplantation and dialysis. Recommended for special libraries.

Gregory, Martha Ferguson. Sexual Adjustment: A Guide for the Spinal Cord Injured. Bloomington, Ill.: Accent on Living, 1974. 73 pp.

Written as a master's thesis by the author, this is basically a literature review. Most of the references are from early 1950's and 1960's. Includes many excerpts from the literature. Discusses paraplegia and not quadriplegia. Divided into four sections: an overview of physical and psychological effects of paraplegia; sexual adjustment; counseling; and the summary and conclusion. Very little mention of female paraplegics. Primary emphasis is on physiological aspects of the male. Not valuable for the layperson. Has bibliography. Recommended for special libraries.

Griffith, Ernest R.; Timms, Robert J.; and Tomko, Michael A. Sexual Problems of Patients with Spinal Injuries: An Annotated Bibliography. Cincinnati, Ohio: Department of Physical Medicine and Rehabilitation, 1973. 58 pp.

Emphasizes physical aspects of sexual dysfunction. Some areas covered are pregnancy, impotence, fertility, and gynecomastia. Contains alphabetic list by author as well as annotations listed alphabetically by author. Includes journals, books, and dissertations with lists of these sources of abstracts. Has list of twenty unobtained articles also. Time span of references ranges from 1917 through 1972 but majority are from 1950-1972. Has some incomplete references. Provides good background for research in this area but limited in clinical setting due to date of most of the material. Recommended for special or research libraries.

Grofs-Selbeck, G., and Doose, H., eds. Epilepsy - Problems of Marriage, Pregnancy, Genetic Counseling: Meeting of the German, Danish, Dutch and Swiss Sections of the International League Against Epilepsy. Regional Conference of Epilepsy International, Kiel (FRG). Stuttgart: Thieme, 1981. 107 pp.

Presents physicians with research currently available on clinical problems in area of epilepsy and pregnancy. Discusses such aspects as pregnancy's effect on the disease and vice versa, effects of anticonvulsive drugs on the fetus, oral contraceptives' effect on disease, abortion, sterilization, genetic counseling, and marital problems of epileptics. Most chapters include an introduction, summary or abstract, and a list of references. Includes a brief index. As a report of a conference, an overview chapter would have been helpful. Contains little overlap of authors with Epilepsy, Pregnancy, and the Child (1980). Some information overlap in report of a Milan study, i.e., risk of abnormalities in children of epileptic parents and antiepileptic drug monitoring. Depth of treatment varies between the two publications, therefore they complement each other nicely. Recommended for medical libraries.

Heslinga, K.; Hastings, K.; Schellen, A. M.; and Verkeryl, A. Not Made of Stone: The Sexual Problems of Handicapped People. Springfield, Ill.: Charles C. Thomas, 1974. 208 pp.

Written by an educator in the field of rehabilitation in collaboration with a gynecologist and rehabilitation specialist, all located in the Netherlands. Emphasizes motor disabilities but also covers chronic conditions, such as cardiovascular disorders and diabetes, quite well. Includes respiratory and dermatologic conditions; these are rarely mentioned in other texts. Covers reproductive systems and disorders, genetics, sex education and ethical considerations, among other topics. Directed at an interdisciplinary audience, primarily professional. Unique features include photographs of diagnostic equipment, sexual aids, amniocentesis and vasectomy procedures, and the sexually stimulated male and female. Other unique features are a chart of sexology of various motor disabilities and chronic disorders and excerpts of counseling sessions. Drawbacks are emphasis on sex within context of marriage and traditional de-emphasis of female sexuality. Includes glossary of medical terms and extensive bibliography. Table of contents appears at end. More thorough and concise than many other texts but some information needs updating. Recommended for special libraries.

Janz, Dieter, et al., eds. Epilepsy, Pregnancy, and the Child. New York: Raven Press, 1982. 552 pp.

Reports for the professional the proceedings of an international meeting held in 1980 to exchange information among research groups in the area of epilepsy and obstetrics. Deals primarily with toxicology and pharmacokinetics of antiepileptic drugs in pregnancy. Includes three major topical divisions: pregnancy, delivery and findings in newborns, and child development. These are subdivided into several topics with each subdivision starting with a literature review. Examples of subtopics include seizure frequency during pregnancy and obstetrical complications, abortion, and stillbirth. References listed at end of each chapter. Well-organized and indexed. Recommended for hospital libraries.

Lancaster-Gaye, Derek, ed. Personal Relationships, the Handicapped and the Community: Some European Thoughts and Solutions. London: Routledge and Kegan Paul, 1972. 150 pp.

Divided into two parts: one on community care, or what is now thought of as independent living facilities, and the other on sex primarily within the context of marriage. Describes advantages and disadvantages of several community care facilities such as those provided by Sweden's Fokus Society and a collective house in Hans Knudsens Plads in Copenhagen. Includes summary of pros and cons of institutional care. Covers United Kingdom, Sweden, Denmark, and Holland. Although emphasis is on cerebral palsied, other mobility impairments are included. Part on sex and marriage discusses personal relationships, genetic counseling, societal attitudes and sex education, among others. Includes chapter written by married cerebral palsied male. Provides a look at European concepts and is thought provoking, even though dated. Unique in that few books discuss sexuality within context of institutional or independent living setting. More helpful than Let There Be Love (Enby, 1975) for its broader perspective. Recommended for special libraries.

Landis, Carney, and Bolles, M. Marjorie. Personality and Sexuality of the Physically Handicapped Woman. New York: Paul B. Hoeber, 1942. 171 pp.

Reports a study of 100 women evenly divided among four disabilities: chronic heart disease, spastic paralysis, epilepsy, and orthopedic disabilities. Participants were primarily non-institutionalized. Emphasizes the emotional and psychosexual development of disabled women on basis of in-depth interview data. Valuable as an early research study in this area; although a small study it appears to have been well-controlled. Another valuable feature is comparisons authors make with their previous study of able-bodied women. Makes comparisons among disabilities studied as well. A 1980 printing of an important work for professionals interested in psychosexual research of disabled. Appendices include evaluation scales, vital statistics of participants, and intervariable comparisons. Has bibliography and index. Recommended for research libraries.

Peterson, Yen. Marital Adjustment in Couples of Which One Spouse is Physically Handicapped. Palo Alto, Calif.: R & E Research Associates, 1979. 116 pp.

Reports results of a detailed study of 43 couples in which one spouse was wheelchair-bound. Indentified factors contributing to stress and cohesion by examining the spouses' approaches to eight tasks central to marriage. Examines relationship of marital adjustment in disabled and able-bodied by sex and in progressive and nonprogressie disabilities. Aimed at the professional and helpful for those in a counseling role. Includes extensive literature review and bibliography. Recommended for special libraries.

Rabin, Barry J. The Sensuous Wheeler: Sexual Adjustment for the Spinal Cord Injured. San Francisco: Multi-Media Resource Center, 1980. 153 pp.

　　For the professional as well as anyone else interested in the topic. Author is well-qualified in this subject area. Meets two purposes: surveys the current information on sexual functioning with emphasis on the spinal cord injured and suggests methods for the individual to attain sexual adjustment. Includes counseling guidelines for the professional, advantages and disadvantages of penile implants, resources for adjustment and an extensive bibliography. Much of the information is presented in tabular format. Well-organized and easily read; an excellent resource on this topic. Recommended for special and public libraries.

Roberts, Gloria A. and McCartney, Julie, comps. Sexuality and the Disabled: An Annotated Bibliography. New York: Katharine Dexter McCormick Library and Planned Parenthood Federation of America, Inc., 1981. 38 pp.

　　Lists approximately 200 annotated references on sexuality and physical, mental, emotional or psychological impairment. Compiled for the International Year of Disabled Persons from the Psychological Abstracts and ERIC (Educational Resources Information Center) databases and other sources. Divided into sections by the broad areas mentioned and listed alphabetically by author within each section. Hearing and visual impairment materials are listed in separate sections. Includes a variety of publication formats, although most are journal articles. Useful as an update to older bibliographies. Recommended for special libraries.

Robinault, Isabel P. Sex, Society, and the Disabled: A Developmental Inquiry into Roles, Reactions, and Responsibilities. Hagerstown, Md.: Harper and Row, 1978. 273 pp.

　　Reviews sexuality as it relates to disability from infancy to maturity. Relates this to sexual development of able-bodied. Has an extensive index and list of references. Has eighteen appendices which contain information useful to laypersons as well as professionals. Several of these appendices are unique to this publication: 1) a table, "Teenages and the Law," covers age of consent for medical care and specific gynecologic/obstetric procedures, 2) precautions for counselors, 3) Catholic code on sex, 4) genetic counseling services by state, and 5) sources for anatomic models for the blind. Would be valuable reference tool even though the text's audience is primarily clinical and/or academic professionals. Recommended for special and public libraries.

Scarlett, Sharon; Thury, Cynthia; and Zupan, Irene, comps. Psychological, Sexual, Social and Vocational Aspects of Spinal Cord Injury: A Selected Bibliography. Minneapolis: Department of Physical Medicine and Rehabilitation, University of Minnesota, 1976. 76 pp.

Intended to be comprehensive on psychological, sexual, social, and vocational aspects of spinal cord injury for professionals in research or clinical practice. Includes a 1977 supplement of eight pages. Mentions future updates but these are no longer handled by the University of Minnesota. The journal Rehabilitation Psychology is to have published an additional supplement. Lists 777 items under each of the four headings; some appear under more than one heading if emphasis warrants it. Primarily contains journal articles but also lists book chapters, dissertations, and proceedings. Appears to be complete but has other useful features as well: author index, index of sports related items and bibliographies included in the text, list of persons and organizations contacted for references, and a list of bibliographies consulted to compile this list. Very useful bibliography; recommended for special libraries.

Sex Education for the Visually Handicapped in Schools and Agencies: ... Selected Papers. New York: American Foundation for the Blind, 1975. 76 pp.

Lack of an introduction or preface to the eight papers leaves them in somewhat of a vacuum. Does not appear to follow a particular progression in the order of the articles. Most discuss sex education programs developed at various institutions for the blind and visually impaired. All but first and last articles have an abstract. There is no index but book does contain margin notes throughout which are very helpful. One of most valuable aspects of this book is the last paper which consists of fairly detailed curriculum suggestions divided into developmental levels. This would be useful reading for teachers and parents interested in sex education. Recommended for education and public libraries.

Sex: Rehabilitations's Stepchild. Proceeding of the Workshop, Continuing Education in the Treatment of Spinal Cord Injuries, June 23, 1973, Indianapolis, Indiana. Chicago: National Paraplegia Foundation, 1974. 37 pp.

Aimed at professionals working with the spinal cord injured. Lists workshop speakers' credentials and contains texts of their presentations. Romano's and Hohmann's talks are much the same as their articles in The Disabled Person and Family Dynamics (Thomason, 1973). Provides unique information on role of the rehabilitation facility in one talk; reports survey of rehabilitation facilities and how sexual information is provided, and suggests guidelines for establishing a sexual counseling service. Other unique information is a chaplain's perspective of religion and sexuality. Lists approximately fifty references in a bibliography. Although presentations are fairly brief, the information on rehabilitation facilities would be useful background for those setting up a counseling service. Recommended for special libraries.

Sha'ked, Ami. Human Sexuality in Physical and Mental Illnesses and Disabilities: An Annotated Bibliography. Bloomington, Ind.: Indiana University Press, 1978. 303 pp.

Intended as a reference source for health professionals. Covers research and clinical literature from 1940 to 1977. Includes various formats of published materials; approximately 15 audiovisuals are extensively annotated in the media chapter. Psychological and nursing literature are included. Scope note or introductions for the chapters (except media) would have been helpful but lengthy annotations provide a good deal of information. Chapters are divided by the type of disability or illness. Includes a general chapter and one on sex education. Includes a selected list of primary sources. Recommended for health science libraries.

Sha'ked, Ami, ed. Human Sexuality and Rehabilitation Medicine: Sexual Functioning Following Spinal Cord Injury. Baltimore, Md.: Williams & Wilkins, 1981. 210 pp.

Combines discussion of both practice and research in one volume. Coverage of the topic is very good and includes chapters devoted to: state-of-the-art; male sexual anatomy, physiology, function and fertility; female sexual anatomy, physiology, function and fertility; counseling; therapy; education; women's sexuality; surgical treatment; and evaluation of rehabilitation programs. Unique information is provided in two chapters on the rehabilitation nurse's and chaplain's roles. Text includes a list of basic sexual rights, discussion of homosexuality, and illustrations and photographs of penile prostheses. References follow each chapter. Has index. Recommended as textbook for course on sexuality and disability.

Shipes, Ellen A., and Lehr, Sally T. Sexual Counseling for Ostomates: A Resource Book for Health Care Professionals. Springfield, Ill.: Charles C. Thomas, 1979. 105 pp.

Excellent handbook for health professionals concerned about sexual function or counseling the disabled. Has a light, readable text with cartoon illustrations. Preface contains brief history and overview of enterostomal therapy. Sections include sexual physiology of the able-bodied; physical and psychological effects of ostomies on sexual function; descriptions of colostomies, ileostomies, and urostomies; definitions of sexuality; and counseling prerequisites and techniques. Unique information includes sections on aged, homosexual and teenage ostomates as well as paraplegic and quadriplegic ostomates. Contains several lists of myths and misconceptions. Has brief glossary, bibliography and index. Recommended for health science and public libraries.

Stewart, W. F. R. The Sexual Side of Handicap: A Guide for the Caring Professions. Cambridge, England: Woodhead-Faulkner, 1979. 208 pp.

Describes various types of disability and their effects on sexual function. Divided into two sections: the first covers general problems and solutions, including legal aspects, counseling and education; the second covers some common disabilities and their sexual, physical, emotional, and social effects, and implications for parenthood. Includes neurologic, cardiovascular, respiratory and mental disabilities. Has definite British slant, particularly in description of legal situations; language seems somewhat convoluted at times. Recommended for special libraries.

Task Force on Concerns of Physically Disabled Women. <u>Within Reach: Providing Family Planning Services to Physically Disabled Women</u>. Everett, Wash.: Planned Parenthood of Snohomish County, Inc., 1977. 48 pp.

Aimed at persons offering health care services to the disabled, primarily women receiving family planning services. Discusses architectural accessibility with clear illustrations of curb cuts, measurements, etc. Describes how clinic services can accommodate disabled patients. Includes discussion of medical aspects of disability as well as brief chapter on Section 504 Regulations. Appendix includes "telephone triage" for receptionist and summary list of implications for female sexuality, reproductive functioning, and contraceptive methods. Has bibliography. Very useful and concise guide for anyone involved in health care services for the disabled. Recommended for special libraries.

United Cerebral Palsy Associations. <u>Human Sexuality</u>. New York: United Cerebral Palsy Association, 1976. 94 pp. in various pagings.

Annotated bibliography equally divided between physical and sociopsychological aspects of sexuality. Includes a few general references on sexuality with the rest concerned with physical disability. Not limited to cerebral palsy; includes special sections for mentally retarded, spinal cord injured and visually handicapped. Covers some training and program aids, audiovisuals and periodicals dealing with sexuality and physical disability. Section on sociopsychological aspects consists primarily of journal article summaries. This appears to be a good basic bibliography although nonevaluative. Especially helpful are the special topics covered, the variety of materials included, and the summaries of the journal articles. Recommended for special libraries.

Vaeth, Jerome M. San Francisco Cancer Symposium, San Francisco, California, March 23-24, 1979. <u>Frontiers of Radiation Therapy and Oncology, Vol. 14 Body-Image, Self-Esteem, and Sexuality in Cancer Patients</u>. Basel, Switzerland: S. Karger AG, 1980. 133 pp.

Includes papers presented at symposium for health professionals. Covers various types of cancers: breast, gynecologic, colon, head and neck, prostate, testis, and penis. Most of the papers are followed by a patient's perspective or audience's participation. The latter are very thought provoking. One paper discusses sexuality in adolescent cancer patients. Emphasizes improved communication between physicians and patients. Recommended for medical libraries.

Veterans Administration Hospital. Sex and the Handicapped: A Selected Bibliography (1927-1975). Cleveland, Ohio: Veterans Administration Hospital, 1975. 55 pp.

Contains approximately 560 references, almost exclusively to the journal literature. Covers burns, aging, drug addiction, and alcoholism in addition to physical disabilities caused by trauma or illness. Has 174 references on spinal cord injury but much less on amputation, arthritis, orthopedic disabilities, poliomyelitis, cystic fibrosis, cerebral palsy, and multiple sclerosis. Contains references to endocrine, cardiovascular, and neurological disorders as well. Although this is a good reference tool, particularly for older material, it lacks an introduction or scope note defining its coverage or the source of the references. Recommended for health science libraries for the breadth of topics covered.

Von Eschenbach, Andrew C., and Rodriguez, Dorothy B., eds. Sexual Rehabilitation of the Urologic Cancer Patient. Boston: G. K. Hall Medical Publishers, 1981. 322 pp.

Aimed at the various professionals working with urologic cancer patients. Emphasizes importance of patient's spouse during the illness and rehabilitation process. Covers both physical and emotional aspects. Includes chapters aimed at the nurse, the clergy and the health care professional. Discusses rehabilitation in framework of team approach. Describes and provides outline for a sexuality assessment. Covers surgical reconstruction and prostheses. Lists references with each chapter, has extensive index. Good review of current concepts in this aspect of rehabilitation. Recommended for hospital libraries particularly.

Woods, Nancy Fugate. Human Sexuality in Health and Illness. 2d ed. St. Louis: C. V. Mosby Company, 1979. 400 pp.

Only about one fourth of this text is devoted to trauma, alterations of body image and chronic illness and how these relate to sexuality. However, the text is excellent in putting sexuality in context with life cycle and life events. Discusses sexual adaptation to hospitalization and illness and covers such topics as mastectomy, diabetes, and hysterectomy. Aimed at the professional and includes section on role of health professional in sexual counseling and sex education. Each chapter includes literature review, summary, general references and references for laypersons. Some chapters include questions for review and media as well. Includes several tables summarizing research on sexual functioning after ostomies and chronic illness. Recommended for health science libraries.

Woodward, James. Signs of Sexual Behavior: An Introduction to Some Sex-Related Vocabulary in American Sign Language. Silver Spring, Md.: T. J. Publishers, 1979. 81 pp.

    For an evaluation of this work, see Chapter 6.

ANNOTATED BIBLIOGRAPHY:
Materials for Laypersons

Baxter, Robert T. Salvaging Our Sexuality: For SCI and Related Disabilities in Distress. East Orange, N.J.: Medical Media Visuals, 1979. 120 pp.

    Written by a quadriplegic. Begins with an extended definition of spinal cord injury which is more complete than most. However, the author makes many bold statements with no accompanying references or statistics to verify them. Briefly discusses costs of rehabilitating SCI individuals. Contains brief list of references and short quiz. There are other books on this subject which are better referenced. Not illustrated. Not recommended.

Becker, Elle Friedman. Female Sexuality Following Spinal Cord Injury. Bloomington, Ill.: Accent Special Publications, Cheever Pub., 1978. 273 pp.

    Written by a disabled woman for both laypersons and professionals. Exposes the reader to the emotional and psychological effects of severe disability. Discusses physical and psychological aspects by way of extensive personal interviews with professionals and other disabled women. Author's husband participates in several of the interviews and these comments are especially valuable. Includes several illustrations, bibliography, and glossary. Definitions of terms are included in text as well. Unique for its presentation of actual comments of the author in initial period after injury and notes in her medical charts made by professionals. Demonstrates the sensitivity and information needed at this traumatic time. Recommended for health science and public libraries.

Binder, Donald P. Sex, Courtship & the Single Ostomate. Los Angeles: United Ostomy Association, Inc., 1973. 20 pp.

    Looks at how ostomies affect relationships with others; discusses morality, lifestyles, whom to tell and how, venereal disease, etc. Superficiality, archaic language and moral tone are pronounced. There are better pamphlets for this purpose. Not recommended.

Bregman, Sue. Sexuality and the Spinal Cord Injured Woman; Guidelines Concerning Femininity, Social, and Sexual Adjustment. Minneapolis: Sister Kenny Institute, 1975. 24 pp.

Summarizes responses of 31 spinal cord injured women interviewed about various aspects of their sexuality. Organized into five sections: setting the mood, techniques, orgasm, physical concerns, and social techniques. Emphasizes similarities among able-bodied and disabled. Much of the information provided is same as for able-bodied person; this could have been summarized and information for disabled could be organized better. Covers the topic superficially and is not really useful as "handbook" as claimed. Not recommended.

Dickman, Irving. Sex Education for Disabled Persons. Pamphlet #531. New York: Public Affairs Committee, 1975. 29 pp.

Devoted in large part to justifying sex education for disabled persons but also covers areas of special concern. Discusses marriage, genetic counseling, child rearing, voluntary sterilization, and the rights of disabled in these areas. Includes resources for teaching blind adolescents about sexuality and lists sixteen organizations from which information is available. Very concise and broad in coverage of the topic. Recommended for public libraries.

Duffy, Yvonne. ... All Things Are Possible. Ann Arbor, Mich.: A. J. Gavin & Associates, 1981. 179 pp.

Author, disabled by polio herself, presents sketches of disabled women's views on various aspects of sexuality. Contains quotes obtained from extensive questionnaire completed by 77 orthopedically disabled women, ages ranging from 19 to 58 years old. Refers to persons as "differently abled" and uses many actual quotes. Author is objective in describing limitations of the information: voluntary responses, limited numbers of blacks, lesbians, unemployed. Covers topics such as parental attitudes, cultural preferences, self-image and child rearing as well as sexuality. Includes chapters on homosexuality, menstruation and masturbation which are not frequently found. Mentions helpful books in several chapters. Includes brief glossary and bibliography. Recommended for public libraries.

Eisenberg, M. G., and Rustad, L. C. Sex and the Spinal Cord Injured: Some Questions and Answers. 2d ed. Cleveland, Ohio: Veterans Administration Hospital, 1974. 44 pp.

Government publication written by two sex educators at Veterans Administration Hospital. Emphasizes male spinal cord injuries and erection, intercourse and ejaculation. This edition was revised to include some information on females. Contains information on adoption of children, particularly foreign children (due to VA slant). Appendix includes statistics on sexual functioning, marriage, divorce, and contraception. Has glossary, references, and illustrations. Some material is dated; other publications present information in more organized fashion. Early example of response to information needs of disabled in this area. Not recommended as there are more current and comprehensive publications.

Enby, Gunnel. Let There Be Love: Sex and the Handicapped. New York: Taplinger Publishing Co., 1975. 65 pp.

Author is disabled Swedish woman who discusses her experiences in Swedish rehabilitation centers. Attempts to enlighten the able-bodied reader to inappropriate reactions to disabled. Suggests improvements which able-bodied and institutions can make to improve conditions of the disabled. Not devoted entirely to discussion of sexuality but rather attitudes and lifestyles in general. Describes archaic attitudes existing in institutions and advocates abolishment of institutional care. Valuable as personal narrative of disabled person's experiences in the Swedish setting. Recommended for public libraries.

Gambrell, Ed. Sex and the Male Ostomate. Los Angeles: United Ostomy Association, Inc., 1973. 23 pp.

Reports some of information provided by questionnaire sent to 95 male ostomates. Provides some of same information as Sex, Pregnancy and the Female Ostomate. Discusses psychological aspects of ostomy as they relate to sexual relationships; especially where sexual difficulties arise. Also discusses sexual impairment of a physical nature. Helpful suggestions cover topics such as penile implants and impotence. Needs to be updated in area of penile prosthesis particularly, but contains a good brief introduction. Recommended for public libraries.

Gordon, Sol. Sexual Rights for the People Who Happen to Be Handicapped. Syracuse, N.Y.: Center on Human Policy, Syracuse University, 1979. 12 pp.

Gives brief overview of the sexual needs of the disabled and how to help them react to these needs. Although author frequently refers to the mentally retarded, this summary is useful for any disabled person. Emphasizes similarity with "normal" persons. It contains references to additional materials which might prove useful to both the professional and layperson. Geared to all people who come in contact with the physically disabled. Although the information is available elsewhere, the reference section makes this a worth-while addition to collections serving the layperson. Uses running titles rather than table of contents or index. Not illustrated. Recommended for public libraries.

Greengross, Wendy. Entitled to Love: The Sexual and Emotional Needs of the Handicapped. London: Malaby Press in Association with National Fund For Research Into Crippling Diseases, 1976. 121 pp.

Attempts to bring the sexual and emotional needs of the disabled into the open. Discusses attitudes of parents, public, and professionals and changes needed. Addressses special problems of the mentally disabled and sex education for the disabled. Although it covers the broad scope of sexuality and disability, author does not discuss nontraditional sexual expression and appears repetitious at times. Recommended for public libraries.

Greengross, Wendy. Marriage Sex and Arthritis. Arthritis and Rheumatism Council, 1973. 28 pp.

This British publication provides brief discussion of wide range of concerns of arthritic persons including adverse effects of drugs, genetic counseling, family planning, and care of the newborn. Although the author mentions that there is often no effect of arthritis on sex and sexuality, and includes many references to "consult your doctor," this pamphlet contains useful information for the layperson. Language level and content recommend it for public libraries.

Hopper, C. Edmund, and Allen, William A. Sex Education for Physically Handicapped Youth. Springfield, Ill.: Charles C. Thomas, 1980. 130 pp.

Although written for the physically disabled adolescent this book would, as the publisher suggests, be a useful reference for parents and teachers as well. Preface is written for parents. Contains information on all aspects of sexuality in language easily understood by adolescents. Contains glossary, but most terms are explained in the text as well. Covers the various aspects of sexuality, including masturbation and fantasizing. Discusses current information on sexually transmitted diseases and genetic counseling. Includes comments of other disabled adolescents about sex and sex education. Lists associations which can provide information on specific genetic diseases and also agencies helping the disabled. Although most mention is made of disabled persons in wheelchairs, this would be a useful book for any disabled youth. The authors take a somewhat extreme view of drugs such as alcohol and tobacco, but otherwise this book is an excellent information source on the topic. Contains bibliography and index. Recommended for education and public libraries.

Johnson, Warren R. Sex Education and Counseling of Special Groups: The Mentally and Physically Handicapped, Ill and Elderly. Springfield, Ill.: Charles C. Thomas, 1975. 213 pp.

Written for the layperson, this text heavily emphasizes the point that disabled persons have just as much interest and need for sexual information as the general public and their concerns are no different. Author is a Professor of Health Education with experience in programs and lectures on sex education for special groups. Most of the information presented could be used with able-bodied as well. Identifies "special groups" as persons with mental or physical disorders or the aged, but disabilities are de-emphasized in the presentation. Reviews literature and presents questions and answers. Discusses primarily sexual behavior rather than physiology. Provides basic, general information. The second edition, 1981, was unavailable for review. Recommended for public libraries.

Life Together: The Situation of the Handicapped. Compiled by Inger Nordqvist. Stockholm: The Swedish Central Committee for Rehabilitation, 1972. 79 pp.

Result of a symposium sponsored by the Swedish Central Committee for Rehabilitation. Not presented as contributed papers but rather a synthesis in the form of answers to questions. Emphasizes the orthopedically disabled, from parents' relationship with the child through parenthood of the disabled person. Discusses sexuality in the home and institutional setting, sex education, contraception, marriage, divorce and living arrangements. Contains sections on sexual physiology for males and females. Has detailed table of contents, summary of measures proposed (three or four per chapter), proposed research, list of participants in symposium, and bibliography. Very readable and well-organized. Some sections need updating, for example, contraceptive methods. Good for developmental perspective on sexuality. Audience could be either lay public or professionals. Recommended particularly for public libraries.

Liskey, Nathan, and Stephens, Phillip. Cerebral Palsy and Sexuality. n.p., 1979. 47 pp.

Uses case studies of two single males, two single females and two married couples to demonstrate similarities of sexual functioning in cerebral palsied and able-bodied. Case studies are lengthy, including discussion of family background, level of disability, early sexual experiences, sex education, if any, and current sexual expression. Uses quotes from the participants. Lack of opportunity for developmement of social skills is a predominant factor discussed. Aimed at the layperson, particularly the cerebral palsied. Consists mainly of emotional support as opposed to factual information. Recommended for public libraries.

Mooney, Thomas O.; Cole, Theodore M.; and Children, Richard A. Sexual Options for Paraplegics and Quadriplegics. Boston: Little, Brown, & Co., 1975. 111 pp.

Discusses and illustrates range of sexual expression and response possible for the spinal cord injured individual. Was prompted by the lack of literature on sexual technique for the disabled and unique feature is clear photographs illustrating the text. Provides explicit information for the professional but text is geared toward the disabled themselves and helping to improve their self-image and feelings toward sexuality. Discussion includes techniques for accommodating appliances, using attendants, penile prostheses, and vibrators. Has detailed glossary and an index. Excellent source of practical information for professionals, disabled, and their able-bodied partners. Recommended for health science and public libraries.

Norris, Carole, and Gambrell, Ed. Sex, Pregnancy & the Female Ostomate. Los Angeles: United Ostomy Association, Inc., 1972. 20 pp.

Provides much better information than Sex, Courtship and the Single Ostomate but for women. Covers a great deal in twenty pages. Discusses results of interviews with 20 ostomates who have had children - their descriptions of how their ostomies affected their pregnancies and deliveries. Stresses that there is little difference from nonostomates. Distinguishes types of ostomies and differences or similarities between them during sex and pregnancy. Good, brief introduction to topic. Recommended for public libraries.

Stoklosa, Jean M; Bullard, David G.; Rosenbaum, Ernest H; and Rosenbaum, Isadora R. Sexuality and Cancer. Palo Alto, Calif.: Bull Publishing, 1980. 18 pp.

Forms part of a series, "A Comprehensive Guide for Cancer Patients and Their Families," and is therefore directed toward the layperson. One of the authors is a clinical specialist in a Veterans Administration Hospital and another is coordinator of a Sex and Disability Training Project. Begins by explaining that there may be no change in sexuality due to illness but if there is, this volume may help in handling these changes. Discusses sexual myths, effects of illness, body image, and specific effects of cancer, e.g., mastectomy, laryngectomy, and ostomy. Includes brief discussion of energy level. Provides list of references for further reading and several resource organizations. Language is clear, simple, and concise, yet sensitive. Recommended for patient or public libraries.

Taggie, Joanne M., and Manley, M. Scott. A Handbook on Sexuality after Spinal Cord Injury. Englewood, Colo.: M. Manley, 1978. 51 pp.

Workbook for spinal cord injured and their partners. Discusses basic understanding of sexuality, physiological aspects, and psychological aspects. Humorous presentation with many illustrations. Stresses similarities to sexuality before injury as well as possible differences and special considerations. Includes short glossary and bibliography. Straightforward language is sometimes simplistic but the book's organization and the amount of information presented make it very useful. Recommended for public libraries.

Task Force on Concerns of Physically Disabled Women. <u>Toward Intimacy: Family Planning and Sexuality Concerns of Physically Disabled Women</u>. 2d ed. New York: Human Sciences Press, 1978. 63 pp.

Very thorough discussion of disabled women's concerns about sexuality. Each section includes list of "possibilities" - possible actions related to that chapter. Covers body image very well and discusses relationship to the health care system. Includes homosexual relationships and relationships with parents; the latter contains useful suggestions for parents of disabled persons. Liberally punctuated with quotations from women with a variety of disabilities. Has brief glossary. One of the better discussions of this topic. Recommended for public libraries.

Thomason, Bruce, and Clifford, Kerry. <u>The Disabled Person and Family Dynamics</u>. Accent on Living: Reprint Series Number 1, 1973. Bloomington, Ill.: Accent Publications, 1973. 24 pp.

Consists of introductory article and two reprints, all written by professional rehabilitation counselors. Introductory article covers impact of disability on the family members, social life, and sexual relationships, among others. A second article discusses the disabled female and such topics as communications and preparation for sexual activity. The third article on the disabled male discusses characteristics and knowledge counselors should possess, sexual activities possible for the disabled and common precautions for counselors. Articles are aimed at the layperson, even though third article was originally written for rehabilitation counselors. Has several weaknesses: introductory article has bias toward male disabled and third article is weak on section of what the patient should be told. However, the publication does serve as a brief introduction to the topic and the overview of the importance of counseling in the area of sexuality and family relationships/adjustments is good. Generally, more indepth information is available in other publications annotated for this chapter. Recommended for public libraries.

11 PHYSICAL EDUCATION, RECREATION, AND TRAVEL

CAROL BATES PENKA/Assistant Reference Librarian and Assistant Professor of Library Administration, University of Illinois Library, Urbana, Illinois

INTRODUCTION

The worldwide participation of millions of physically disabled individuals in recreational activities is the result of several converging factors. Disabled veterans returning home after World War II were determined to live as normal a life as possible. Secondly, the discovery of antibiotics and new methods of medical treatment led to the lengthening lifespan of those with spinal cord injuries. No longer did 80% die within three years of being injured.(1) Thirdly, when the civil rights movement for the disabled arose in the 1970s, laws were enacted which assured access to school physical education programs and community recreation programs which receive federal funds. Finally, the number of trained rehabilitation personnel has increased dramatically with the advent of college programs which produce adaptive physical education teachers, therapeutic recreators, occupational therapists, music and dance therapists, and other rehabilitation therapists.

The literature in this chapter has arisen from the diverse informational needs of these rehabilitation professionals, in addition to those of disabled consumers and their families. The majority of the literature in this chapter is directed toward professionals who work with the mobility impaired. A few books are geared to the special informational needs of those working with hearing or visually impaired persons. Relatively few works are directed toward disabled consumers or their families.

Although millions of disabled persons do participate in recreational activities, access to recreational programs and facilities remains a problem. Therefore, several important works concern attitudinal and architectural barriers. Local governments officials, faced with shrinking budgets, are often reluctant to support community-based programming for a minority of the population. This occurs despite the provisions of Section 504 of the Rehabilitation Act of 1973 which state that

> "No otherwise qualified handicapped individual in the United States ... shall solely by reason of his handicap, be excluded from participation in, be denied the benefits of, or be subjected to discrimination under any program or activity receiving federal financial assistance."

Two excellent general works both published in Canada, cover the philosophical basis of community involvement for the disabled participant. Peter Witt's Community Leisure Services and Disabled Individuals provides guidance to municipal officials who may be initiating leisure services to the disabled population. Hutchinson and Lord's Recreation Integration focuses on the integration of the disabled into the community as a societal process. Another important work, Arts and the Handicapped: an Issue of Access reports on cultural and educational programs—museum displays, painting classes, natural trails—in which solutions to both architectural and attitudinal barriers are being developed.

While attitudinal barriers often hinder participation, architectural barriers may totally prevent it. Making Physical Education and Recreation Facilities Accessible to All, an annotated bibliography, published by the Physical Education and Recreation for the Handicapped Information and Research Utilization Center (IRUC), is intended to serve as a beginning resource for both professionals and the general reader. Sports Centres & Swimming Pools by Felix Walter offers an overview of architectural design features, and it can be used by architects and building committees while they are planning accessible indoor sports facilities. Austin's Playground and Playspaces for the Handicapped establishes design criteria for planning outdoor playgrounds which can be used by disabled children. These guidelines are intended for planners, therapists, and administrators, although the work will be useful for parents as well. Other works on accessibility are included in the chapters on "Barrier Free Design" and "Federal Publications." In addition, books on particular sports usually cover the design of the facilities necessary for that particular sport.

For children, recreational needs are often met in the physical education program at their school. The Education for All Handicapped Children Act (P.L. 94-142) assures accessibility by stating that specically designed instruction must be conducted in physical education classes as well as in the academic classroom. Some students may have little difficulty participating in the regular program. Others, more severely disabled, may participate only because the activities have been modified or adapted to their individual functional level. Current emphasis in the field is on the integration of as many disabled children as is possible into the regular program where they can interact with their able-bodied peers. Several college-level textbooks provide an overview of the types of disabilities usually found in the public school population and the functional level of those afflicted with these disabilities. Wheeler and Hooley's Physical Education for the Handicapped and Arnheim, Auxter, and Crowe's Principles and Methods of Adapted Physical Education and Recreation are good examples of this type of basic text.

Other works on children emphasize enjoyable activity by putting value on the therapeutic nature of play. This type of publication appeals to a broader audience and can be useful for parents, scout leaders, or classroom teachers. Physical Education for Special Needs, edited by Groves, bridges the gap between play and physical education. It discusses the physical education experience for disabled children and includes essays by experts on pleasurable activities such as swimming, outdoor adventure, and dance. Cratty and Breen's Educational Games for Physically Handicapped Children and Geddes' Physical Activities for Individuals with Handicapping Conditions outline games and activities which can be both enjoyable and therapeutic. Two works by Dr. Charles Buell, Physical Education for the Visually Handicapped and Physical Education for Blind Children, discuss the special need of the visually impaired child for rigorous physical exercise.

One publication which deals solely with equipment for use in the adaptive physical education program is the Handbook of Adapted Physical Education Equipment and Its Use. In this work Michael Sosne provides basic information on adapting, constructing, and purchasing physical education equipment for physically impaired individuals.

An important recreational activity which is taken for granted by most Americans is travel. Disabled travelers have often been hindered by educational barriers. Often they simply did not know what could be accomplished, or they found that it was difficult to obtain accurate information from travel agents. Fortunately, several publications written within the last six years present accurate and practical information for disabled consumers. The most comprehensive treatment is Lois Reamy's TravelAbility, which is limited in scope to travel in the United States. This book covers all aspects of travel: planning the trip, locating lodgings, selecting the mode of transportation, and choosing a destination. Weiss' Access to the World includes information regarding international travel. A different approach is taken by Atwater in Roll'On. This book provides carefully planned itineraries for tours of major cities in the U.S. A fourth indispensible work is Annand's The Wheelchair Traveler, which rates hundreds of motels and hotels in the United States, Canada, and Mexico regarding their accessibility to the mobility impaired traveler. For travelers who have not "done it themselves" the personal account of someone who has can be both informational and inspirational. John Nelson provides such a work in Wheelchair Vagabond, a readable account of van camping across the United States.

The disabled traveler should not overlook standard sources of travel information. The Mobil Travel Guide Series includes mention of attractions and accomodations with special equipment or design for the convenience of travelers in wheelchairs. For the international traveler, Michelin Red Guides designate hotels with bedrooms accessible to wheelchairs, and tour guides such as those written by Stephen Birnbaum, Eugene Fodor and others include travel tips for disabled travelers.

Additional sources of information specifically designated for the disabled traveler include membership in the Society for the Advancement of Travel for the Handicapped. Membership is open to disabled consumers as well as to professionals in the travel industry. Members receive a monthly newsletter and information on tour operators and travel agents. Magazines for the disabled consumer such as Paraplegia News(2) and Accent on Living(3) feature articles on various aspects of travel. Another useful source is the Travel Information Center at Moss Rehabilitation Hospital, a free service designed to help the disabled person plan trips.

The many federal laws and regulations mandating accessibility of public areas have given rise to a wealth of travel information which can be found in the chapter entitled "Federal Publications." Among these titles are Highway Rest Areas for Handicapped Travelers, Access Amtrak, National Parks: a Guide for Handicapped Visitors, and Access Travel: Airports a Guide to Accessibility of Terminals.

NOTES

1. Jackson, Robert W., and Fredrickson, Alex. "Sports for the Physically Disabled. The 1976 Olympiad (Toronto)." American Journal of Sports Medicine, vol. 7 (1979): p. 293.

2. Paraplegia News Phoenix, Ariz.: Paralyzed Veterans of America 1946- . Monthly.
3. Accent on Living, Bloomington, Ill.: Cheever Publishing, 1956- . Quarterly.

ANNOTATED BIBLIOGRAPHY

Access Chicago: A Guide to the City. Chicago: Rehabilitation Institute of Chicago, 1982. 62 pp.

For the mobility impaired Access Chicago: A Guide to the City gives detailed information on how to enter buildings, stadiums, theaters, restaurants, sports facilities, etc. The establishments listed are not rated, and the listings were chosen on a random basis.

Adams, Ronald C.; Daniel, Alfred N.; and Rullman, Lee. Games, Sports, and Exercises for the Physically Handicapped. 3rd ed. Philadelphia: Lea & Febiger, 1982. 400 pp.

This book is designed as a basic text for adaptive physical education teachers, physical education teachers, physical therapists, and therapeutic recreators who work with disabled children in schools and hospitals. The authors concentrate on programs, procedures, and equipment that have been tested in actual situations. Following a brief history of therapeutic exercise and of wheelchair sports, the authors survey prevalent defects and prescribe therapeutic exercises for those afflicted with these disabilities. A major portion of the book describes adapted sports, games, and activities and gives detailed rules for both ablebodied and for disabled participants. The chapter on posture evaluation will be of particular interest to school personnel. Recommended for professional collections.

Allen, Anne. Sports for the Handicapped. New York: Walker and Co., 1981. 80 pp.

Written for the lay audience, this popularized account of sports for the disabled relates biographical sketches of athletes and coaches. The sports are skiing, wheelchair basketball, swimming, track and field, football, and horseback riding. The book is liberally illustrated with black and white photographs. An appendix lists a selection of sports organizations serving the disabled. The book will be of value for laypersons wanting to know more about sports for the disabled and may also be of use in counseling the disabled consumer.

Alvin, Juliette. Music for the Handicapped Child. 2d ed. London: Oxford University Press, 1976. 150 pp.

The author, Juliette Alvin, is a pioneer in the field of music therapy. In her book she promotes the value of music to the disabled child. She discusses at length the correlation between the different stages of maturation of disabled children and their musical development. She also discusses the kind of musical experiences which can help the child's social and emotional integration and influence his attitudes toward work and play, toward himself, and others. She addresses the special problems of the psychologically impaired and the physically disabled, as well as of those children with sensory impairments. Although much of the material is based on the author's own experiences, she relates it to the work of others in the field. The book should be of interest to anyone concerned with a disabled child, as well as of interest to music therapists and teachers.

Annand, Douglass R. The Wheelchair Traveler. Rev. ed. Milford, N.H.: Douglass R. Annand, 1979. 300 pp.

The author, a healthy paraplegic with a 26" wheelchair, rates motels, restaurants, hospitals, and park visitor centers according to their accessibility to the paraplegic traveler. Criteria for accessibility include the width of doors, the height of beds, the presence of support bars in the bathroom and the size of the bathroom. Listings are arranged by state or province, subdivided by city. Listings for Mexico and Canade are included. The preface gives hints on travel, and the six-page bibliography lists guides to individual cities and helpful pamphlets. Contributions from readers are solicited. One of the most useful travel publications available for the mobility impaired.

Anderson, William. Teaching the Physically Handicapped to Swim. London: Faber and Faber, 1968. 84 pp.

This book is for swimming teachers, physical therapists, and physical educators. The author discusses disabilities due to paralysis and those caused from physical defects. He indicates the type of swimming strokes that those suffering from these afflictions can perform. The chapter on general disabilities discusses teaching the blind and the deaf. Separate chapters cover swimming strokes and group teaching techniques. A typical sequence of lessons and exercises is outlined. The final chapter outlines desirable design features for a swimming facility. Recommended for physical rehabilitation collections.

Arnheim, Daniel D.; Auxter, David; and Crowe, Walter C. Principles and Methods of Adapted Physical Education and Recreation. 4th ed. St. Louis, Mo.: C. V. Mosby, 1981. 524 pp.

This college textbook is designed for the elementary and secondary school physical educator and the recreation specialist in adaptive physical education. As such, it serves as an introduction to the diverse and complex nature of all types of disabilities and contrasts the physical development of the disabled with the physical development of the able-bodied. The authors present both an academic and a practical approach in sections on teaching and therapy skills, programming for specific problems, and the organization and administration of a program of adaptive physical education.

Arts and the Handicapped: An Issue of Access. New York: Educational Facilities Laboratories and the National Endowment for the Arts. 1975. 78 pp.

Accessibility to the arts implies the removal of barriers which hinder or exclude potential patrons. These include architectural barriers (steps, curbs, lack of elevators, etc.) and attitudinal barriers such as fixed admissions requirements, literacy tests, insurance requirements, or simply preconceived notions about the safety and desirability of involving disabled participants. Today a disabled person's choice of accessible arts activities is very limited, but this report focuses on 131 programs which are developing solutions to the problems. For each program a contact person, pertinent associations, and resource organizations are listed. Recommended for general collections.

Atwater, Maxine H. Roll'on. New York: Dodd, Mead & Co., 1978. 290 pp.

Roll'on contains general travel tips, plus detailed accessibility information about hotels, restaurants, restrooms, and sights. It includes detailed itineraries of tours of Chicago, Honolulu, New York, Philadelphia, San Antonio, San Diego, San Francisco, Washington, D.C., and highlights of five additional cities. The bibliography lists tour guides for individual cities. The list of operators of tours for the disabled is of special interest. Even though information on hours of operation and restaurant recommendations may become dated, the tour itineraries should remain useful.

Austin, Richard L. Playground and Playspaces for the Handicapped. Manhattan, Kan.: Ag Press, 1974. 62 pp.

This study establishes design criteria for developing free play recreational environments for disabled children. These guidelines direct site analysis, site organization, equipment selection and construction, and program orientation for planners, therapists, and administrators. The book discusses the classification of disabled children according to their disability and functional level: and it discusses the implication of the particular disability on play activities. Black and white photographs depict play areas and structures. An appendix highlights applicable standards.

Avedon, Elliott M. Therapeutic Recreation Service: an Applied Behavioral Science Approach. Englewood Cliffs, N. J.: Prentice-Hall, 1974. 254 pp.

    This work is a specialized textbook for those planning to enter the practice of therapeutic recreation service. Section One reviews the historical roots of therapeutic recreation, skims contemporary developments, and offers a philosophical rationale for practice. Section Two examines the required knowledge and skills required for practice. Section Three takes a detailed look at program planning, organization, and content from a social and behavioral point of view. Throughout the text the author has used actual case material to illustrate the theoretical concepts. The final chapter offers the readers an opportunity to respond to questions posed by case studies. Recommended for specialized collections.

Brooks, Howard, and Oppenheim, Charles J. Horticulture as a Therapeutic Aid. New York: Institute of Rehabilitation Medicine, New York University Medical Center, 1973. 47 pp.

    The authors describe some of the methods used in the therapeutic horticulture program developed at the Institute of Rehabilitation Medicine in New York. Recognizing that each project must fit its own particular situation, they do not give a blueprint for successful programs. Instead they provide certain guidelines which will help establish functional programs. Routines that have been successful, procedures that are useful in structuring activities, and benefits that derive from this work have been set down. Professional jargon has been avoided. The books, pamphlets, and sources listed give more specific information. An excellent presentation suitable for any type of library.

Buell, Charles Edwin. Physical Education and Recreation for the Visually Handicapped. Rev. ed. Washington, D.C.: American Alliance for Health, Physical Education and Recreation, 1982. 84 pp.

    Dr. Charles Buell is a physical education teacher for visually handicapped students. He has written this book to meet the needs of persons working with visually impaired participants in community recreation programs and in physical education classes in public schools. The book will also be used by personnel in residential facilities or in specific programs for the visually impaired. The book is divided into three parts: (1) What Physical Educators and Recreation Specialists Should Know About Blindness, (2) Activities for Visually Handicapped Children, and (3) Bibliography.

Buell, Charles E. Physical Education for Blind Children. Springfield, Ill.: Charles C. Thomas, 1966. 24 pp.

    This manual is written especially for teachers and administrators in public and residential schools for the blind. It describes the ingredients for a well-rounded program of vigorous physical education. The author discusses equipment, historical developments, leisure-time activities, contests, games, and competitive activities. Brief biographical sketches of blind athletes are included.

Clark, Cynthia A., and Chadwick, Donna M. Clinically Adapted Instruments for the Multiply Handicapped; a Sourcebook. Westford, Mass.: Modulations Company, 1979. 192 pp.

The use of traditional instruments have long been included in music therapy programs, but for the physically disabled client their use often has been frustrating and impossible. Therefore, many programs for the profoundly handicapped have stressed passive listening to music rather than active listening or learning. The authors, both music therapists, provide the reader with designs for modified musical instruments which are clinically designed for specific physical purposes and intended for use in a course of live creative therapy.

Emphasis is placed on the team approach in the treatment of clients. This is an excellent presentation of practical know-how accompanied by theroretical concepts. It is profusely illustrated. The resource section lists equipment companies and suppliers and includes a bibliography and a glossary.

Colson, John H.C. Progressive Exercice Therapy in Rehabilitation and Physical Education. 3rd ed. Bristol, Eng.: John Wright & Sons, 1974. 260 pp.

This book deals with the application of progession in specific exercise therapy. It provides a comprehensive collection of free exercises for all parts of the body. There exercises are graded and progress in strength and mobility from the simplist to the most strenuous movement. Assisted movements are not included in this book. One section covers the exercise treatment of various surgical and orthopedic conditions. Other sections cover the modern approach to circuit training and exercises to music and the use of music and movement and activities useful in the treatment of the developmental disabled and the mentally ill. The book is useful to specialists in the field of exercise therapy. Recommended for professional collections.

Cordellos, Harry C. Aquatic Recreation for the Blind. Washington, D.C.: Physical Education and Recreation for the Handicapped, Information and Research Utilization Center, 1976. 126 pp.

Harry Cordellos, a blind swimmer, highlights some of the many aquatic activities which are possible and practical for the blind and partially sighted. He first discusses design features for swimming pools to be used for blind swimmers. He then discusses the modifications of basic teaching techniques whch are necessary in order to teach blind students. The aquatic activities covered are swimming, diving, water skiing, skin and scuba diving. Other activities are survival swimming, boating and sailing, recreational swimming, and water games. In discussing how these activities can be taught with a minimum of problems and with no increased risk in personal safety, Mr. Cordellos has created a book which is useful for adaptive physical educators, coaches, and volunteers.

Cratty, Bryant J., and Breen, James E. <u>Educational Games for Physically Handicapped Children</u>. Denver, Colo.: Love Publishing Co., 1972. 91 pp.

This volume was written to spell out ways in which the capacities of the orthopedically impaired child may be extended by motivating him to use larger muscles in the playground setting. The activities covered fall into two subdivisions: (1) lead up activities, which require relatively moderate effort and involve chiefly effort of the smaller muscles with the total of the child's body fixed in space (2) vigorous activities, requiring greater effort and in which the child must move his total body in space, through his own efforts, or with the assistance of mechanical devices (crutches, wheelchairs, etc.). Games chosen for inclusion use a minimum of special equipment and require the child's intellectual involvement whenever possible.

The book is graphically illustrated with line drawings. It is clearly written and includes descriptions of the games and the intended results. Although aimed at physical educators, the book will be useful for anyone dealing with the mobility impaired child in a recreational setting. Recommended for general and professional collections.

Croucher, Norman. <u>Outdoor Pursuits for Disabled People</u>. London: Disabled Living Foundation, 1981. 192 pp.

Norman Croucher is a skilled rock climber and mountaineer who has had both legs amputated below the knee. In this report, he details ways in which the physically disabled can be encouraged to take part in outdoor pursuits. Visual handicaps, deafness, epilepsy, and diabetes are considered along with mobility impairments. Safety, insurance, competition, and prosthetic devices are discussed in the introduction. A few of the less common activities mentioned are spelunking, gliding, rock climbing, snorkelling, orienteering, and waterskiing. The author lists only British organizations and publications. Recommended for rehabilitation collections.

Dixon, Jess Thomas. <u>Adapting Activities for Therapeutic Recreation Service: Concepts and Applications</u>. San Diego, Calif.: Campanile Press, 1981. 74 pp.

This book presents thirty-two illustrated examples of ideas for modifying recreational activities for individuals with various handicapping conditions. Included are such activities as Twister adapted for the blind, an auditory jump rope, an adapted Etch-a-Sketch, and a snowplay device for a prosthetic hand. The text discusses the theory and social impact of making leisure opportunities accessible to disabled individuals. Although the book is intended for students in therapeutic recreation and for practicing rehabilitation professionals, parents and classroom teachers will find the imaginative techniques useful.

The Easy Path to Gardening. London: Reader's Digest Association, 1972. 88 pp.

The first part of the work deals with tools and techniques that make work easier and more stimulating for the disabled home gardener. The advice given also applies to patients in a hospital garden. The Gardening as Therapy section was written by doctors and occupational therapists as a manual for use in hospitals. The final chapter addresses problems unique to children's hospitals. Special projects are suggested. There is no bibliogrpahy or index; however, there is a detailed table of contents. Contains excellent illustrations.

Edwards, Eleanor M. Music Education for the Deaf. South Waterford, Maine: The Merriam-Eddy Co., 1974. 248 pp.

Music Education for the Deaf is divided into two parts. The first section is a fairly complete historical study of materials in the area of music and rhythm with the deaf and hard-of-hearing. The main body of the articles which are cited were published in American Annals of the Deaf and in The Volta Review. Other material is scattered in various periodicals, in chapters of books, and in unpublished papers and theses. The earliest article cited was written in 1848 and the latest dates from 1971. The remaining section outlines a program of music education for the deaf. The justification and goals of such a program are articulated. Specific techniques for teaching rhythm, tempo, melody, dynamics, harmony, and tone color are given. The author draws from her experiences as a music educator at the Crotched Mountain School for the Deaf in Greenfield, New Hampshire. An extensive bibliography with an author index is provided. The depth of coverage makes this book especially valuable for the music educator of the deaf and hard-of-hearing. Recommended for professional collections.

Funk, Deborah. Travel Agent Guidelines for Travel Planning for the Physically Handicapped. Washington, D.C.: Hawkins and Assoc. 1979. 37 pp.

This practical booklet is designed for use by travel agents. The first section describes several of the most prevalent physical disabilities: blindness, deafness, ambulatory limitations, respiratory ailments, kidney disease, and diabetes. The extent of travel assistance required by those affected with disabilities is then outlined. The author discusses special the arrangements required when traveling by ship, air, rail, or rented car. A questionnaire for use in interviewing the client is reproduced. An extensive bibliography enhances the usefulness of the pamphlet. Recommended for general collections.

Gault, Elizabeth, and Sykes, Susan. <u>Crafts for the Disabled</u>. New York: Thomas Y. Crowell, 1979. 120 pp.

Using methods they developed in their own work with disabled, the authors have adapted basic craft techniques for persons suffering from varying degrees of disability. They use easily available household items and have kept the gadgetry to a minimum and assume the person attempting the craft has never done anything like it before. The book is designed to help disabled people become independent and in the practice of knitting, crocheting, chair caning, canvas embroidery, and making soft toys. Each chapter begins with a list of the necessary materials and equipment and includes a list of craft suppliers in England. The book should be of interest to the disabled individuals, to teachers, friends, or relatives, or to staff in residential homes or day centers.

Geddes, Dolores. <u>Physical Activities for Individuals with Handicapping Conditions</u>. 2d ed. St. Louis, Mo.: Mosby, 1978. 150 pp.

Dolores Geddes presents a noncategorical approach to modifying physical education and recreational activities for individuals with handicapping conditions. She directs the text toward students who are taking adapted physical education or therapeutic recreation courses, as well as toward leaders of physical activity programs. The handicapping conditions dealt with are subaverage intellectual function, learning disabilities, visual impairments, hearing problems, orthopedic conditions, and emotional disturbances. To facilitate evaluation, she includes a chapter on examples of behaviors that might be developed in participants and a list of references for evaluation criteria. For each handicapping condition a brief overview is followed by general suggestions for teaching participants. Specific activity suggestions for primary level, intermediate level, and adolescent level, and young adult level are given. She does not include standard descriptions of physical activities and sports. Although the book is directed toward a professional audience, some of the general suggestions will be useful to parents and others.

Gilbertson, Kristina. <u>Physical Education, Recreation and Sports for Individuals with Hearing Impairments</u>. Washington, D.C.: Physical Education and Recreation for the Handicapped, 1976. 122 pp.

This annotated bibliography includes journal articles and books on a variety of topics such as art, recreation, drama, music, sports, and swimming for individuals with hearing impairments. Multiple handicaps involving hearing impairment are beyond the scope of the publication. Other sections of the book cover integration of the hearing impaired into regular programs, program descriptions, physical education, and motor development. The second half of the book reprints articles and lessons from the John Tracy Clinic Correspondence Course for Parents of Preschool Deaf Children. Special chapters cover audiovisual materials and resource organizations and personal contacts. An excellent resource despite the lack of an index.

Gould, Elaine, and Gould, Loren. <u>Arts and Crafts for Physically and Mentally Disabled: the How and Why of It</u>. Springfield, Ill.: Charles C. Thomas, 1978. 348 pp.

"This volume, a happy medium between popular crafts books and specialized scholarly works, is presented for the lay craft worker, the volunteer, the program director, and the professional. Detailed, illustrated instructions for over 120 projects compromise the bulk of the book. However, the authors also include discussions on the overall craft program, availability of supplies, organizational plans, methods for motivating patients to participate, and techniques for working with a variety of disabilities."

The authors do not attempt to explore in-depth all the techniques of the various crafts described or the detailed therapeutic methods of working with specific disorders. The tips on managing a craft program will be useful for anyone using crafts with a group. Recommended for general collections.

Groves, Lilian, ed. <u>Physical Education for Special Needs</u>. Cambridge: Cambridge University Press, 1979. 154 pp.

This collection of articles written by British experts presents information about physical education and sport for disabled children. The authors make no attempt to detail types of disabilities, and the emphasis in the book is on enjoyable activitiy rather than therapeutic manipulation. Most activities suggested in the book can be enjoyed by children with varying needs and abilities. Throughout the book, emphasis is given to ways of integrating disabled individuals or groups into regular programs of physical education. It includes a selected bibliography, list of films, a list of useful British addresses, and an index.

Gunn, Scout Lee. <u>Basic Terminology for Therapeutic Recreation and Other Action Therapies</u>. Champaign, Ill.: Stipes Pub. Co., 1975. 83 pp.

This is a glossary of the basic terminology which is used in settings where therapeutic recreators work. The glossary is divided into such categories as mental retardation and gerontology. Some terms are cross-listed. The definitions are clear and concise. A bibliography and a list of symbols used in charting and record keeping are included. Recommended for professional collections.

Guttman, Ludwig. <u>Textbook of Sport for the Disabled</u>. Aylesbury, England: Wiley, 1976. 184 pp.

Professor Guttman, a renown British expert in the field, surveys the historical development of sports for the disabled. He discusses the physiological aspects of training and conditioning. He also includes basic rules, classification, and techniques for specific sports. The disabilities covered are amputation, blindness, cerebral palsy, deafness, and spinal paralysis. Profusely illustrated, this comprehensive manual is recommended for both laymen and professionals because of the breadth of knowledge presented. It is a classic work in the field.

Hamill, Charlotte M., and Oliver, Robert C. <u>Therapeutic Activities for the Handicapped Elderly</u>. Rockville, Md.: Aspen Systems Corporation, 1980. 295 pp.

The majority of this manual (174p.) describes craft projects for use in a therapeutic program for adults, particularly the handicapped elderly. Specific instructions, clear illustrations, and adaptations for the visually handicapped are given for each craft. Charts list a variety of disabilities in four categories: social-psychological, physical, sensory, and perceptual. For each disability appropriate kinds of activities are indicated. The remaining portions of the book discuss the physical facilities and equipment needed to operaate such a therapeutic program. Other chapters discuss such issues as the use of volunteers, the motivation of participants, and education of the staff. Useful appendices list sources for supplies and equipment. Highly recommended for general collections.

Hedley, Eugene. <u>Boating for the Handicapped: Guidelines for the Physically Disabled</u>. Albertson, N.Y.: Human Resources Center, 1979. 114 pp.

The purpose of these educational guidelines is to maximize recreational boating opportunities for the physically disabled by informing disabled consumers of the recreational boating opportunities available to them. For rehabilitation and recreational professionals who counsel and teach handicapped persons, they provide basic guidance and support. The genesis of the guidelines was a strategy paper <u>National Recreational Boating for the Physically Handicapped</u>. (Human Resources Center, 1978) which was developed for the U.S. Coast Guard and which reflected the state-of-the-art in recreational boating for the physically handicapped. It is assumed that the reader is already familiar with basic boating concepts and terminology. One chapter is in braille. Recommended for public libraries and rehabilitation collections.

Hill, Kathleen. <u>Dance for Physically Disabled Persons: A Manual for Teaching Ballroom, Square, and Folk Dances to Users of Wheelchairs and Crutches</u>. Washington, D.C: American Alliance for Health, Physical Education and Recreation, 1976. 114 pp.

The author describes step-by-step procedures for teaching folk, square, and ballroom dancing to individuals in wheelchairs or on crutches. The dances included are fairly easy to teach and follow as closely as possible the moves that a leg dancer would do. The book contains diagrams and illustrations, reprints of articles, an extensive bibliography. In addition, descriptions of the facilities required for teaching dance are included.

Holidays for the Physically Handicapped, 1980. London: The Royal Association for Disabilitiy and Rehabilitation, 1980. 580 pp.

Holidays for the Physically Handicapped is an annual listing of accessible nursing homes and hotels in England, Ireland, Scotland, Wales, and the Channel Islands. For each tourist region, addresses, publications, and ideas for places to visit are given. Special sections include the following: special interest holidays, cruises, sports vacations, youth hostels, work-camps, and camping. The Holidays Abroad section expands the coverage to include transportation, lodging, and travel guides to countries outside the United Kingdom. Symbols indicate the range of disability catered to by each establishment. Listings are primarily for the mobility impaired.

Human Resources Center. National Recreational Boating for the Physically Handicapped: Strategy Paper and Annotated Bibliography. Albertson, N.Y.: Human Resources Center. 1978. 42 pp.

This report, a "state-of-the-art" of recreational boating for the physically disabled, contains recommendations in four areas: safety, independence afloat, emergency procedures, and access to and from boating facilities and boats. Boat manufacturers, marinas, yacht clubs, organizations and individuals with physical disabilities were surveyed. The information is presented clearly and concisely in a readable style. No prior knowledge on the part of the reader is assumed. The extensive bibliography includes books, journal articles, and publications from such organizations as the American Red Cross. The annotations are concise and useful. The report is designed by and for professionals engaged in various aspects of rehabilitation and/or boating.

Hutchinson, Peggy, and Lord, John. Recreation Integration: Issues and Alternatives in Leisure Services and Community Involvement. Ottawa: Leisurability, 1979. 152 pp.

Many communities are having difficulty integrating the disabled into existing recreational programs. This comes as no surprise to the authors given the dominant assumptions, values, and priorities which exist in most communities toward those who are different and toward the process of recreation. This book will serve as an indispensable manual for anyone concerned with community recreation programs: disabled consumers, parents of disabled children, community leaders, and recreation professionals. The authors have combined a philosophical concern for society's values with practical guidelines. In articulating a model to guide recreation practice, the authors explore: Process of Recreation in the Community, Upgrading Personal and Community Settings, Educating Consumers, Volunteers, Parents and Professionals, and Implementing and Evaluating a Recreation Integration Plan. Because people need to work together to make integration happen, consumer groups and activist disabled consumers will become more influential in the future. The primary focus of integration must be on the transformation of social values; only secondary is there a concern for technical solutions.

<u>Involving Impaired, Disabled, and Handicapped Persons in Regular Camp Programs</u>. Washington, D.C.: American Alliance for Health, Physical Education, and Recreation, 1976. 121 pp.

This publication is intended to provide some broad guidelines for camp personnel who serve disabled children in nonspecialized or regular day and residential camps. Case studies are included to illustrate the guidelines. The information is divided into three basic areas. The first section discusses practical issues as matching camps and campers, adapting activities, and facilitating adjustment to camp. For each section an extensive annotated bibliography analyzes pertinent literature. A separate chapter annotates audiovisual materials. Forms used to obtain information about campers are reprinted. Recommended for professional collections.

Kay, Jane G. <u>Crafts for the Very Disabled and Handicapped</u>. Springfield, Ill.: Charles C. Thomas, 1977. 205 pp.

The author presents a compilation of craft projects based on her own real-life experiences working with the disabled, the aged, and the mentally handicapped. However, in this book she is primarily concerned with nursing home residents. The projects are intended to hold the interest of adults, and can be completed in a one-hour session utilizing readily available and inexpensive materials. Each project is graded according to the level of difficulty; and all crafts are limited to a low level of difficulty. Detailed patterns and diagrams are accompanied by explicit direction. Projects are such practical items as salt beads, wind chimes, Christmas ornaments, recipe card holders, and potato print greeting cards. The book is designed for use by volunteers and by occupational therapists. A separate chapter discusses craft therapy. Useful for general collections and public libraries.

Kelly, Jerry D., ed. <u>Recreation Programming for Visually Impaired Children and Youth</u>. New York: American Foundation for the Blind, 1981. 160 pp.

Leaders from the fields of recreation and vision have pooled their knowledge to bring the reader a text on recreation programming for children who experience visual limitations. The book is designed primarily for the recreation consultant or trainer who is concerned with assisting the community recreation leader in his efforts to provide recreation programs and services for the visually impaired child. Built around a theme of what the recreation leader would need to know to be an effective programmer, the book attempts to look at questions and issues from an applied perspective, utilizing a "how-to" approach. Background material includes the history of educational and recreational services to visually impaired persons, an overview of federal legislation which mandates a policy of integration, and an introduction to visual impairments. Chapters on programming concerns discuss relations with parents, integration of disabled children into existing programs, and administrative concerns. Special consideration has been given to the topics of finance, safety, liability, and staff training. The final chapter provides further sources of information with annotated listings of resources at the national, state, and local levels.

Making Physical Education and Recreation Facilities Accessible to All: Planning, Designing, Adapting. Washington, D.C.: American Alliance for Health, Physical Education and Recreation, 1977. 138 pp.

This comprehensive annotated bibliography serves as a resource to enable readers to plan accessible facilities or to remove architectural barriers in existing facilities which are designed for physical education, recreation, and sports. The preface and the introductions to each chapter present overviews of the architectural standards for accessible playgrounds, outdoor recreation facilities, and swimming pools. The references are to books, journal articles, pamphlets, and reports from governmental and other sources. Separate chapters cover architectural accessibility legislation, travel, and tourism. Appendices list organizations, equipment suppliers, and laws. Highly recommended for libraries serving architects, community planners, adaptive physical educators, and therapeutic recreators.

Materials on Creative Arts (Arts, Crafts, Dance, Drama, Music and Bibliotherapy) for Persons with Handicapping Conditions. Rev. Washington, D.C.: American Alliance for Health, Physical Education and Recreation, 1977. 100 pp.

This annotated bibliography provides references for persons who include art, crafts, dance, drama, and music in programs for individuals with various handicapping conditions. The basic criteria for inclusion in the bibliography was the general applicability of the described activity to creative art programs for the disabled. These materials are appropriate for education programs, recreational activities, rehabilitation efforts, or therapeutic purposes. Certain activities are designed for structured or formal settings while others are more appropriate for creative or informal settings. The materials come from a variety of sources and from personnel with a variety of backgrounds, experiences, and training. Materials are divided into five sections: State-of-the-Art, Printed References, Audiovisual Materials, People and Organizations, Equipment and Material Suppliers. Within the Printed Materials section the book, journal, and other types of citations are divided by type of activity. Recommended for rehabilitation collections.

Midwest Symposium on Therapeutic Recreation, St. Louis, 1975. Expanding Horizons in Therapeutic Recreation: Selected Papers from the 1975 Symposium. Columbia, Mo.: University of Missouri, 1976. 103 pp.

This is a selection of thirteen papers presented at the 1975 Midwest Symposium on Therapeutic Recreation. The papers cover a wide range of topics within the broad area of therapeutic recreation. Of special interest here are those on "Recreation for the Deaf-Blind," "Trails, "Playgrounds and Activities for the Handicapped," and "European Programming for the Handicapped." A separate chapter on "Audiovisual Instructional Materials" lists audiocassettes, films, filmstrips, transparencies, and videotapes useful for educators in therapeutic recreation. Recommended for rehabilitation collections.

Miller, Arthur G., and Sullivan, James V. Teaching Physical Activities to Impaired Youth. New York: John Wiley & Sons, 1982. 242 pp.

This book is designed for students, teachers, and supervisors in the fields of elementary, secondary, special, and adapted physical education. The book is organized into three parts. Part I, "Learning About Impaired Youth," has an introduction, descriptions of various types of impairments, and information on self-concept and body image. Part II, "Evaluating and Planning Activity Programs." familiarizes the reader with pupil evaluation, individualized educational planning, the mainstreamed program, the adapted program, and adapted activities. Part III, "Instructing Impaired Youth," provides information on the team approach, tactics for instruction, teaching approaches, and suggestions. Parents and other family members will find that the book provides information on what physical activities are appropriate and how to teach them to impaired children.

Muller Henrik, and Rolen, Gosta. Airlines and Disabled Traveller. Stockholm: ICTA Information Centre, 1977. 54 pp.

Disabled persons utilizing the international air transportation system meet with varying degrees of success depending on the type and extent of their disability. This investigative study surveys air terminals, aircraft, and passenger services; and, it formulates proposals to increase the ease and safety of disabled air travelers. Fifteen experienced disabled travelers relate their experiences. From these case studies, a summary table of the actions an air traveler must undergo in order to complete his journey has been developed. Descriptions of terminal facilities and aircraft are presented with complete diagrams. Useful for engineers, architects, and planners.

Nelson, John G. Wheelchair Vagabond: a Guide and a Goad for the Handicapped Traveler. Santa Monica, Calif.: Project Press, 1975. 132 pp.

John Nelson, who suffers from multiple sclerosis and heart problems, writes a personal narrative of his numerous camping trips in the United States. He outlines his "drive and rest" technique of van camping. He includes complete information on choosing a vehicle, storing gear, planning the itinerary, and purchasing equipment. The author's suggestions, based on his own experience, include things he would have done differently and why. The suggestions are mostly for those traveling on a limited budget. A unique chapter tells where to meet the "natives" and get acquainted during necessary rest periods. This is a realistic and thoroughly practical account, written in a readable direct style. The book contains line drawings, checklists, and appendices which list tourism offices, campground guides, camping equipment catalogs, and camping publications.

Newman, Judy. Swimming for Children with Physical and Sensory Impairments: Methods and Techniques for Therapy and Recreation. Springfield, Ill.: Charles C. Thomas, 1976. 187 pp.

In this volume Judy Newman shares her techniques and technical know-how to help other teachers use swimming, aquatics, and water environments for therapy, recreation, and fun. In the first chapter she discusses swim patterning, the method whereby the development of the disabled child can be aided through the use of a series of coordinated movement patterns. Clear descriptions and simple illustrations provide practical and functional information and direction for using this technique. Separate chapters deal with specific applications of swim patterning and other proven teaching methods for children with spina bifida, traumatic paraplegia, multiple handicaps, spastic and athetoid cerebral palsy, and junior rheumatoid arthritis, as well as for those who are blind or deaf. Additional chapters detail how to organize and conduct swim shows, swim meets, and fun days. The final section provides answers to questions most often posed at workshops, institutes, and classes.

O'Morrow, Gerald S. Therapeutic Recreation: A Helping Profession. 2d ed. Reston, Va.: Reston Publishing Co., 1980. 336 pp.

Therapeutic Recreation: A Helping Profession is an introductory text intended for students in their first two years of college. In addition, it can be adapted for use in in-service training programs within health and correctional agencies and institutions. Overall, the book explores with the student the profession

of therapeutic recreation, what demands the profession will make
of him, and whether he possesses the talents and abilities to
meet those demands. The first section offers an overview of the
following topics: the importance of recreation, the prevalence
and characteristics of special populations, the attitude of society toward special populations, the agencies and institutions
that offer rehabilitation and special services to special populations, and historical base of rehabilitation and therapeutic recreation. The second section considers the philosophical orientation toward therapeutic recreation as a process and as a service.
The third section explores the competencies necessary to be a successful therapeutic recreation specialist. Suggested reading are
listed at the end of each chapter. The appendices included medical terminology, drug therapy progress note guidelines, professional standards, and a listing of voluntary and professional organizations involved in rehabilitation. Recommended for professional collections.

Oppelt, Kurt. Oppelt Standard Method of Therapeutic and Recreational Ice Skating. State College, Pa.: Kurt Oppelt, 1974. 38 pp.

The author, a former Olympic gold medal winner, introduces
his own tested method of teaching ice skating to the disabled or
the beginning recreational skater. Written for teachers and students with little or no previous skating experience, the book is
a text on the technique of teaching both individuals and groups.
As such, it may be useful in pre-service and in-service training
for physical educators, recreational therapists, and skating instructors involved in recreation and therapeutic ice skating programs. The text is profusely illustrated with black and white
photographs. Recommended for general collections.

Overs, Robert P.; O'Connor, Elizabeth; and Demarco, Barbara.
Avocational Activities for the Handicapped. Springfield, Ill.:
Charles C. Thomas, 1974. 178 pp.

This text is designed to bring to the field of avocational
counseling tools and techniques comparable to those developed in
vocational counseling. The book presents descriptive information
about a selected group of avocations. The avocations are classified and coded according to the classification system in the Avocational Activities Inventory. The descriptions in this book are
written from the point of view of a person searching for avocational activities and they are designed for use in avocation
counseling by counselors, recreation therapists, occupational
therapists, and social workers. This volume does not attempt to
give all of the information necessary to set up and supervise an
activity; therefore, detailed game rules are omitted. Information
about each avocational activity is presented in two ways. A check
list section includes a listing of the environmental factors and
social-psychological factors associated with the activity. It

estimates whether the activity is within the physical and/or mental capacity of an individual with a given type of impairment, and it gives an estimated range of energy expenditure expressed in METS (energy expenditure unit). Following the checklist, each activity is described in narrative form. The emphasis in the narrataive is on the phenomenological and other psychological dimensions of the activity, the interpersonal relationships involved, and the social setting in which it occurs. Recommended for professional collections.

Owen, Edward S. Playing and Coaching Wheelchair Basketball. Urbana, Ill.: University of Illinois Press, 1982. 320 pp.

Edward S. Owen has played wheelchair basketball since 1961 and he has coached the game since 1972. He provides a brief history of the sport. His main concentration, however, is on coaching techniques and the philosophy and the development of player skills. This comprehensive and heavily illustrated book will be valuable to both players and coaches.

Physical Education and Recreation for Impaired, Disabled and Handicapped Individuals...Past, Present and Future. Washington, D.C.: American Alliance for Health, Physical Education, and Recreation, 1976. 424 pp.

This report is based on State of the Art: Physical Education and Recreation for Handicapped Individuals, Part One of the final report for the Information and Research Utilization Center in Physical Education and Recreation for the Handicapped (IRUC). Experts in the field address the following issues: professional preparation, physical education for individuals with various handicapping conditions, and program organization and administration. Priorities for the profession are established in these areas, and extensive bibliographies are listed.

Reamy, Lois. TravelAbility; a Guide for the Physically Disabled Travelers in the United States. New York: Macmillan, 1978. 298 pp.

Lois Reamy has written the most comprehensive travel book for those with limited physical mobility who need special arrangements when they travel. Information useful to blind, deaf, or mentally retarded travelers has been included when available. In order to provide a detailed approach to travel, this book is limited to the United States, with only an occasional reference and an appendix of international sources. Sections cover how to plan a trip, how to go, where to go, and where to stay. The chapter on "Medical Questions and Answers" is written by Arthur S. Abramson, M.D., chairman of rehabilitation medicine at Albert Einstein College of Medicine and a disabled traveler himself. Hundreds of addresses are given for obtaining additional travel information. This is an excellent presentation of practical advice on all aspects of travel.

Robinson, Frank M. Therapeutic Re-Creation: Ideas and Experiences. Springfield, Ill.: Charles C. Thomas, 1974. 181 pp.

This work is a compilation of papers written by graduate students who are studying for a Master's degree in recreation and who are employed in a variety of therapeutic settings. Work with the physically disabled, the mentally retarded, the emotionally and socially maladjusted, and the elderly is related. Additional sections of the book cover approaches and concerns in the field of therapeutic recreation. The papers present a practical approach from a personal point of view.

Savitz, Harriet May. Wheelchair Champions: A History of Wheelchair Sports. New York: Thomas Y. Crowell, 1978. 117 pp.

Utilizing the files and resources of Sports 'n Spokes magazine, plus other sources, the author has compiled a short history of wheelchair sports from the beginnings in the 1940's to 1977. Biographical sketches of athletes are included. Although the writer's style is a bit inspirational in tone, the book contains information that may be difficult to find elsewhere. The lack of any tabular data of sports records limits its usefulness, however. Recommended for public libraries.

Sherrill, Claudine, ed. Creative Arts for the Severely Handicapped. 2d. ed. Springfield, Ill.: Charles C. Thomas, 1979. 286 pp.

This work, the collaborative effort of twenty-seven experts in the field, consists of articles on proven practical techniques for teaching music, dance, drama, art, and creative expression to the severely disabled. Articles provide a review of research in the field, present the state-of-the-art, and describe the severely disabled population. The authors, who write clearly and avoid jargon, have produced an excellent introduction to the field, as well as comprehensive manual for the practitioner. The book includes an extensive combined bibliography (31 pp).

Shivers, Jay S., and Fait, Hollis F. Therapeutic and Adapted Recreational Services. Philadelphia: Lea & Febiger, 1975. 366 pp.

"This book is designed for use in preparing recreationists whose future employment will be in the therapeutic program of a treatment center or in recreational service in a community setting." An overview of the therapeutic and adapted recreational services in these two settings is presented first. Subsequent chapters deal with the medical and pyschological aspects of physical and mental disabilities, the organization of treatment settings, and the administration of recreation programs. The authors include techniques and methods developed from their personal experience in working with the disabled. Separate chapters on the performing and graphic arts, camping and nature-oriented activities, and games and sports relate techniques for conducting specific activities. The philosophical premise of the book is that each handicapped person should be treated as an individual who has certain abilities as well as certain limitations. Recommended for special collections.

Sosne, Michael. Handbook of Adapted Physical Education Equipment and Its Use. Springfield, Ill.: Charles C. Thomas, 1972. 210 pp.

The primary focus of the manual is the use of adaptive physical education equipment by the physically and mentally handicapped student. Geared toward the regular classroom teacher, as well as to special education and physical education teachers, the book describes techniques of adapting and constructing equipment. Of special interest are the two appendices listing sources for equipment and supplies. Other appendices list audiovisual materials useful in teaching sports techniques.

Sport and Physical Recreation for the Disabled. London: Disabled Living Foundation, 1970. 22 pp.

This study is a report of a panel charged by the Disabled Living Foundation "to investigate the existing participation in recreational activities with particular reference to physical recreation by the disabled and in light of these findings to pursue means of extending this participation." Written totally with a view to facilities and activities in Great Britain, this inquiry is useful only for international comparative study. Recommended for professional collections.

Walberg, Franette. Dancing to Learn: a Contemporary Dance Curriculum for Learning and Physically Handicapped Adolescents. Novato, Calif.: Academic Therapy Publications, 1979. 104 pp.

The author utilizes disco dance as an approach to building self-esteem, motor skills, and body-image in learning-disabled and physically disabled teens. The majority of the book describes dance steps; and the text is illustrated with excellent photographs. A separate chapter recounts current research on self-esteem. Because no information is given as to how to adapt the dance steps for the use of the mobility impaired students, the book is primarily useful for teaching the developmentally disabled or students with learning disabilities.

Walter, Felix. Sports Centres & Swimming Pools. Edinburgh: The Thistle Foundation, 1971. 39 pp.

Access to public buildings, including sports and recreational facilities is a prerequisite for the social integration of the disabled. In this book, Mr. Walter presents design elements which building committees and architects concerned with such buildings should consider for the disabled. Many of these same features also benefit the able-bodied and can be incorporated at little or no cost if included at the planning stage. Mr. Walter bases his recommendations on his survey of existing facilities in the United Kingdom and on the continent. This is an excellent overview and should be consulted by anyone planning a sports center. Clear illustrations and a comprehensive index enhance the usefulness of the book. Recommended for professional collections.

Weiss, Louise. Access to the World: a Travel Guide for the Handicapped. New York: Chatham Square Press, 1977. 178 pp.

This basic travel guide includes chapters on tips for traveling by airplane, bus, automobile, train, and ship. It includes a list of domestic and international destination and access guides, plus a list of tour operators. Selective lists of accessible hotels and motels give the criteria that hotel and motel chains use to designate their firms' rooms as accessible. The chapter on air travel lists policies of 24 airlines regarding disabled travelers and includes a guide to the accessibility of airport terminals. Much of the information included is covered by other guides such as Annand's.

Wheeler, Ruth Hook, and Hooley, Agnes M. Physical Education for the Handicapped. 2d ed. Philadelphia: Lea & Febiger, 1976. 385 pp.

This basic textbook is designed for the professional training of adaptive physical education teachers and therapeutic exercise teachers. As such, it cover such topics as the nervous system, mechanical and muscular efficiency, and common deviations of posture. The authors recommend activities for persons afflicted by fifteen different diseases and conditions found in school populations. These include mental retardation, learning disabilities, deviations of posture, cerebral palsy, and the orthopedically handicapped. The authors discuss the management of the integrated physical education program within the school setting. Of special interest is the chapter "Camping for the Handicapped" which may be used by parents in selecting a camp for a disabled child. Recommended for professional collections.

Witt, Peter A., Community Leisure Services and Disabled Individuals. Rev. ed. Washington, D.C.: Hawkins, 1979. 134 pp.

This book gives an overview of the fundamental problems in planning, developing, and delivering leisure services for the disabled at the municipal level. Elected officials and others are often reluctant to initiate or to expand leisure services for that minority of the community which is disabled. This book attempts to counter that reluctance by providing guidance on such issues as a philosophy of service, transportation, community responsibility, and architectural barriers. Reprints of twelve articles from the Journal of Leisurability are included. Article titles range from "How to Fire a Volunteer" to "Emerging Leisure Counseling Concepts and Orientations." Recommended for general collections.

12 THE DISABLED CHILD

BETSY K. BAKER/Reference Librarian, Northwestern University Library, Evanston, Illinois

INTRODUCTION

In recent years strides have been made in identifying and studying the special needs of disabled children. As a result, there have been many books written which may be useful to the professional who works with the disabled child and his family. The works which are reviewed in this chapter were chosen because they provide the professional with information necessary for counseling the child and those who interact with the child.

A child can be considered disabled if he, through some anomaly, varies from his peers. Disabled children may be motor handicapped or otherwise physically disabled, suffering from brain dysfunction, or motor handicapped with a brain disorder. The anomoly is such that special services are required to meet the needs of the child. Current estimates show that more than nine million children and youth from infancy to age 20 are considered to be disabled in some way. The National Foundation for March of Dimes estimates that six percent, or one in every 14 babies is born with a significant birth defect and that 250,000 children are born in the U.S. each year with a handicapping defect.(1)

As such, the study of disabled children is a broad field and encompasses psychologic, social, intellectual, medical and physical problems of the child. Because of the extremely broad nature of this topic, the special problems of the disabled child treated here have been limited to two areas: physical development and functioning of the child; and emotional and social development of the child. Although the works selected deal primarily with these topics, many of them address other aspects of the disabled child as well. Titles dealing specifically with special education have been excluded.

There is extensive literature on the physical, behavioral and social adjustment of disabled children. A good introduction and survey of the literature completed in the 1950's and 1960's is Solnit's _Physical Illness and Handicaps in Childhood_. The papers included in this anthology have contributed to the understanding of what a child experiences when he is ill. These papers also address the problem of how parents and others can enable the child to achieve psychological adjustment as well as physical rehabilitation. A more recent review of research in the field can be obtained in Cruickshank's _Psychology of Exceptional Children and Youth_. Now in its fourth edition, this compilation reflects new trends and developments in the field. An excellent overview of the disabled child is Gliedman and Roth's _The Unexpected Minority: Handicapped Children in America_. Virtually every aspect of disability is examined with specific discussion concerning the ways that society misconstrues the abilities of the handicapped child.

A number of other titles reviewed also provide a general overview of the educational, physical, psychological, and social problems of disabled children. The titles which follow resemble texts in format and content and may serve as a professional introduction to the field of disabled child psychology. For example, _The Handicapped Child_ by Bowley and Gardner addresses the specific needs of the disabled child and suggests how they can be met. A work which emphasizes the physical aspects of childhood disability is _The Child With Disabling Illness_ by Downey and Low and covers selected illnesses in children, disorders of the neuromuscular system, and disorders of the musculoskeletal system. This work is a good source of technical information. Henderson's _Disability in Childhood and_

Youth gives a balanced treatment of the physical and psychological aspects of the subject.

The physical, psychological, and social adjustment to the environment is discussed at length in the chapter on Mobility Impairment and Barrier Free Design. However, there are several works reviewed here which address environmental issues of the disabled child. Halliday and Kurzhal provide specific ideas for teachers and parents to aid them in developing an environment which is conclusive for learning in Stimulating Environments for Children Who are Visually Impaired. They stress that a child's understanding of the environment is a prerequisite to learning. Calhoun and Hawisher in Teaching and Learning Strategies for Physically Handicapped Students provide guidelines for barrier free school facilities. Another title providing similar information is Edington's The Physically Handicapped Child in Your Classroom. Susan and Andrew Dibner in Integration or Segregation for the Physically Handicapped Child explore the social and psychological issues of integrative and segregative social structures by studying disabled children attending integrative summer camps and segregative summer camps. It was found that both structures offer positive and negative aspects for the child. A collection of readings by Loring and Burn entitled Integration of Handicapped Children in Society addresses the issue of integrating handicapped children in traditional schools.

Although visually and hearing impaired individuals are treated indepth in other chapters of this book as well, several titles are included here which address the special problems faced by children. Chapman's Visually Handicapped Children and Young People provides a theoretical overview of the subject. Freeman's Understanding the Deaf/Blind Child describes practical suggestions for pre-school activities to help parents and teachers of the deaf/blind child better assist in the development of the child.

Research has recently explored the parents influence on the psychological adjustment of the child and how important it is for parents and children with disabilities to receive competent counseling. A number of titles reviewed here address this issue specifically, Webster's <u>Professional Approaches with Parents of Handicapped Children</u>, Seligman's <u>Strategies for Helping Parents of Exceptional Children</u>, Noland's <u>Counseling Parents of the Ill and the Handicapped</u>, Buscaglia's <u>The Disabled and Their Parents</u>, and Tymchuk's <u>Parent and Family Therapy</u>.

The field addressed in this chapter is one of very active research. Increasingly sophisticated methods of early disability identification have been developed along with tactics of early intervention. With society's increased awareness of the problems of these children, more programs and services are in existance today than ever before. Even with recent declines in federal spending, activity in the field should continue. New works are introduced regularly which extend our present knowledge and understanding of the problems of disabled children. The books described below provide a view of the state of the art as it exists today.

NOTES

1. Brewer, Garry A. and James S. Kakalik. <u>Handicapped Children: Strategies for Improving Services</u>. New York: McGraw-Hill, 1979. 611 pp.

ANNOTATED BIBLIOGRAPHY

Allen, K. Eileen; Holm, Vanja A.; Schiefelbusch, Richard L. <u>Early Intervention: A Team Approach</u>. Baltimore, Md.: University Park Press, 1978. 489 pp.

The text "explains and describes the professional activities of an interdisciplinary team working to guide developmentally delayed or impaired children." The efforts of the team are considered in relation to early intervention activities of teachers whose efforts are influenced by the recommendations of the team. The continuing activities, in turn, produce feedback to the team. Team diagnosis is combined with an individualized instructional program. The book begins with an introductory section on normal and abnormal child development and early childhood education followed by a review of the philosophy and tactics of interaction. Individual chapters deal with the developmental team and examine the clinical nurse, pediatrician, therapist, nutritionist, psycholgist, communications specialist, social worker and the early childhood educational specialist. The book concludes with a section covering specific aspects of intervention: organizing program implementation, developing a curriculum for early intervention and specifying teaching strategies. This work should serve as a valuable aid to those professionals interested in interdisciplinary training.

Anderson, Elizabeth M. The Disabled Schoolchild: A Study of Integration in Primary Schools. Fakenham, Norfolk: Cox and Wyman, Ltd., 1973. 377 pp.

The author studied ninety-nine disabled children who were in traditional schools, first measuring the extent of their handicaps and then looking at the social, emotional, and educational problems they met using their classmates as the control group for comparison. This study found that the likelihood of success for a physically handicapped child in a traditional school depends on social class, size of family, intelligence level and a child's extent of neurological damage. The author is research officer at the University of London, Institute of Education. An excellent book for teachers and researchers. Research data, case history material, and references to literature, are included.

Bergsma, Daniel, and Palver, Ann E. Developmental Disabilities: Psychologic and Social Implications. New York: Alan R. Liss, 1976. 188 pp.

This collection of proceedings from the 1976 National Foundation March of Dimes Conference on Developmental Disabilities includes papers which discuss the medical aspects of the developmental disabled, pre-adult disability, individual and family needs, and society's reaction to the handicapped. The list of contributors is impressive with all actively involved in the medical, social psychological or educational problems of the handicapped. Richardson's review of the research dealing with the social consequences of physical disability and Hewett's presentation of some of the problems of research concerning the families of children who suffer from cerebral palsy or mental retardation should be of particular interest to those individuals interested in research of disabled children.

Bowley, Agatha H., and Gardner, Leslie. The Handicapped Child. London: Churchill Livingstone, 1980. 242 pp.

Bowley and Gardner provide a compact, yet comprehensive text on the educational, psychological and social problems of handicapped children and suggest how their special needs can be met. The volume begins with a chapter on handicapped people in general and their position in society. A look at the psychological effects of handicap is presented. The authors then discuss the child with physical handicaps. Emphasis in this section is primarily on the child with cerebral palsy. Cerebral palsy has been researched extensively as it is the most frequently encountered disabling condition in children. The authors state that knowledge gained in this area has shown to be applicable in other handicaps. A chapter on work with the handicapped in developing countries has been included in this edition. Brief case studies are distributed through the work. An excellent overview on the subject and should be a useful addition to professionals and students.

Bricker, Diane D. <u>Intervention with At-Risk and Handicapped Infants: From Research to Application</u>. Baltimore, Md.: University Park Press, 1982. 317 pp.

This publication contains a collection of readings focusing on the need to expand communications between researchers and practitioners concerning handicapped and at-risk infants. The readings evolved from a conference entitled "Handicapped and At-Risk Infants: Research, and Application" which was held in the Asilomar Conference Center, Pacific Grove, California, in May 1980. A primary goal of this volume is to establish a foundation for increasing useful exchanges between practitioners and researchers. The contributors to the volume have addressed the research/practitioner issue through a variety of topics. The first section discusses theory to practice concerns. A primary concern is the neglect of theory in the area of handicapped and at-risk populations resulting in a literature that is difficult for practitioners to apply. Section two addresses assessment issues and contains four papers. A review of assessment strategies for infants is provided, problems confronting interventionists are described, hazards of central tendency measures are outlined, and a warning against adoption of only one assessment strategy is presented. Section three is devoted to a discussion of problems encountered with assessing at-risk and handicapped children. Section four and five deal with environmental, social, and developmental issues. The final section suggests direction and content for intervention. This is a very useful publication for the educator, theorist, student, and practitioner. In one volume, a variety of issues central to the issue of early intervention are presented. Practical systems, strategies, and procedures for intervention are provided. The papers have been contributed by experts in the field, educators, and field researchers. This should be a welcome addition to the literature in the field.

Brown, Sara L., and Moersch, Martha S. <u>Parents on the Team</u>. Ann Arbor: University of Michigan Press, 1982. c1978. 192 pp.

This publication is the result of two programs that were funded between 1973-1976 by the "Frist Chance" Network of the Handicapped Children's Early Education Program, Bureau of Education for the Handicapped to support parents as primary treatment providers for handicapped children and to provide in-service training and consultation to school systems and agencies wishing to develop early intervention programs for handicapped children. Parents were assigned active roles in all phases of the development of their handicapped children in these programs. This book was written to help parents assume the active role and to point out to professionals the roles parents can play in securing services for their child. An excellent publication for parents and professionals. Included is an extensive bibliography.

Buscaglia, L. The Disabled and Their Parents: A Counseling Challenge. Thorofare, N.J.: Charles B. Slack, Inc., 1975. 393 pp.

The primary objective of this book is to help disabled persons and their families understand the nature and implications of a disability. For this understanding to occur, professional counseling is crucial. However, the current lack of conclusive research is an impediment to good counseling. Buscaglia hopes to make the professional community more aware of the importance of counseling disabled children and their families and have this awareness reflected by research. A review of the literature about the guidance of disabled children and their parents is included. A general bibliography is provided, along with a list of suggested readings. A highly recommended book for parents and professionals.

Caldwell, Bettye M., and Stedman, Donald J. Infant Education: A Guide for Helping Handicapped Children in the First Three Years. New York: Walker & Co., 1977. 167 pp.

Research has suggested that infancy is the best time to begin working with disadvantaged children. The papers included in this book review the work of the last few years in this area. Chapter 1 presents evidence supporting early intervention programs and identifies problems with existing programs. Chapter 2 explores the implications of early detection of children with handicapping conditions. Assessment of the handicapped infant is considered in Chapter 3. Existing infant programs are described in the remaining chapters. These case studies provide practical information and would be a resource for consultation by other professionals considering the development of programs for infants.

Calhoun, Mary Lynne, and Hawisher, Margaret F. Teaching and Learning Strategies for Physically Handicapped Students. Baltimore, Md.: University Park Press, 1979. 362 pp.

This text is written for school personnel to assist them in their efforts to expand or establish programs for physically handicapped children. The practical issues of establishing a classroom program, developing teaching materials, and working with other professionals are discussed. The appendices include a list of agencies for sharing teaching ideas, guidelines for barrier-free school facilities, media for in-service education, and a listing of organizations and agencies serving persons with physical handicaps.

Chapman, Elizabeth K. Visually Handicapped Children and Young People. Boston: Routledge & Kegan, 1978. 162 pp.

Elizabeth Chapman discusses numerous aspects of the visually handicapped child in this work. The first two chapters review the nature and implications of visual handicaps and the concerns of the parent. The following chapters focus on the educational issues of the disabled child. The book concludes with an examination of the social and personal development of the blind child and blind adolescent. A substantial bibliography is included. The work is primarily intended for those who teach or are studying to teach visually handicapped children. However, it should also be of assistance to other educators, psychologists or social workers who have contact with visually handicapped children.

Cratty, Bryant J., and Sams, Theressa A. The Body-Image of Blind Children. New York: American Foundation for the Blind, 1968. 72 pp.

The Body-Image of Blind Children is a research report sponsored by the University of California and the American Foundation for the Blind. The purpose of the study was to measure body perception in blind children. The authors state that in order to assist the blind child grasp spatial concepts it is imperative that he first learn about himself and his body. The investigation attempted to develop an assessment device for the evaluation of blind children's body image; to evaluate the body image of a select group of blind children; to make comparisons within the group on the basis of size, age, IQ, etc.; and to develop tasks related to body image training of visually impaired children. The data analysis revealed that it is feasible to assess the blind child's ability to identify body parts and other concepts relative to body image.

Creer, Thomas L., and Christian, Walter P. Chronically Ill and Handicapped Children. Champaign, Ill.: Research Press, 1976. 183 pp.

This book addresses the problem of chronically ill and handicapped children. Statistical data is presented that points out the extent to which such conditions are prevalent. Doctors Creer and Christian describe how "social learning principles can be applied to manage and rehabilitate youngsters who suffer from a chronic disease." Elements common to various applications of behavior modification are discussed. The book focuses on how children can be taught to live productive lives despite a chronic illness. An extensive bibliography supplements the material presented. A good overview of the subject that would be beneficial to students in the health, psychological, and child development fields.

Cruickshank, William M. Psychology of Exceptional Children and Youth. 4th ed. Englewood Cliffs, N.J.: Prentice-Hall, 1980, 595 pp.

Now in its fourth edition, this work provides an excellent overview of the field of psychology of exceptional children and youth. Each chapter for this edition has been prepared by one or more authorities in the field. "The phrase exceptional children and youth means those who by reason of a physical or intellectual variance, are considered unique among their peers". Chapters deal with the psychology or the intellectually superior, as well as those with inferior intellectual ability. The material reflects the trends and the results of recent research. The text is organized in four parts with part one discussing foundation concepts, part two examining the psychological components of language and sensory disabilities, part three commenting on psychological components or physical disabilities, and part four outlining psychological factors in intellectual, perceptual and emotional disabilities.

Curtis, Scott; Donlon, Edward T.; and Wagner, Elizabeth. Deaf Blind Children: Evaluating Their Multiple Handicaps. New York: American Foundation for the Blind, 1970. 172 pp.

For an evaluation of this work, see Chapter 2.

Dibner, Susan Schmidt, and Dibner, Andrew S. Integration or Segregation for the Physically Handicapped Child. Springfield, Ill.: Charles C. Thomas, 1973. 201 pp.

This study explores the social and psychological effects of integrative and segregative social structures on camp children. It developed from an interest of the Massachusetts Easter Seal Society to evaluate their extensive integrated camp program for handicapped children. After conducting a series of preliminary studies to determine if the society's approach was positive, an intensive field study was conducted in two integrated camps and one segregated camp. A small sample was necessary due to the nature of the subject and the method of investigation used. The researchers found in the study that both the integrated and segregated social structures have positive and negative aspects in terms of social interaction, sole behavior, productivity level, and cooperative behavior. They advocate the alteration of some aspects of both types of camps and make some recommendations for improving camp. The study is written in layman language and should be of interest to planners of services for handicapped children, educators, and recreation instructors.

Downey, John A., and Low, Miels L. The Child with Disabling Illness. 2d ed. New York: Raven Press, 1982. 638 pp.

In its second edition, this text, covers selected chronic medical illnesses, disorders of the neuromuscular system, disorders of the musculoskeletal system and injuries, psychosocial aspects, and dentistry for the handicapped. A textbook for professionals seeking specific information concerning a childhood disability.

Doyle, Phyllis, B. Helping the Severely Handicapped Child: A Guide for Parents and Teachers. New York: Crowell, 1979. 150 pp.

For an evaluation of this work, see Chapter 2.

Drouillard, Richard, and Raynor, Sherry. Move It!: A Guide for Helping Visually Handicapped Children Grow. Washington, D.C: AAHPER, 1977. 93 pp.

This booklet has been prepared to assist parents, teachers, and others who interact with the visually disabled child. Specific suggestions for learning activities are presented to keep in the physical and educational development of the child.

Edington, Dorothy. The Physically Handicapped Child in Your Classroom: A Handbook for Teachers. Springfield, Ill.: Charles C. Thomas, 1976. 75 pp.

With increasing numbers of physically handicapped children being integrated into the regular classroom, many teachers are facing a situation which is unfamiliar and for which they may have had no training. This handbook has been compiled to give these teachers an understanding of some of the more common physical disorders that affect children. It deals specifically with cerebral palsy, spina bifida, muscular dystrophy, cystic fibrosis, epilepsy, and Leggperthes disease. The author stresses that the emotional needs of handicapped children are the same as those of all human beings and that it is teacher's attitude that will set the tone of the teacher-student relationship. The guide is easy-to-read, illustrated, and provides a short bibliography at the end of each chapter.

Featherstone, Helen. A Difference in the Family; Life with a Disabled Child. New York: Basic Books, 1980. 262 pp.

Through personal experiences, research and case studies Helen Featherstone explores the ways a handicapped child affects the family. The emotional responses of fear, anger, loneliness, and guilt are examined in the first four chapters. Stress areas in the marital relationship are identified and discussed. The remainder of the book focuses on the parent/professional relationship and the need for getting and giving help. Parents of disabled children will appreciate this frank discussion of the child's affect on family life.

Fine, Peter J., ed. Deafness in Infancy and Early Childhood. New York: Medcom Press, 1974. 232 pp.

This collection of readings covers virtually all issues associated with deafness in early childhood. Dr. Robert J. Ruben discusses medical aspects of deafness and describes the procedures used to diagnose diseases associated with hearing loss. Psychological aspects of deafness are discussed by Dr. Kenneth Z. Altshuler who has had extensive clinical experience in detailing the effects of deafness on the child. McCay Vernon, a professor of psychology, addresses the psychological aspect of diagnosing deafness in a child. General educators explore education issues. David Denton, Richard Brill, Margaret Kent and Nancy Swaiko trace the history of educating deaf children. Dr. Brill describes an educational system known as Total Communication which is designed to use all the communication possibilties left to the deaf child. Mr. Louie Fant, Lecturer in Special Education describes the various forms of sign language and details what he feels is the best communication system for deaf people. The final section of the book is devoted to a discussion of the effect of parent's deafness on hearing children. All contributors to this publication draw upon extensive backgrounds and experience in deaf education. The book is written in a language which is understandable and clear to the lay person as well as the professional. The references included are direct supplements to the readings in the book.

Freeman, Peggy. Understanding the Deaf/Blind Child. London: Heinemann, 1975. 126 pp.

For an evaluation of this work, see Chapter 2.

Gitler, David, and Vigliarolo, Diane. The Handicapped Child and His Family. New York: Institute of Rehabilitation Medicine, New York University Medical Center, 1978. 99 pp.

"This monograph is a result of a conference on "The Handicapped Child and His Family" presented by the staff of the Children's Service of the Institute of Rehabilitation Medicine for the members of the New York City Affiliate of the Association for the Care of Children in Hospitals, 1978." Papers selected for this work include an examination of the implications of disability on the parent-child relationship, a discussion of the self-image of the adolescent, a review of the educational and development concerns of the pre-school child, a social work perspective on the handicapped child and the family, and a paper devoted to determining the physical therapy needs of the handicapped. A brief annotated bibliography on the handicapped child is included.

Gliedman, John, and Roth, William. The Unexpected Minority: Handicapped Children in America. New York: Harcourt, Brace, Jovanovich, 1980. 525 pp.

In this volume, Gliedman and Roth discuss virtually every aspect of disability. Much of the discussion focuses upon the ways that society misconstrues the abilities of the handicapped child. In Part one, they explore the social situation of handicap and ask why society has failed to view the handicapped as an oppressed social group. Part two focuses on the traditional methods used by psychologists to study the development of the handicapped child. Alternatives to these methods are provided and recommended. Part three outlines services available to the handicapped. The potentials and dangers of federal and state legislation designed to "mainstream" handicapped children are explored. The employment situation for the handicapped is described in Part Four. Various social service issues are discussed in the appendices. The authors are addressing a broad audience of specialists and nonspecialists. An extensive use of notes to expand the arguments is presented in the text.

Halliday, Carol, and Kurzhals, Ina W. Stimulating Environments for Children Who are Visually Impaired. Springfield, Ill.: Charles C. Thomas, 1976. 142 pp.

This text provides specific ideas for teachers and parents to aid them in developing an environment which is conducive to learning the importance of a child's understanding of the environment. The role of the parent is reviewed. The necessity of correct educational program placement is stressed and the desired classroom environment is described. Outdoor related activities are discussed at length. Included in the appendices is such practical information as guidelines for designing a day program, a list of nature-focused activities, and sample forms for evaluating the school camp experience. The authors are both professional educators of visually impaired children.

Heward, William; Dardig, Jill C.; and Rossett, Alison. Working with Parents of Handicapped Children. Columbus, Ohio: Charles E. Merril Publishing Co., 1979. 299 pp.

This textbook provides practical information for professionals who have contact with parents of handicapped children. "Its focus is on using behavioral strategies to improve the frequency and quality of parent-professional communication and to increase the productivity of the parent-child relationship." The authors provide information on a behavior change process for parents, a behavior management systems for the home, opportunities parents have to be effective, and the need for parent education. An extensive resource directory is included.

Hart, Verna. Beginning with the Handicapped. Springfield, Ill.: Charles C. Thomas, 1974. 128 pp.

This book was written for parents, teachers, and paraprofessionals who work with young children in activities which will help them attain higher levels of functioning. Teaching techniques are presented in the areas of self-care skills, motor development training, adaptive behavior, and language development. A task analysis approach is used and sample charts are provided for recording levels of functioning as well as for determining task objectives.

Henderson, Peter. Disability in Childhood and Youth. London: Oxford University Press, 1974. 198 pp.

This book provides an "introduction to, not a textbook on, some of the disabilities and difficulties of children and young people that affect their development and education." The disabilities covered include visually handicapped children; partially-hearing and deaf children; children with language and speech disorders not due to deafness; educationally subnormal children; emotional and behavior difficulties and disorders; children with physical disorders; and socially deprived children. This book should benefit teachers and social workers.

Illinois State Office of Education. Bureau of Education for the Handicapped. *Preschool Learning-Activities for the Physically Disabled: A Guide for Parents.* Washington, D.C.: Computer Microfilm International Corporation, 1974. 101 pp.

This publication is intended for parents of disabled children and suggests learning activities for children three to six years of age. The material is presented in five sections: learning to move; self-care skills; learning to think and communicate; developing self awareness; and activities to help a child learn to like himself and others. The importance of play is stressed and the variety of specific suggestions focusing on play activities would benefit teachers of disabled children as well as parents.

Charts covering the stages of normal development from birth to six years of age can be found in the appendix. These charts are suggested to be used as a guide for identifying the child's stage of development once this has been determined, activities can be planned to help him develop from that level. A list of readings is included in the publication.

Karnes, Merle B., and Lee, Richard C. *Early Childhood.* Reston, Va.: Council for Exceptional Children, 1979. 109 pp.

In this monograph, the authors have examined components which they feel are necessary for quality and effective programming activities for the pre-school handicapped child. Each component is discussed in a separate chapter and include identification, parent involvement, mainstreaming, teacher behavior, promoting self concept of the child, ongoing assessment, individualization of instructor, role of the paraprofessional, and promoting generalization. The authors have provided basic research studies associated with each component and directions for implementing the components into existing preschool programs. While the work is primarily of value to school personnel it should also serve as an educational aid to prospective preschool teachers.

Kolodny, Ralph L. *Peer-Oriented Group Work for the Physically Handicapped Child.* Boston: Charles River Books, 1976. 230 pp.

The publication is intended for social workers who interact with disabled children. The author draws upon his affiliation with the Department of Neighborhood Clubs of Boston Children's Services Association (1952-1966) to describe issues encountered in integrated group work of physically disabled and normal children and discusses techniques employed to deal with them. In the Department of Neighborhood Clubs, integrated group work involved establishing a club around a disabled child who was referred to the Department of Counseling with the other members of the club being drawn from among his physically normal peers. This approach is based on the theory that association with normal children under professional leadership can provide many disabled children with a positive emotional experience resulting in the integration of the disabled child into the social life or his peers.

The author stresses the importance adequately preparing not only the child for the new experience but preparing the family of the child. He then describes the criteria used in club formation and provides treatment considerations in the use of programming activities for the club. The social worker's understanding of the strains and tensions that are subject to these special groups is felt to be imperative by the author.

Lear, Roma. Play Helps: Toys and Activities for Handicapped Children. London: Heinemann Health Books, 1977. 150 pp.

Roma Lear uses the experience she gained as a Hospital Teacher, Home Tutor, and organizer of the Kingston Toy Library for handicapped children in the preparation of this book. The creative toys and activities for use with handicapped children are arranged under the names of the five senses: sight, hearing, touch, taste and smell. While the book has been written primarily for parents, counselors, teachers and other individuals interacting with handicapped children should find it useful.

Loring, James, and Burn, Graham. Integration of Handicapped Children in Society. Boston: Routledge & Kegan Paul, 1975. 217 pp.

This collection of readings addresses the issue of integrating handicapped children in ordinary schools. The social aspects of integration, designing for physically handicapped children, the problems of the multiple-handicapped child, and the special school as a normalizing agency are aspects of the issue which are discussed in this work.

McMichael, Joan K. Handicap: A Study of Physically Handicapped Children and Their Families. Pittsburgh, Pa.: University of Pittsburgh Press, 1971. 208 pp.

In this monograph Dr. McMichael reports the findings of a study "dealing with the personal and social circumstances of fifty severely handicapped children, all of whom were pupils in a special primary school for the physically handicapped." At the time of the study, Dr. McMichael was school doctor. The study presents information on the difficulties and problems faced by these children with severe physical handicaps. The problems of parents and families was also obtained in the study and the lack of counseling available for families was discovered.

Mindel, Eugene. They Grow in Silence: the Deaf Child and His Family. Silver Spring, Md.: National Association of the Deaf, 1971. 118 pp.

For an evaluation of this work, see Chapter 3.

Morrison, Delmont; Pothier, Patricia; and Horr, Katy. Sensory-Motor Dysfunction and Therapy in Infancy and Early Childhood. Springfield, Ill.: Charles C. Thomas, 1978. 261 pp.

This book reflects an interdisciplinary approach to sensory-motor dysfunction and therapy in infancy and early childhood. The authors include a physical therapist whose specialty is handicapped children, a child psychiatric, nurse, and a child clinical psychologist. Considerable attention has been given in this work to the various methods of assessing and treating sensory-motor dysfunction. Case presentations support the discussion. The relationship between sensory-motor and emotional development is also discussed. This text should be of interest to "anyone" interested in the role that sensory-motor experience plays in psychopathological development in infancy and early childhood and the treatment of this psychopathology through sensory-motor techniques.

Moses, Harold Alton. Counseling with Physically Handicapped High School Students: A Dissertation. Columbia, Mo.: University of Missouri, 1974. 128 pp.

This dissertation, completed at the University of Missouri, investigated the critical job requirements of high school counselors when working with disabled students on problems related to their disability. A survey of high school counselors was conducted to determine the number of physically handicapped students attending regular classes; extent of counseling services; and type of handicap. A follow-up survey was conducted on counselors who reported four or more cases with disabled students. The investigator asked that these counselors provide additional information concerning two counseling cases, one effective and one ineffective. This data was analyzed and critical job requirements of counseling with disabled students were determined. Briefly, it was found that counselors with disabled students felt that this activity was an important aspect of their duties. However, the counselors felt that they approached the disabled student with more apprehension due to inexperience and lack of knowledge. Interaction seemed to be the most important role the counselor must be able to perform.

Mullins, June B. A Teacher's Guide to Management of Physically Handicapped Students. Springfield, Ill.: Charles C. Thomas, 1979. 405 pp.

This book discusses physical handicapping conditions and health problems from the viewpoint of the school. With mainstreaming, more children are being placed in the classroom on the basis of learning need rather than on the basis of disabilities and a need exists for teachers to understand the special problems of the child with a disability. The objective of this book is to fill the need. The book is organized by section including information on skeletal and muscle problems, central nervous problems, systemic disorders, stress related disorders, life threatening diseases and sensory disorders. Emphasis is placed on the psychological environment as well as the physical environment that the classroom provides. An extensive appendix is included which lists resources and organizations which are available to disabled persons, their families and to teachers.

Murray, Joseph N. Developing Assessment Programs for the Multihandicapped Child. Springfield, Ill.: Charles C. Thomas, 1980. 304 pp.

With legislation from the seventies mandating a free education to all children, including disabled children, educational programming provided for the disabled child must be specifically designed to meet his special needs. A knowledge of functional diagnostic assessment is crucial for this programming to be effective. This book provides the reader with information dealing with every facet of the assessment process as it relates to the severely and/or multiply handicapped population. Instrumentation available for use with deaf or hearing impaired, language impaired, blind or visually impaired, physically handicapped, and multiple handicapped individuals is described. Vocational evaluative issues are also discussed. This work is primarily directed to the student who is training to work with disabled individuals.

Noland, Robert L. Counseling Parents of the Ill and the Handicapped. Springfield, Ill.: Charles C. Thomas, 1971. 606 pp.

This collection of articles is devoted to the topic of counseling parents of ill or handicapped children. The volume is divided into seven sections. Part 1 is intended as an orientation to the area of parent-child-therapist interaction and the implication of a disability. Part 2 is concerned with counseling parents of the mentally retarded child. Part 3 focuses on the counseling of parents of children with epilepsy and cerebral palsy. Part 4 contains articles on counseling parents of children with speech, hearing and visual handicaps. This section also includes articles on individual, group, and genetic counseling. Part 5 briefly provides information on counseling parents of children with cardiac, diabetes, hemophiliac, and asthmatic handicaps. Part 6 includes articles on counseling parents of children with severe and terminal illnesses. Part 7 deals with genetic counseling and parents of children with handicaps. This work contains many references to the existing literature and should serve as a useful source of information for counseling parents.

Parker, Clyde A. Psychological Consultation: Helping Teachers Meet Special Needs. Minneapolis: Leadership Training Institute/Special Education, University of Minnesota, 1975. 270 pp.

This publication is the compilation of papers presented at the 1974 Leadership Training Institute/Special Education Conference. The papers included examine the concept of psychological consultation in the schools. Specific emphasis is given to specific methods of psychological consultation currently in use.

Prensky, Arthur L., and Palkes, Helen Stein. Care of the Neurologically Handicapped Child: A Book for Parents and Professionals. New York: Oxford University Press, 1982. 331 pp.

This book is written for parents of neurologically handicapped children and for professionals who work with neurologically handicapped children. The authors discuss "the types of training given to members of each of the major disciplines concerned with serving the neurologically handicapped child, why a child would be placed under their care and what services these professionals can be expected to supply." The book begins with an overview of normal and abnormal development and discusses the discovery of a neurological handicap. The following chapters review the services offered by the family physician, the medical specialist, the psychologist, the educator, the therapist, the nurse, the speech pathologist, the social worker, the nurse, and the lawyer. The authors conclude the book with a discussion of the most common neurological handicaps. A detailed index is included in the publication.

Routledge, Linda. Only Child's Play. London: William Heinemann Medical Books, 1978. 150 pp.

Written primarily to aid occupational therapists in their day-to-day contact with handicapped children but also well suited for anyone working with handicapped children. The recommendations for establishing a toy library would be beneficial for a school or public librarian. Ms. Routledge discusses the importance of play in a child's development and focuses on how play can be used to develop the capacities of handicapped children. She describes the different kinds of handicaps one is likely to encounter and presents methods of assessing the capabilities and needs of the child. Special equipment designed to allow the child more independence at home is discussed.

School Nurses Working With Handicapped Children. Kansas City, Mo.: American Nurses' Association, 1980. 7 pp.

This publication consists of a position statement issued by the American Nurses' Association Divisions on Nursing Practice, the American School Health Association, and the National Association of School Nurses in Response to the Education of all Handicapped Children Act of 1975 (P.L.94-142). This statement was developed "to assist educators, school nurses, administrators of school nursing services and school physicians as they consider the impact of this law on schools and on the community." The position statement expresses concern that quality health care cannot be administered to handicapped students in the current climate of school nursing and funding shortages. The risks involved in directing other school personnel for delivery of school health services are ackowledged. A six-step plan toward solution of the problems identified is recommended. The plan recommends 1) school health services to handicapped children be provided by school nurses; 2) the initial evaluation of handicapped students should include a comprehensive health and developmental history as well as a health assessment; 3) individual nursing care plans for handicapped children requiring special health services; 4) a safety program should be determined for each handicapped student; 5) children, parents, teachers, and school nurses should work together as a team in providing assistance to students with handicaps; 6) a nationwide program of continuing education for school nurses should be instituted.

Seligman, Milton. Strategies for Helping Parents of Exceptional Children. New York: Free Press, 1979. 240 pp.

This book was written for parents and teachers of handicapped children. The author feels that a greater understanding by the teachers of the "paths often taken when a disabled child is born, of the dynamics operating both within the family and between family and community and of the attitudes of professionals is necessary in order to understand the life circumstances confronting such parents." Issues discussed in the book include an examination of the teacher and facilitator and understanding the dynamics of families with an exceptional child. Specific strategies for working with parents of exceptional children are provided as well as strategies for working with problem parents. The book includes an appendix which lists resources to help teachers help parents. Also included is an extensive bibliography.

Solnit, Albert J. Physical Illness and Handicap in Childhood. New Haven, Conn.: Yale University Press, 1977. 321 pp.

The papers included in this anthology emphasize the role and importance of therapeutic work by psychoanalysts in helping the physically ill or handicapped child. These psychoanalysts have contributed to a better understanding of how children react to injury and to the therapy administered. The papers selected for this work are presented in three parts. The volume begins with a paper by Freud on "The Role of Bodily Illness in the Mental Life of Children." Following this is a discussion on hospitalization of children. This is followed by papers focusing on the psychological reactions and therapeutic services to children and their parents. These papers were written between 1952-1963 and provide insight into the gains reached during this decade.

Soyka, Patricia W. Thursday's Child has Far to Go. New York: National Council for Homemaker-Home Health Aide Services, 1979. 123 pp.

This book is the final phase of a project undertaken by the National Council for Homemaker-Home Health Aide Services and financed by the American Legion Child Welfare Foundation designed to gather information about homemaker-home health aide services provided to disabled children and their families. Through national platforms, the Council presented the information gathered and encouraged agencies to expand existing programs and/or develop new programs. This publication deals with the major areas of disability identified in the project and describes community efforts "aimed at countering the effects of handicapping condition on children and their families." Numerous case studies are presented. Two papers are included in the appendix which were presented at a national conference reacting to "A Child is Born," a paper proposed by the Council.

Stewart, Jack. <u>Counseling Parents of Exceptional Children</u>. Columbus, Ohio: Merrill, 1978. 152 pp.

This textbook provides a discussion of the theoretical as well as practical aspects of counseling giving specific attention to developing effective working relationships between the professional and parents of exceptional children. The book is divided into two parts. Part one deals with professional counseling and covers such issues as counselor attitudes, counselor process, and approaches in counseling. Part two is devoted to the subject of counseling parents of exceptional children. Chapters in this section include discussions of counseling parents of children with speech, hearing and visual handicaps, counseling parents of children with learning disabilities, and counseling parents of the physically handicapped child. In this section, the author's primary goal is "to raise some basic issues, indicate appropriate research findings and to suggest additional study."

This brief text was written to serve as a resource for professional personnel as a guide for students entering programs in special education fields or counselor education. Problems for individual study and class discussion follow each chapter.

Stratton, Josephine. <u>The Blind Child in the Regular Kindergarten</u>. Springfield, Ill.: Charles C. Thomas, 1977. 88 pp.

This book provides guidelines for educating the blind child in a regular classroom. The early physical and social development of the blind child is discussed and implications for education are presented. A list of kindergarten activities coded for use with a blind child is included. The author believes that the regular classroom teacher can effectively reverse the approach to the education of blind children from one that is "blind oriented" to one that is "child-oriented." The book includes an index and a list of suggested readings for teachers.

<u>Testing for Impaired, Disabled, and Handicapped Individuals</u>. Washington, D.C.: American Alliance for Health, Physical Education and Recreation, 1975. 110 pp.

This publication is "designed to provide information about physical fitness tests, perceptual-motor scales, and developmental profiles for use with impaired, disabled and handicapped persons so that valid and informed decisions can be made in selecting instruments for prescriptive and diagnostic persons." The guide includes a general introduction to the values and uses of testing;

background information to help in selecting tests; summaries of various physical fitness tests, psychomotor scales and development profile. This publication by the American Alliance for Health, Physical Education and Recreation (AAHPER) should serve as a valuable aid for physical education teachers, or therapists. The AAHPER provides numerous publications designed to help professionals and volunteers provide better physical education to the disabled.

Thain, Wilbur S.; Casto, Glendon; and Peterson, Adrienne. Normal and Handicapped Children: A Growth and Development Primer for Parents and Professionals. Boston: John Wright, 1980. 258 pp.

The authors discuss and describe the average growth and development of children and problems of abnormal growth and development. The book is written in language suited for the lay or professional person. Sources for obtaining help in particular situations are presented. A bibliography and glossary are included.

Thomas, David. The Social Psychology of Childhood Disability. London: Methuen, 1978. 165 pp.

This book is written with the intent of providing teachers, social workers, physiotherapists and others working with disabled children information concerning social behavior and handicaps in children. An overview of social psychology and handicap opens the discussion with subsequent chapters focusing on handicapped children, attitudes and the handicapped, personality and self-image, socialization of the handicapped child, the family and the handicapped children, and schools and handicapped children. The author addresses areas that require urgent attention and reviews recent positive developments which enable the disabled to better become part of the community. A lengthy bibliography is provided.

Tymchuk, Alexander J. Parent & Family Therapy. New York: SP Medical & Scientific Books, 1979. 278 pp.

This book proposes an integrative approach to working with parents of developmentally disabled children. The work opens with a theoretical rational for adopting the integrative approach to parent therapy. The various components for the utilization of parent therapy are addressed. The importance of considering parental dynamics is stressed. The remainder of the book presents an explanation of the different aspects of parent therapy.

The book is intended for use by all professionals who work with the families of developmentally disabled children. A Reference Guide to Brochures for parents and professionals is included in the appendix and is particularly comprehensive.

Varma, Ved P., ed. Stresses in Children. London: University of London Press, 1973. 165 pp.

This book discusses some of the problems exceptional children must face. The content of this publication includes chapters on blind children, injury-prone children, slow-learning children, handicapped children in the ordinary school, deaf and partially-hearing children, and children with physical handicaps. This work was written for "teachers, parents, social workers and others who need to be aware of the special problems posed by handicapped children and imposed on them." It was also written to alert readers to the existence of other groups of children; bereaved children, delinquent children, immigrant children, whose special problems and stresses need to be more recognized. A most informative and readable book.

Voysey, Margaret. A Constant Burden. London: Boston Routledge & Paul, 1975. 244 pp.

This study is an examination of the effects of a disabled child on family life. The study is based on parents' responses to questions. The researcher explores the issue of why parents say what they say when interviewed and if such responses portray an accurate picture of family life with a disabled child. It is argued in the publication that parents' responses do not provide an accurate picture. Information contributing to the selection is presented. Many references to the existing literature are cited plus an extensive bibliography. This well-organized book will provide valuable information to the researcher.

Webster, Elizabeth J. Counseling with Parents of Handicapped Children. New York: Grune & Stratton, 1977. 155 pp.

In this volume Elizabeth Webster draws on her experience as a professional who has worked with the parents of handicapped children for many years. Guidelines for improving communication between parent and counselor are presented. The book is divided into three parts. Part 1 focuses on parent counseling as interpersonal communication. Part 2 deals with improving counselor communication. Information in this section includes establishing the counselor-parent contract and a discussion on the mechanics of beginning and terminating a series of sessions. Part 3 describes the helpful function counselors provide for parents. Their functions consist of receiving information from parents, giving information to parents, assisting parents in the clarification of ideas and emotion, and helping parents to change behavior.

Webster, Elizabeth J. Professional Approaches With Parents of Handicapped Children. Springfield, Ill.: Charles C. Thomas 1976. 268 pp.

The objective of this collection of readings is "to provide an indepth look at several models of interaction with parents." It is felt that such a presentation of models of interaction will help professionals and students build a rationale for work with parents and assist in planning procedures to use in counseling parents. The contributors to this publication represent such professions as social work, speech pathology, and special education. While this work is intended for use by professionals or students, parents of disabled children will find it informative.

13 FEDERAL GOVERNMENT PUBLICATIONS

SUSAN E. BEKIARES/Documents Librarian, University of Illinois Library, Urbana, Illinois

INTRODUCTION

The United States Government Printing Office (GPO) is the world's largest printing house, and its products in the field of physical disability cover a broad range of subject areas; there is literally something for everyone. The literature published by the federal government is unique because of its diversity and availability. The published materials cover everything from mainstreaming children with hearing impairments to living with arthritis. Titles range from highly technical information for health care professionals or architects to purely informative booklets for parents of disabled children or for the disabled themselves. Books for the disabled include information on services provided by government and private agencies, and accessibility on college campuses and in national parks, while publications for professionals cover demographic statistics and accessibility standards.

While other chapters in this book and other bibliographies tend to focus on a particular impairment, or a single aspect of disability, this chapter is a representative sample of the thousands of titles available from the federal government on the broad topic of physical disabilities. To see the extent of titles available, it is possible to request an online computer search of the Monthly Catalog of Government Publications, the basic bibliography of all titles from GPO. Using the general terms "handicapped" and "disabled or disability", such a search would retrieve well over 1500 titles, published between 1976 and 1982. This chapter represents a sample of titles from many agencies on the subject of physical disabilities which reflect the variety of subjects covered and the various audiences these materials address. It illustrates the general types of materials from the federal government, mentions the agencies that are responsible for these materials, and illustrates what they produce, and finally describes how one learns of these titles and how to obtain them.

Because of recent legislation regarding the rights of the physically disabled (described in the chapter "Legal Rights: Advocacy, Legislation, Litigation, and Programs"), the federal government financially supports programs in all areas of disability research, and many supported programs are required to issue reports and other informational publications. As indicated in this chapter there is ongoing research into the causes, prevention, detection, treatment, and cures of many diseases, as well as investigations in the fields of barrier free design, specially designed or modified housing, and accessible transportation. Among the reports issued as a result of government funded research, we find: Family Planning Services for Disabled People; A Manual for Service Providers (HE 20.5108:F21/7), Study and Evaluation of Integrating the Handicapped in HUD Housing (HH 1.2:H19/2), and An Evaluation of Making Rail Transit Systems Accessible to Handicapped Persons (TD 7.2:H19/3). These are primarily of interest to professionals in the field, usually architects, planners, social workers, and educators. Other specialized reports which are of particular interest to professionals include statistical reports, such as: Disability Survey 72 (HE 3.49:56), and Digest of Data on Persons with Disabilities (HE 23.2:D63).

FEDERAL GOVERNMENT PUBLICATIONS 371

Besides those publications directed specifically to or about physically disabled individuals, the general publications such as reports from the 1980 Census of Population and Housing will give some detailed demographic characteristics of disabled persons, and statistics can frequently be found in Statistical Abstract of the United States(1) and in various reports from the Vital and Health Statistics Series.(2)

In the field of education for handicapped children and adults, there are many excellent publications available. The titles provide very specific information on numbers of students served, laws regarding accessibility, and practical suggestions for how best to integrate the special students, both physically and socially. Professional educators who work directly with handicapped students at various age and grade levels should be aware of these titles: Mainstreaming Preschoolers (HE 23.111: various numbers), The Status of Handicapped Children in Head Start Programs (HE 23.112:977), Development of Individualized Education Programs (IEPs) for the Handicapped in Vocational Education (HE 19.143:144) and Least Restrictive Alternative for Handicapped Students (HE 19.143:143).

As a result of extensive research in many areas, government agencies have amassed knowledge which is useful to the disabled individual and to his family. The materials range from very simple, plain language pamphlets which cover the causes, symptoms, and treatments for various disabilities (How to Cope with Arthritis: HE 20.3302:Ar7/2/981) to conference proceedings which address the emotional and mental health of the disabled person (The Deaf Child and His Family: HE 1.602:D34). Other titles for the disabled which focus on different aspects of living include: Recreation and Leisure for Handicapped Individuals (ED 1.8:R26/2) and Access National Parks (I 19.9/2:H19/2).

There are many federal agencies which sponsor research in this field and which publish various kinds of materials. Among them are: The Department of Education, the Department of Health and Human Services (formerly Health, Education and Welfare) and its subagencies, especially the Public Health Service, the National Institutes of Health, the Office for Handicapped Individuals, the Department of Housing and Urban Development (HUD), the Library of Congress and its National Library Service for the Blind and Physically Handicapped, the President's Committee on Employment of the Handicapped, the Department of Transportation (DOT), and the Veterans Administration. There are also hundreds of titles issued by Congress as committee prints, hearings, reports, and documents, but these are not included here, as they are more appropriately placed in the chapter on "Legal Rights: Advocacy, Legislation, Litigation, and Programs."

This chapter is arranged by the Superintendent of Documents (SuDoc) classification number, a number which appears in most standard indexes of government publications, and which is used in many libraries for classification and shelving. This arrangement will group all publications by a particular agency, which will give the reader an appreciation for the types of publications issured by each agency and will also tend to group the publications by subject or audience. For example, all of the HUD publications deal with housing for the elderly and handicapped, such as: Mobile Homes; Alternative Housing for the Handicapped (HH 1.2: M71/6), while the DOT titles tend to focus on public transportation accessibility for the elderly and handicapped (Conceptual Study of Handicapped Facilities for the New Subway Station Designs: TD 7.11:DC-06-0182-80-1).

As mentioned earlier, government publications are unique because they are so readily available. In most large public and academic libraries, the user will find several basic bibliographies which are invaluable for identifying materials from the government. The most comprehensive of these is the Monthly Catalog of Government Publications.(3) This title goes back to the early twentieth century and the citations from July, 1976 to date can be searched by use of computerized literature retrieval systems.

FEDERAL GOVERNMENT PUBLICATIONS

The Catalog lists all titles published by GPO from pamphlets to conference proceedings. The Monthly Catalog is supplemented by several other GPO publications. The Subject Bibliographies, including The Handicapped (GP 3.22/2:037) and Hearing and Hearing Disability (GP 3.22/2:023) among others, furnish the reader with a list of recent titles which are in stock and for sale. The citations include bibliographic information, a brief annotation and the ordering information including price and stock number. The Publications Reference File (PRF)(4) is a current list, in microfiche, of all titles in print and for sale by GPO. PRF includes an index by keyword, and indexes by Superintendent of Documents classification number, and by stock number. The information in PRF would enable the user to find the item in a library or to order the publication from the Government Printing Office.

There are several basic bibliographies which are commercially produced, and which are found in large research libraries. These are Congressional Information Service's CIS/Index(5) and American Statistics Index (ASI).(6) They are specifically designed for the user who needs legislative or statistical information. Their ease of use, and very complete abstracts make them invaluable research aids.

Other important bibliographies which are produced by the government, but which are not restricted to government titles, are Index Medicus(7), an index to the medical literature, Resources in Education(8), an index which covers journals, dissertations, books, and reports which, in some cases, relate to the education of the disabled, and Government Reports Announcements and Index.(9) The last title is issued by the Department of Commerce, National Technical Information Service (NTIS), and gives abstracts of reports resulting from government funded research. The basic bi-weekly abstract journal can be supplemented by various "Current Published Searches", online searches which NTIS executes, prints and sells for $30.00. Relevant titles include: Blindness, Housing for the Handicapped, Transportation for the

Elderly and Physically Handicapped, and Rehabilitation of the Physically Handicapped. Index Medicus, Resources in Education, and Government Reports Announcements and Index can all be searched online as well as in their printed forms.

All titles listed in this chapter, and indeed, most listed in Monthly Catalog and other bibliographies, will be available in a large government depository library. In many libraries, they will be arranged by the SuDoc number given here; in others they will be classified by whatever system that library uses. In the past, many titles published by the government were available free by requesting them from the issuing agency. This is becoming less true, however, and the Government Printing Office is now selling more titles and is keeping them in print longer by printing them in microfiche.

In summary, this chapter is not meant to be an exhaustive survey of the literature, but rather a sampler of recently published titles. The reader should scan these in order to appreciate the variety of materials, then consult the printed or online computer bibliographies in order to do an in-depth literature search. Titles listed in this chapter do not appear in other chapters of this book.

NOTES

1. Statistical Abstract of the United States. Washington, D.C.: Department of Commerce, Bureau of the Census. For sale by the U.S. Government Printing Office.

2. Vital and Health Statistics (various series). Bethesda, Md.: Department of Health and Human Services, Public Health Service, National Center for Health Statistics. For sale by the U.S. Government Printing Office.

3. U.S. Superintendent of Documents. Monthly Catalog of United States Government Publications. Washington, D.C.: U.S. Government Printing Office.

4. Publications Reference File. Washington, D.C.: U.S. Government Printing Office, Sales Management Division, Records Branch. For sale by the U.S. Government Printing Office.

FEDERAL GOVERNMENT PUBLICATIONS

5. CIS/Index. Washington, D.C.: Congressional Information Service.
6. American Statistics Index. Washington, D.C.: Congressional Information Service.
7. Index Medicus. Bethesda, Md.: Department of Health and Human Services, Public Health Service, National Institutes of Health. For sale by the U.S. Government Printing Office.
8. Resources in Education. Washington, D.C.: Department of Education, National Institute of Education, Education Resources Information Center. For sale by the U.S. Government Printing Office.
9. Government Reports, Announcements and Index. Springfield, Va.: Department of Commerce, National Technical Information Service.

ANNOTATED BIBLIOGRAPHY

ED 1.2:V85. Status Report of Interagency Linages at the State Level: Vocational Education Models for Linking Agencies Serving the Handicapped. Wisconsin Vocational Studies Center, University of Wisconsin-Madison. Washington, D.C.: U.S. Dept. of Education, Office of Vocational and Adult Education, 1981. 86 pp.

The project is designed to assist states in meeting vocational needs of students at secondary, post secondary and adult levels. The report describes interagency communication at the federal, state and local levels in Maryland, Virginia and New Jersey. The goals of this project are to identify and describe federal programs and their relationships to states, report on state level agencies, develop a model for cooperative agreements, and develop a resource manual. This volume mainly reports methodology rather than results. It includes sample forms and summary responses from worksheets.

ED 1.8:Ar2. Architectural Barriers Removal. Washington, D.C.: U.S. Dept. of Education, Office of Special Education and Rehabilitative Services, Office for Handicapped Individuals, 1980. 34 pp. For sale by: Supt. of Docs. U.S. G.P.O. $2.50.

This guide is intended to meet the information needs of persons working to remove and prevent architectural barriers. It lists available information resources, existing federal publications, and funding sources. It is only national level information and does not include private foundations, state agencies or community organizations. The section on funding lists agencies and their programs, assistance available, eligibility requirements, and application procedures. Information is excerpted from the Catalog of Federal Domestic Assistance. Included is a list of publications available from federal sources and mailing addresses for ordering federal publications. This guide would be useful in the absence of other more comprehensive tools such as The Catalog of Federal Domestic Assistance, or the Monthly Catalog.

ED 1.8:R26. Rehabilitation Engineering and Product Information: Information Resources, Funding Guide, Publications Available from Federal Sources. Washington, D.C.: U.S. Dept. of Education. Office for Handicapped Individuals, 1980. 149 pp. For sale by: Supt. of Docs., U.S. G.P.O. $3.75.

Rehabilitation Engineering is defined as the application of science and technology to improve the quality of life for persons with disabilities. Resources included have information on sensory, mobility, and communication technology which assist handicapped individuals in daily activities. The guide, which is intended for professionals, gives information on federal and private information sources (the organization, services provided and how to use them), general information sources (name, address, and 2-5 line description), financial assistance and loans for aids and equipment, funding guide, and an annotated publication list.

ED 1.8:R26/2. Recreation and Leisure for Handicapped Individuals: Information Resources, Funding Guide, Publications Available From Federal Sources. Washington, D.C.: U. S. Dept. of Education, Office of Special Education and Rehabilitative Services, Office for Handicapped Individuals, 1981. 102 pp. For sale by: Supt. of Doc. U.S. G.P.O. $4.75.

This resource guide was created to meet information needs of those working in the area of recreation programs for the handicapped. It includes sources for program information, funding resources, and governmental publications. Information for funding resources includes program description, uses, eligibility, application procedure, examples of funded projects, and information contacts.

ED 1.202:H19/2. Directory of National Information Sources on Handicapping Conditions and Related Services. Washington, D.C.: U.S. Dept. of Education, Office of Special Education and Rehabilitative Services. Clearinghouse on the Hanicapped. 1982. 270 pp. For sale by: Supt. of Docs. U.S. G.P.O. $8.00.

This is the third edition of a standard reference work for information providers in the field of service to the disabled. The directory documents, at the national level, information resources existing for disabled persons and those working in their behalf. It contains abstracts on 285 organizations. Abstracts cover: handicapping conditions served, the organization (affiliations, direct services provided, eligibility for services), and information services (information, education, seminars, publications and contacts). It is an essential reference source, made even more useful by its detailed subject index.

FEDERAL GOVERNMENT PUBLICATIONS

ED 1.210: Annual Report of the Rehabilitation Services Administration to the President and the Congress on Federal Activities Related to the Administration of the Rehabilitation Act of 1973, As Amended. Washington, D.C.: United States Rehabilitation Services Administration, 1981.

This series of annual reports provides information on program activities which are funded by the Rehabilitation Act of 1973. The report cited covers the period October 1, 1980 through September 30, 1981. The 1981 report emphasizes efforts for more efficient use of limited resources because of the potential numbers of individuals who require services and because the services were considerably expanded by a 1978 amendment to the Act.

GP 3.22/2:023. Hearing and Hearing Disability. Washington, D.C.: U.S. Government Printing Office, Superintendent of Documents, 1981. 4 pp. Free from Supt. of Doc. U.S. G.P.O.

GP 3.22/2:037. The Handicapped. Washington, D.C.: U.S. Government Printing Office, Superintendent of Documents, 1981. 14 pp. Free from Supt. of Doc. U.S. G.P.O.

These two titles appear in a series of over 300 Subject Bibliographies. Each bibliography lists items which are for sale by the G.P.O. Citations include title, issuing agency, price, SuDoc number, and in many cases, a descriptive annotation. The Subject Bibliographies are updated regularly and are found in most depository libraries. The reader can request a free copy of the index to the series, or copies of the individual bibliographies from G.P.O.

HE 1.6/3:D63/2. Pocket Guide to Federal Help for the Disabled Person. Produced by the Office of Resources for the Handicapped, Department of Health, Education, and Welfare. Washington, D.C.: Dept. of Health, Education and Welfare, Office of Information and Resources for the Handicapped, 1979. 20 pp. For Sale by: Supt. of Docs. U.S. G.P.O. $1.00.

This brochure is intended for handicapped individuals or their parent/guardian. Its intent is to make individuals aware of principal federal government services for which they may be eligible. It does not treat specific disabilities, but rather types of services available, such as education, transportation, and rehabilitation. It does include many agency addresses and should be used as a starting point for those in need of federal services.

HE 1.602:D34. The Deaf Child and His Family: Proceedings of National Forum VI, Council of Organizations Servicing the Deaf, March 14-16, 1973. Williamsburg, Virginia. Glenn T. Lloyd, Editor. Washington, D.C.: U.S. Dept. of Health, Education, and

Welfare, Office of Human Development, Rehabilitation Services Administration, 1973. 90 pp. For sale by: Supt. of Docs. U.S. G.P.O. $1.55.

The Forum report is an important contribution to the available literature on deafness, especially on family involvement in the vocational rehabilitation of deaf people. This conference was unique because of its focus on family relationships and emotional concerns, rather than on clinical, vocational or research aspects. Papers give a personal viewpoint to the problem of being deaf in a hearing world, being a hearing child with deaf parents, and having multiple handicaps. The papers themselves are practical, yet moving, the discussions are lively and varied, and the bibliographies and notes are useful. Recommended reading for a deaf person and his family.

HE 3.2:Se2/4/979. The Supplemental Security Income Program for the Aged, Blind, and Disabled: Selected Characteristics of State Supplementation Programs as of January, 1982. Washington, D.C.: Dept. of Health, Education and Welfare, Social Security Administration, Office of Research and Statistics, 1982. 99 pp. For sale by: Supt. of Docs. U.S. G.P.O. $3.00.

The Federal Supplemental Security Income (SSI) Program provides basic assistance payments to needy aged, blind, and disabled persons. SSI legislation also provides for supplementation of the basic federal payment by states. The information presented here covers selected charateristics of state programs, as of October 1, 1979 and one or two pages of information for each state. Updated reports will be published periodically.

HE 3.49:56. Disability Survey 72: Disabled and Nondisabled Adults: A Monograph. Compiled by Donald T. Ferron. Washington, D.C.: U.S. Dept. of Health and Human Services, Social Security Administration, Office of Policy, Office of Research and Statistics, 1981. 45 pp. For sale by: Supt. of Docs. U.S. G.P.O. $9.50

This survey, conducted by the Census Bureau in mid-1972, of 18,000 persons, was designed to update prior estimates of the extent and severity of disability in the U.S. population. Data are presented on major topics as demographic and family characteristics (disabled are more likely to be older, poorer, less educated, divorced, separated or widowed), the prevalence of chronic disease, injury or work disability (most frequently musculoskeletal or cardiovascular conditions), health care and coverage (generally require outside assistance) economic factors, government programs, and adjustment factors. Charts and tables have extensive coverage and are very specific. This is an essential reference work for a library or anyone interested in demographic characteristics of the disabled.

HE 19.102:D63/2. Disability: Our Challenge: A Distinguished Lecturer Series, Sponsored by the Project for Handicapped College

FEDERAL GOVERNMENT PUBLICATIONS

Students, Teachers College, Columbia Univeristy. John P. Hourihan, editor. Washington, D.C.: Dept. of Health, Education, and Welfare, Education Division, Office of Education, Bureau of Education for the Handicapped, 1979. 190 pp.

This book presents all of the lectures in a series presented by the Regional Education Programs for Handicapped College Students at Teachers College, Columbia University. The lecturers, themselves disabled persons, presented role models to students and examples to teachers and administrators. They lectured on employment, civil rights, education, social aspects, recreation, and leisure. The monograph includes biographies and addresses of lecturers.

HE 19.143:143. Least Restrictive Alternative for Handicapped Students. Written by Lloyde W. Tindall and John J. Gugerty, University of Wisconsin-Madison. Washington, D.C.: Dept. of Health, Education, and Welfare, Education Division, Office of Education, Bureau of Occupational and Adult Education, 1979. 40 pp. For sale by: Supt. of Docs. U.S. G.P.O. $1.80.

This publication examines the origin and current status of the concept of least restrictive alternative approach to vocational education of the disabled. It summarizes vocational programs which attempt to provide alternatives for handicapped students. Representative models of service delivery and diverse recommendations are made which translate this concept into concrete ideas.

HE 19.132:144. Development of Individualized Education Programs (IEPS) for the Handicapped in Vocational Education. Written by Lorella A. McKinney. National Center for Research in Vocational Education and Donna M. Seay, APC Skills. Washington, D.C.: Dept. of Health, Education, and Welfare, Education Division, Office of Education, Bureau of Occupation and Adult Education, 1979. 60 pp. For sale by: Supt. of Docs. U.S. G.P.O. $2.40.

This publication is intended for vocational educators who are developing an IEP for handicapped persons. Its purpose is to provide information which will extend awareness and understanding of educators and demonstrate the diversity of needs of the disabled. References, planning charts and sample forms are included as appendices.

This title and the preceding one are two in a series of 16 papers produced by NCRVE which are concentrated in four areas: special needs subpopulations, sex fairness, planning, and evaluation in vocational education. These books will be of interest to all vocational educators and administrators, researchers, and others.

HE 19.143:146. Job Placement and Adjustment of the Handicapped: An Annotated Bibliography. Compiled by Carol P. Kowle. Washington,

D.C.: Dept. of Health, Education, and Welfare, Education Division, Office of Education, Bureau of Occupational and Adult Education, 1979. 24 pp. For sale by: Supt. of Docs. U.S. G.P.O. $1.40.

This bibliography has been produced to assist special educators and vocational educators in obtaining information on job placement and career adjustment of various handicapped populations. It has been compiled from two computer assisted searches of the Educational Resources Information Center (ERIC) collection. It covers documents and journals from 1966-1978 and reproduces ERIC citations with abstracts.

HE 20.2752:F32/973. Feeding the Child With a Handicap. Washington, D.C.: U.S. Dept. of Health, Education and Welfare. Maternal and Child Health Services, 1973. 19 pp. For sale by: Supt. of Docs. U.S. G.P.O.

This pamphlet makes suggestions on how to meet the feeding needs of certain handicapped children. It describes techniques of feeding and specially designed implements that are adapted to these children. It discusses the principles of child growth and development that apply to all children and includes suggested menus and meals plans.

Principles in this pamphlet will help parents understand the child's special needs and encourage self-feeding and proper nutrition.

HE 10.3002:Ar7/4. Arthritis Research and Education in Nursing and Allied Health: A Forum. Sponsored by the National Arthritis Advisory Board. Bethesda, Md.: U.S. Dept. of Health and Human Services, Public Health Service, National Institutes of Health, 1980. 114 pp. For sale by: Supt. of Docs. U.S. G.P.O. $4.75.

The National Arthritis Advisory Board (NAAB) supported this invitational conference of outstanding experts in nursing, physical therapy and occupational therapy to assess the current state of the art and needs for future action in arthritis related research and education. The papers address the obvious and urgent need to identify and correct any deficiencies in preparation of nurses and therapists to effectively provide clinical services to arthritis patients. The participants gave specific examples of programs, projects, and recommendations for action. The proceedings are condensed, but cover a full range of useful information and the forum served as a guide for future planning for the NAAB.

HE 20.3008:Ar7. Thru the Arthritis Maze: A Guide to Federal Legislation Authorizing Services for the Chronically Ill: A Report. By the National Arthritis Advisory Board. Bethesda, Md.: Dept. of Health and Human Services, Public Health Service, National Institutes of Health, 1980. 84 pp.

Twenty-two federal laws which affect persons with arthritis and the services they authorized are reviewed in this guide.

FEDERAL GOVERNMENT PUBLICATIONS 381

Section I is a checklist of services authorized by law; section II summarizes the laws in chart form and provides information of interest to individuals and government agencies; section III is a narrative description of each law.

HE 20.3302:Ar7/2. How to Cope with Arthritis. Prepared by National Institute of Arthritis, Metabolism, and Digestive Diseases. Bethesda, Md.: U.S. Dept. of Health, Education, and Welfare, Public Health Service, National Institutes of Health, National Institute of Arthritis, Metbolism, and Digestive Diseases, 1976. 27 pp.

One of many pamphlets designed for the patient. It describes arthritis in its many forms, gives a little informatin on therapy, treatment and research and lists the drugs used to treat arthritis. It can be used as a guide for a discussion between physican and patient.

HE 20.3316:Au2. Audiovisual Materials Catalog: Arthritis Information Clearinghouse. Bethesda, Md.: U.S. Dept. of Health and Human Services. Public Health Service. National Institutes of Health. National Institute of Arthritis, Metabolism and Digestive Diseases, 1980. 192 pp.

Arthritis information Clearinghouse maintains a computerized database of inforamtion on materials concerning arthritis and related diseases. This catalog represents the information processed in the first year. It includes indexes for print materials, nonprint materials, subjects and authors. The catalog has 1050 bibliographic citations with no annotations. Materials listed are for use in patient, public, and professional education, but the reader must be the judge of which audience is best served by each title.

HE 20.3321:979. The Arthritis Program: Annual Report of the Director. National Institute of Arthritis, Metabolism, and Digestive Diseases. Bethesda, Md.: Public Health Service, National Institutes of Health, 1980. 72 pp.

This is the third annual report of the National Institute of Arthritis, Metabolism and Digestive Diseases (NIAMDD). Over 31 million Americans suffer from arthritis and related diseases, with symptoms ranging from discomfort to total disability. This report describes government supported research currently being performed and highlights programs and progress for that year. Not intended for a specific audience, this is the annual report submitted to the President and the Congress.

HE 20.3502:Am9. Amyotrophic Lateral Sclerosis: Lou Gehrig's Disease: Research Strikes Back. Bethesda, Md.: Dept. of Health, Education, and Welfare, Public Health Service, National Institutes of Health, 1977. 19 pp. For sale by: Supt. of Docs. U.S. G.P.O. $1.40.

HE 20.3502:Ep4/2. The NINCDS Research Program. Epilepsy. National Institute of Neurological and Communicative Disorders and Stroke. Bethesda, Md.: Dept. of Health and Human Services, Public Health Service, National Institutes of Health, 1980. 23 pp.

HE 20.3502:F11. Fact Book - National Institute of Neurological and Communicative Disorders and Stroke. Bethesda, Md.: Dept. of Health, Education and Welfare, Public Health Service, National Institutes of Health, National Institute of Neurological and Communicative Disorders and Stroke, 1979. 27 pp.

HE 20.3502:M91/980. The NINCDS Research Program. Multiple Sclerosis. Bethesda, Md.: Dept. of Health, Education and Welfare. Public Health Service. National Institutes of Health, National Institute of Neurological and Communicative Disorders and Stroke, 1980.

HE 20.3502:Sp4/2/980. The NINCDS Research Program. Spinal Cord Injury and Nervous System Trauma. National Institute of Neurological and Communicative Disorders and Stroke. Bethesda, Md.: U.S. Dept. of Health and Human Services, Public Health Services, National Institutes of Health, 1980.

HE 20.3502:Sp4/3. The NINCDS Research Program. Spina Bifida and Neural Tube Defects. Bethesda, Md.: U.S. Dept. of Health, Education and Welfare. Public Health Service, National Institutes of Health. 1980.

HE 20.3502:St8. The NINCDS Research Program, Stroke. Bethesda, Md.: Dept. of Health and Human Services, Public Health Service, National Institutes of Health, 1981.

The seven titles listed above are examples of a large and diverse series of pamphlets prepared by the National Institutes of Health. The series is designed for the patient and his family and most titles are updated annually. Generally, they describe the disease in plain language, and give symptoms, treatments, prognosis, and a description of ongoing research. Some titles include a section on where to find additional information. These are useful for a physician to use as a discussion guide, and should be included in public library collections.

HE 20.3517:N39/3. National Research Strategy for Neurological and Communicative Disorders. Bethesda, Md.: U.S. Dept. of Health, Education, and Welfare. National Institutes of Health, National Institute of Neurological & Communicative Disorders and Stroke, 1979. 171 pp.

The National Institute of Neurological and Communicative Disorders and Stroke has developed this National Research Strategy as a means of deciding how to allocate its resources in the best possible way and how to help relieve the burden of illness and disability imposed on victims of neurological disorders. The Institute called together seven panels of experts to address questions concerning health problems and research in various subject areas such as convulsive disorders, pain, and communicative disorders. In addition, task forces were formed and public forums were held. This volume is the basic summary of concrete research goals and their fiscal and manpower needs. Additional volumes cover individual panel and task force reports and the summary of the public forum. This report is recommended for research and medical libraries.

HE 20.5108:F21/7. Family Planning Services for Disabled People: A Manual for Service Providers. Rockville, Md.: U.S. Dept. of Health and Human Services, Public Health Service, Health Services Administration Bureau of Community Health Services, 1981. 185 pp. For sale by: Supt. of Docs. U.S. G.P.O. $6.50.

This document is the result of a year-long project to develop a demonstration model for the improvement of family planning services to disabled persons in Seattle, Washington. This manual can be used to help other communities duplicate the accessibility demonstrated here. This is a "how-to" manual for making service accomodations. Chapters cover fundamentals of etiquette and communication, the clinic visit including reception, counseling, choice of contraceptive, laboratory procedures, and the physical examination, staff training, architectural access, and medical aspects of disability.

HE 20.5108:R22. Moore, Coralie B. And Kathryn G. Morton. A Reader's Guide for Parents of Children with Mental, Physical or Emotional Disabilities. Washington, D.C.: U.S. Dept. of Health, Education and Welfare. Public Health Service, Health Services Administration, 1979. 144 pp. For sale by: Supt. of Docs. U.S. G.P.O. $3.50.

This publication is an outgrowth of "Selected Reading Suggestions for Parents of Mentally Retarded Children," prepared by the Children's Bureau in 1967 and revised in 1970. The scope has been greatly expanded to cover the whole range of mental, emotional, and physical handicaps. This is an annotated bibliography which covers: 1. basic reading; 2. books that tell how to teach, train, and play at home; 3. books written by parents and others who have "lived it", and 4. books which deal intensively with a particular issue of a problem. Arrangement is by subject or disability. Also included are books for children about disabled children and lists of further sources of information, organizations, agencies, directories, and journals. Annotations are succinct, and bibliographic citations include the price. Its usefulness is enhanced by the list of publishers addresses, and an author and title index.

HE 20.8127:1,2,3. Mental Health in Deafness. Washington, D.C.: Dept. of Health, Education, and Welfare. Public Health Service, Alcohol, Drug Abuse, and Mental Health Administration, National Institute of Mental Health, Saint Elizabeths Hospital, 1977. For sale by: Supt. of Docs. U.S. G.P.O. $2.00.

The only issues received were experimental iussue no. 1, 2, and 3 and the articles included were on the President's Commission on Mental Health, epidemiology of mental health and deafness, treatment of emotionally disturbed deaf children, statewide planning of coordinated mental health services for deaf persons, and legal change in mental health care for the deaf. This periodical would be useful for general awareness in the area of the mental health of the deaf because it includes news briefs, meetings announcements, and book reviews. It appears to have been discontinued.

HE 22.108:L85. Activities Coordinator's Guide: A Handbook for Activities Coordinator in Long-Term Care Facilities. John Philip Bachner. Washington, D.C.: Dept. of Health, Education, and Welfare. Health Care Financing Administration, Health Standards and Quality Bureau, 1978. 126 pp. For sale by: Supt. of Docs. U.S. G.P.O. $3.00.

This guide has been prepared as a reference work and as a basic course text for those who are or who are learning how to be activities coordinators in long-term facilities. All aspects of activities are covered, including basic concepts, program evaluation, activities development, and resources and management. Appendices include lists of activities, glossary, health problems, attitudes, lists of relevant national organizations and suggested reading.

HE 23.2:D63. Digest of Data on Persons with Disabilities. Prepared under contract to the Congressional Research Service, Library of Congress by Rehab Group, Incorporated. Washington, D.C.: Dept. of Health, Education, and Welfare, Office of Human Development Services, Office for Handicapped Individuals, 1980. 141 pp. For sale by: Supt. of Docs. U.S. G.P.O. $4.75.

This publicatioin provides data which gives an overview of the size and characteristics of the disabled population. It also explains and clarifies some confusion of "definitions and labels." It provides summary tables, charts and explanatory notes for the following subjects: impairments and developmental disabilities, work disabilities, limitation of activity, occupation and employment, and federal programs. Detailed tables and explanatory notes cover the following subjects: income, employment, and education; health status and activity limitations; residential status; veteran status and mental health. Appendices include a glossary, discussions of primary sources, selected list of resources for statistical data, and a bibliography. The statistics and definitions are excellent and usefulness is increased by the subject index matrix.

HE 23.2:H19. Federal Assistance for Programs Serving the Handicapped. Washington, D.C.: Dept. of Health, Education, and Welfare, Office of Human Development Service, Office for Handicapped Individuals, 1980. 366 pp. For sale by: Supt. of Docs. U.S. G.P.O. $7.00.

This directory is for use by fund developers and service providers. Most listed programs provide assistance to disabled people and to people working with or for them, and are from the Catalog of Federal Domestic Assistance. Appendices include: List of resources for funding information, bibliography, and addresses of state agencies serving the disabled.

HE 23.2:Y8. Youth Volunteers and the Disabled: Getting It Together. Prepared by The National Institute for Advanced Studies; Edited by Jowava M. Leggett. Wahington, D.C.: Dept. of Health, Education, and Welfare, Office of Human Development Services, Office of Handicapped Individuals, 1979. 31 pp.

The report of a 14 month project entitled "The Development of an Active Liaison With Key Organizations Servicing the Handicapped." Chapter I is a discussion of the role of Office of Handicapped Individuals in promoting programs and activities to benefit the disabled. Chapters II and III provide an overview of 4-H and Girl Scout Seminars. The project involves meeting the needs of disabled individuals through services provided by youth volunteers, and more importantly, involving disabled youth as participants in youth volunteer organizations.

HE 23.1012: Annual Report of the U.S. Department of Health, Education, and Welfare to the Congress of the United States on Services Provided to Handicapped Children in Project Head Start. Washington, D.C.: Dept. of Health, Education, and Welfare, Office of Human Development Services, Administration for Children, Youth, and Families. 1979. For sale by: Supt. of Docs. U.S. G.P.O.

The Head Start, Economic Opportunity, and the Community Partnership Act of 1974 (PL 93-644) requires that 10% of the enrollment opportunities in Head Start programs shall be available for handicapped children. Eligible children have a permanent disability, are between 3 years of age and school age, and are from low income families. This survey provides data on the children involved, the services available to them, information on mainstreaming, and an evaluation of the program.

HE 23.1110:H35. Mainstreaming Preschoolers: Children With Hearing Impairment: A Guide for Teachers, Parents, and Others Who Work With Hearing Impaired. Washington, D.C.: Dept. of Health, Education and Welfare, Office of Human Development Services,

Administration for Children, Youth and Families, Head Start Bureau, 1978. 131 pp. For sale by: Supt. of Docs. U.S. G.P.O. $3.25.

HE 23.1110:Or8. Mainstreaming Preschoolers: Children With Orthopedic Handicaps: A Guide for Teachers, Parents, and Others Who Work With Orthopedically Handicapped Preschoolers. Washington, D.C.: Dept. of Health. Education, and Welfare, Office of Human Development Services, Administration for Children, Youth and Families, Head Start Bureau, 1978. 141 pp. For sale by: Supt. of Docs. U.S. G.P.O. $3.50.

HE 12.1110:Sp3. Liebergott, Jacqueline and Aaron Favors, Jr. Mainstreaming Pre-Schoolers: Children with Speech and Language Impairments: A Guide for Teachers, Parents, and Others Who Work With Speech and Language Impaired Preschoolers. Washington, D.C.: Dept. of Health, Education, and Welfare, Office of Human Development services, Administration for Children, Youth and Familes, Head Start Bureau, 1978. 167 pp. For sale by: Supt. of Docs. U.S. G.P.O. $3.75.

HE 23.1110:V82. Alonso, Lou. Mainstreaming Preschoolers: Children With Visual Handicaps: A Guide for Teachers, Parents, and Others Who Work With Visually Handicapped Preschoolers. Washington, D.C.: Dept. of Health Education, and Welfare, Office of Human Development Services, Administration for Children, Youth and Families, Head Start Bureau, 1978. 127 pp. For sale by: Supt. of Docs. U.S. G.P.O. $3.25.

The four titles listed here are in a series of guides designed to help parents and teachers understand the concepts of mainstreaming and of various types of disabilities. The publications define concepts in simple terms and use specific examples of classroom situations, activities, and techniques in mainstreaming. Each includes a section on funding resources and specialists, and an annotated bibliography. Each is a useful, well-designed guide for teachers, parents and others who work with disabled preschoolers.

HH 1.2:B86/3. Steinfeld, Edward; Schroeder, Steven and Marilyn Bishop. Accessible Buildings for People With Walking and Reaching Limitations. Washington, D.C.: Dept. of Housing and Urban Development, Office of Policy Development and Research, 1979. 169 pp. For sale by: Supt. of Docs. U.S. G.P.O. $4.75.

This title, and the next three listed are parts of a series of six reports which are the result of research undertaken to develop American National Standards Institute (ANSI) Standard A117.1, "Making Buildings and Facilities Accessible to and Usable by the Physically Handicapped."

This report contains photographs, diagrams and tabular information relating to anthropometrics, wheelchair maneuvers, ramps, bathroom and kitchen facilities, doorways, elevators, telephones, and mailboxes. Findings are compared with previous research, and the scope does not include the environments of young children. Includes a list of references.

HH 1.2:B86/4. Aiello, James and Edward Steinfeld. Accessible Buildings for People With Severe Visual Impairment. Washington, D.C.: Dept. of Housing and Urban Development, Office of Policy Development and Research, 1979. 113 pp. For sale by: Supt. of Docs. U.S. G.P.O. $4.00.

This project attempts to determine whether the usability of buildings for people with severe visual impairments can be enhanced through design. The report covers background, study methods, discussion of testing phases, presentation of data, design recommendations, and suggestions for further research.

HH 1.2:B86/5. Schroeder, Steven A. and Edward Steinfeld. The Estimated Cost of Accessible Buildings. Washington, D.C.: Dept. of Housing and Urban Development, Office of Policy Development and Research, 1979. 153 pp. For sale by: Supt. of Doc. U.S. G.P.O. $4.75.

The purpose of this study is to assist in determining the construction costs for redesign of new buildings and renovation of existing buildings to be in conformance with the proposed American National Standards Institute's A117.1 standard (1978). This report is a detailed analysis of renovation and design of nine buildings, complete with diagrams, references, and cost estimates.

HH 1.2:En8/4. Access to the Built Environment: A Review of the Literature. Washington, D.C.: Dept. of Housing and Urban Development, Office of Policy Development and Research, 1979. 150 pp. For sale by: Supt. of Docs. U.S. G.P.O. $4.75.

Chapters in this volume include a summary description of the purpose of the series (to revise and improve the existing American National Standards Institute's ANSI A117.1 Standard); an analysis of the history of the civil rights of the disabled; a description of the disabled population; current accessibility codes and regulations; an analysis of the scope of barrier-free design (including a problem identification matrix); a description of the origins and scope of human factors research; an essay on the impact of inaccessibility; and a description of the possibilities of changing attitudes through design. Each chapter includes a list of references; but the excellent narration of this publication makes this much more than a literature review.

The last four titles can be used as resources for making buildings accessible to and usable by the physically disabled. The series has won a research award from Progressive Architecture and is highly recommended.

HH 1.2:E12/10. U.S. Housing Developments for the Elderly or Handicapped. Prepared by Office of Multifamily Housing Development. Washington, D.C.: Dept. of Housing and Urban Development, Office of Housing, 1979. 119 pp.

A listing of all housing developments funded under Sections 202, 231, and 236 prior to enactment of the Housing and Community Development Act of 1974. Sections 202, 231, and 236 are described as they apply to construction, services and facilities, or mortgage and rent for low income handicapped and elderly. Most of the volume is an alphabetic list by state and city of housing developments, their address, number of units, and project type.

HH 1.2:E12/11. Nathanson, Iric. Housing Needs of the Rural Elderly and Handicapped. Washington, D.C.: U.S. Dept. of Housing and Urban Development, 1980. 36 pp. For sale by: Supt. of Docs. U.S. G.P.O. $2.25.

Elderly people in rural areas have special problems; housing assistance is often not readily available to them because their communities may lack the network of housing services and programs found in most urban areas. This report analyzes the housing needs of the rural elderly and handicapped, and examines alternative approaches for meeting those needs.

HH 1.2:H19/2. Study and Evaluation of Integrating the Handicapped in HUD Housing. By Battelle's Columbus Laboratories for Office of Policy Development and Research, Dept. of Housing and Urban Development. Washington, D.C.: Dept. of Housing and Urban Development, Office of Policy Development and Research, 1977. 290 pp. For sale by: Supt. of Docs. U.S. G.P.O. $4.50.

This report documents the increased cost of construction necessary to make rented housing accessible to handicapped persons with differing degrees of disability. It does not address the cost of retro-fitting existing housing. Data were collected from four HUD-subsidized housing projects and from interviews with 80 disabled persons. The study concludes that additional construction costs range from .25 to 4.7%, and modifications are useful to able-bodied as well as disabled persons. Includes methodology, definitions, detailed cost analysis, and recommendations for implementation. An annotated bibliography that would be useful for architects and building managers is included.

HH 1.2:M71/6. Mobile Homes: Alternative Housing for the Handicapped. Washington, D.C.: Dept. of Housing and Urban Development, Office of Policy Development and Research, 1977. 47 pp. For sale by: Supt. of Docs. U.S. G.P.O. $1.80.

Describes an experiment set in Laurinburg, North Carolina to test the mobile home as a solution to the problem of safe, mobile and accessible housing for the disabled. It gives the study background, description of laboratory units (including floorplans), a detailed description of the demonstration unit (room by room), a safety analysis, and site considerations. Photographs and excellent graphics are used as illustrations.

HH 1.2:P69/books1,2, and 3. A Playground for All Children. City of New York. Washington, D.C.: Dept. of Housing and Urban Development, Office of Policy Development and Research, 1978. 3 volumes. For sale by: Supt. of Docs. U.S. G.P.O. $2.30 (V. 1) $1.60 (v.1) $3.50 (v.3).

A three volume detailed description of the development, by the City of New York, of the first outdoor public playground especially designed for integrated play between disabled and able-bodied children. Book 1, User Groups and Site Selection, describes the underlying research studies, site analysis and criteria, and special play needs for able-bodied and disabled children from the ages of three to eleven. Appendices include lists of consultants and major correspondence.

Book 2, Design Competition Program, details the design competition used by the City of New York to encourage a creative and varied approach to playground design. Included are descriptions of playground feature specifications and construction procedures.

Book 3, Resources Book, deals with the processes and products of the playground development. Includes surveys of existing playgrounds, four winning designs, and descriptions of new and innovative concepts in design and playground components.

Highly recommended for special educators, recreation specialists and archtectural designers. A brief bibliography of books, pamphlets, reports, periodicals and films is included in Book 3.

HH 1.6/3:H19/Inst. Management of Housing for Handicapped and Disabled Persons: Instructor's Guide. Washington, D.C.: Dept. of Housing and Urban Development, Office of Policy Development and Research, 1980. 248 pp. For sale by: Supt. of Docs. U.S. G.P.O. $6.50.

The instructor's guide to accompany HH 1.6/3: H19/part. follows the textbook and gives additional introductory information, methodology for each section, answers and grading information, and a list of national organizations.

HH 1.6/3:H19/part. Management of Housing for Handicapped and Disabled Persons: Participant's Workbook. Washington, D.C.: Dept. of Housing and Urban Development, Office of Policy Development and Research, 1980. 129 pp. For sale by: Supt. of Docs. U.S. G.P.O. $4.75.

This workbook is part of a housing-management curriculum developed by HUD in conjunction with Temple University. It provides students with an understanding of the special needs of disabled persons and considers how their needs affect the role of manager of specialized housing facilities. The text covers background, objectives and exercises dealing with disabilities, independent living, barriers, legislation, and other topics.

HH 1.36:11/11. HUD Challenge: Special Issue on the Handicapped. Washington, D.C.: Dept. of Housing and Urban Development, The Assistant Secretary for Administration, Publications and Information Division, Office of General Services, 1977. 28 pp.

This special issue of Challenge! highlights some examples of how the use of HUD programs broadens opportunities for disabled people to participate fully in their communities. Topics covered include: opportunities for independent living in private and public housing, and community housing for people with chronic mental illness.

I 29.912:H19/2. Access National Parks: A Guide for Handicapped Visitors. Washington, D.C.: Dept. of the Interior, National Park Service, 1978. 198 pp. For sale by: Supt. of Docs. U.S. G.P.O. $3.50.

This handbook of accessibility for handicapped visitors to the National Park System shows evidence of progress toward the goal of making our parks comfortable and enjoyable for everyone. The guide has an alphabetic index and regional maps, and is arranged by state. Information covers facilities, programs, location, medical or special services, and information contacts. It is an essential reference for libraries and for handicapped travelers.

I 70.2:B86/2. Parrott, Charles A. Access to Historic Buildings for the Disabled: Suggestions for Planning and Implementation. Washington, D.C.: U.S. Dept. of the Interior, Heritage Conservation and Recreation Service, Technical Preservation Services Division, 1980. 86 pp. For sale by: Supt. of Docs. U.S. G.P.O. $4.25.

This publication is intended to assist in providing barrier free access to historic buildings through methods that are in conformance with the Secretary of the Interior's Standards for Historic Preservation Projects. It discusses relevant laws and building codes, and through photographs and descriptions examines methods being used to provide access. Includes selected bibliography, list of State Historic Preservation Officers, and the Secretary of the Interior's Standards for Rehabilitation. It should provide useful background information to architects, historic site managers, and planners.

L 37.8/4:Or8. Interviewing Guides for Specific Disabilities: Orthopedic Disabilities. Washington, D.C.: Dept. of Labor, Employment and Training Administration, 1979. 17 pp. For sale by: Supt. of Docs. U.S. G.P.O. $1.00.

FEDERAL GOVERNMENT PUBLICATIONS

This interviewing guide is designed to acquaint employment counselors and interviewers with the nature of orthopedic disabilities and to assist in understanding the implication for employment. Part I describes various orthopedic disabilities. Part II lists factors in evaluating work capacity. Part III is a glossary. Part IV lists cooperating agencies. The guide will be useful in assessing the applicant's physical capability in relation to a suitable field of work or a specific job.

LC 3.4/2:63. Reproduction of Copyrighted Works for the Blind and Physically Handicapped. (circular R63) Washington, D.C.: Library of Congress, Copyright Office, 1977. 3 pp.

This publication describes the new simplified procedure by which a copyright owner, (author) can make his works available to the National Library Service for the Blind & Physically Handicapped (NLS) for transcription to braille or phonorecord editions.

LC 19.6/2:B27. Planning Barrier Free Libraries. Washington, D.C.: Library of Congress, National Library Service for the Blind and Physically Handicapped. 1981.

This guide suggests how to establish a new building or renovation program for a network library. The "ideal" is discussed, but practical information in the forms of diagrams and checklists is given for space requirements, equipment and furniture. the appendices which give time schedules, requirements for space, personnel and restrooms, and the accessibility checklist are extremely valuable for librarians and architects.

PM 1.8:Se4. Handbook of Selective Placement of Persons with Physical and Mental Handicaps in Federal Civil Service Employment. Washington, D.C.: Office of Personnel Management, 1981. 72 pp. For sale by: Supt. of Docs. U.S. G.P.O. $2.80.

This handbook outlines concepts and procedures that can and should be used to provide equal employment opportunity for all qualified handicapped applicants and employees. The information summarized here is from the Federal Personnel Manual, and most publications cited are available from the Office of Personnel Management. The handbook gives guidelines for personnel directors, agency coordinators, and counselors regarding equal employment opportunity, job sites, career development and publicity, and offers imformation about provisions for special groups such as blind, deaf, mobility impaired, and those with hidden handicaps. The publication is useful for the disabled individual, so that he understands his rights as an employee, and is essential for personnel managers.

PrEx 1.10/8:H43/977. Highway Rest Areas for Handicapped Travelers. Washington, D.C.: President's Committee on Employment of the Handicapped, 1977. 77 pp.

The Federal Highway Administration and The American Association of State Highway Officials are determined that all newly constructed rest areas shall be accessible. The 1977 edition of this guide lists over 800 accessible rest areas complete and under construction in 48 states. The guides enables handicapped travelers to plan their trips and avoid the inconvenience of inaccessible rest areas. The directory is by state and lists the route, direction served, location, and milepost. It is recommended for all libraries and would be invaluable to the handicapped motorist.

PrEx 1.10/8:St9. Smith, Lynn M. The College Student with a Disability: A Faculty Handbook. Washington, D.C.: The President's Committee on Employment of the Handicapped, 1980. 35 pp. For sale by: Supt. of Docs. U.S. G.P.O. $2.50.

Designed as a reference work for faculty, this publication provides a set of guidelines for making classroom activities accessible. It includes a glossary and practical tips such as the manual alphabet, information on large print typewriters, curb cuts or ramps, and physical limitations of students with ostomies. Includes references and resources list.

PrEX 1.10/9:R26/982. Schwab, Lois O. Rehabilitation for Independent Living, a Selected Bibliography, 1982. Washington, D.C.: President's Committee on Employment of the Handicapped, 1982. 47 pp.

This compilation of materials is a carefully selected sample of information thought to be useful to the disabled and their advocates. Most materials are recommended for inclusion in a basic library for independent living. The bibliography covers in print materials, includes cost, and has a complete list of publishers addresses in Section C. Includes books, pamphlets, and films, most of which are privately published. The bibliography is easy to use and the brief annotations are informative.

PrEx 1.10/9:V85. Hippolitus, Mona L. Resources for the Vocational Preparation of Disabled Youth. Washington, D.C.: President's Committee on Employment of the Handicapped, 1980. 44 pp. For sale by: Supt. of Docs. U.S. G.P.O.

This document contains descriptions of materials gathered at the "National Forum on Pathways to Employment" in 1976 and 1979, sponsored by the President's Council on Employment of the Handicapped. Each entry includes: title, address, cost, and short narrative description of the material's content.

TD 1.2:E12/3. Transportation for the Elderly and Handicapped: A Literature Capsule. Cambridge, Mass.: Department of Transportation, Transportation Systems Center, Technology Sharing Program Office, 1977. 83 pp.

This title is designed to make the literature in transportation concerning the elderly and handicapped more accessible to users. The capsule is organized as follows: an introduction to the literature which highlights the scope of current research and planning; selected summaries of five detailed studies which cover a wide range of topics; and the annotatead bibliography of literature from 1970-77. The annotated bibliography is arranged by broad subject (overview, needs, programs, planning, and policy), includes an author index, and has a list of suggested periodicals and other sources of current information. This title is recommended for government officials and planners who are concerned with transportation for the elderly and handicapped.

TD 1.2:E12/4. Conference on Transportation for the Elderly and Handicapped, 6th, 1977. Transportation for the Elderly and Handicapped: Programs and Problems. Washington, D.C.: U.S. Dept. of Transportation, Transportation Systems Center. Technology Sharing Program Office, 1978. 145 pp.

This document includes papers presented at the Sixth Annual Conference on Transportation for the Elderly and Handicapped at Florida State University. Papers cover planning and implementation, examples of state and local programs, and driver training and equipment selection. It includes a glossary and list of authors with addresses and phone numbers.

TD 1.2:E12/5. Transportation for the Elderly and Handicapped: Programs and Problems II. Washington, D.C.: U.S. Dept. of Transportation, Office of the Secretary, Office of the Assistant Secretary for Governmental Affairs, Research and Special Programs Administration, Transportation System Center, Technology Sharing Office, 1981. 193 pp. For sale by: Supt. of Docs. U.S. G.P.O. $6.00.

This report is a companion piece to TD 1.2:E12/3 and TD1.2:E12/4, and is a compilation of condensations of papers presented at the Seventh Annual Conference on Transportation for the Elderly and Handicapped. The papers reflect an emphasis in implementation rather than planning and in the ongoing problems of recently established systems. Papers cover accessibility, coordination and brokerage, demand, and related issues such as insurance, labor, and vehicles. It also includes a list of names and addresses of authors.

TD 1.8:P69. Carter, Goble, Robert, Inc. Joint HEW-UMTA Evaluation of Elderly and Handicapped Transportation Services in Region IV: Planning and Coordination Manual. Washington, D.C.: Dept. of Health, Education and Welfare, U.S. Dept. of Transportation, 1979. 330 pp.

This is a "how-to" manual intended for use by persons responsible for planning and/or operating specialized transportation systems, such as paratransit, elderly, and handicapped transportation services. The manual is lengthy and draws upon experience of numerous systems and their directors. It includes illustrations, statistics, sample reporting forms, and a glossary.

Development phases covered are: how to start, advance planning, operations planning and programming, implementation and development, auditing, reporting and evaluation.

TD 1.30:79-146. Templer, John A. and Jean D. Wineman. The Feasibility of Accommodating Physically Handicapped Individuals on Pedestrian Over and Undercrossing Structures: Final Report. Washington, D.C.: U.S. Dept. of Transportation, Office of Research and Development, Environmental Division, 1980. 98 pp. For sale by: Supt. of Docs. U.S. G.P.O. $4.50.

The objective of this study was to determine the feasibility of accommodating physically handicapped pedestrians on over and undercrossing structures. Of 124 crossing structures evaluated, 86% had at least one major barrier. Alternative solutions were developed and examined for cost effectiveness.

TD 7.2:E12/7. Elderly and Handicapped Transportation: Local Government Approaches. Prepared by Public Technology, Inc. Secretariat to the Urban Consortium for Technology Initiatives. Washington, D.C.: Dept. of Transportation, Urban Mass Transportation Administration, 1979. 60 pp. For sale by: Supt. of Docs. U.S. G.P.O. $2.50.

This publication describes how a number of localities provide public transportation to handicapped or elderly citizens. Among the systems described, some are federally funded, some are locally initiated. Some modify conventional services and others are specifically designed for a special user group. Included is a list of city contacts. This title is useful for planners, engineers, and city officials who are working to make public transportation accessible.

TD 7.2:H19/3. An Evaluation of Making Rail Transit Systems Accessible to Handicapped Persons: A National Summary of Cost Estimates and Comments on Desirability. Washington, D.C.: U.S. Dept. of Transportation, Urban Mass Transportation Administration (UMTA), 1981. 114 pp.

This report summarizes studies on making fixed-guidance and light rail and commuter rail systems accessible to disabled individuals. It is intended to estimate the magnitude of minimum cost solutions so that Congress and Urban Mass Transportation Administration can decide on appropriate legislation. Several representative systems were studied and analyzed.

TD 7.11:DC-06-0182-80-1. Collins, William and Delon Hampton. Conceptual Study of Handicapped Facilities for New Subway Station Designs. Washington, D.C.: U.S. Dept. of Transportation, Urban Mass Transportation Administration, Office of Technology Development and Deployment, 1980. 53 pp. For sale by: NTIS.

FEDERAL GOVERNMENT PUBLICATIONS

This report analyzes seven new subway station concepts developed from similar types in Canada, Mexico, and Europe and identifies what modifications could be in corporated into their design to facilitate use by handicapped persons. Most modifications include relocation or addition of elevators. The assumption is that stations exist in high density areas.

VA 1.20/2:Se9. Sex and the Handicapped: A Selected Bibliography. Washington, D.C.: U.S. Veterans Administration, 1975. 55 pp. For sale by: Supt. of Docs. U.S. G.P.O. $1.45.

This selected bibliography deals with the sexual life of the disabled and is divided into the following subject areas: sex education, marriage and family life; drug addiction; alcoholism; amputations; trauma; burns; arthritis and orthopedic problems; spinal cord injury; poliomyelitis; cystic fibrosis; cerebral palsy; multiple sclerosis; urogenital disorders; renal transplantation and dialysis; ostomy patients; neoplasms; neurological, cardiovascular, endocrine and mental disorders; and the aged. Films and miscellaneous pamphlets are listed separately. The "selection" criteria for inclusion is not given and no evaluative information is provided.

VA 1.22:11-31. A Source Book Rehabilitating the Person with Spinal Cord Injury. Washington, D.C.: Veterans Administration, Department of Medicine and Surgery, 1972. 58 pp. For sale by: Supt. of Docs. U.S. G.P.O. $1.85.

The rehabilitation of veterans who have suffered disabling injuries to the spinal cord is one of the programs of which the Veterans Administration is most proud. This book outlines methods and techniques for rehabilitating injured veterans physiologically, socially, and psychologically so they can make an easier readjustment of normal life.

VA 1.22:11-63. Spinal Cord Injury: A Selected Bibliography Supplement, 1971-1975. Washington, D.C.: Veterans Administration, Central Office Library, 1977. 248 pp.

The Veterans Administration provides a comprehensive treatment plan of Spinal Cord Injured (SCI) veterans including acute care and rehabilitation. Through the SCI bibliography, the VA demonstrates its continued support of all phases of treatment. The bibliography has 3897 entries, in a broad subject arrangement, with author index. Items listed are mainly journals, with some books and dissertations included.

VA 1.22:11. Handbook of Hearing Aid Measurement. Washington, D.C.: Veterans Administration, 1980. 212 pp. For sale by: Veterans Administration.

The Veterans Administration and the National Bureau of Standards evaluate hearing aids, electroacoustically, which have been voluntarily submitted by the manufacturer. Test data are presented, in alternate years, for special purpose hearing aids (1983) and for regular instruments (1982). The information provided is too technical for the consumer, but is useful for the professional who provides hearing aids.

Y 3.B17/2:D46. Designing for Everyone... Access America. Washington, D.C.: Architectural and Transportation Barriers Compliance Board, 1981. 8 pp. For sale by: Supt. of Docs. U.S. G.P.O.

Brief descriptions and scale drawings indicate minimum space requirements and design features for curbs, ramps, toilet, and restroom facilities. Drawings also indicate basic design factors for range of reach and clearance for wheelchairs and canes.

Y 3.B17/2:D63. Cotler, Stephen R. Architectural Accessibility for the Disabled on College Campuses. Albany, N.Y.: Architectural and Transportation Barriers Compliance Board, 1976. 133 pp.

This report was developed by an architect and a University Administrator who is disabled. It is an update of the 1967 and 1974 guides. It very specifically describes such things as ramps, restrooms, drinking fountains, and alarm systems as to their necessity, construction, and rationale. Its emphasis is to ensure the accessibility of all to college campuses.

Y 3.W58/18:1/977v.1,v.2 pts. A, B, C, v.3. The White House Conference on Handicapped Individuals. Washington, D.C.: White House Conference on Handicapped Individuals, 1977. For sale by: Supt. of Docs. U.S. G.P.O. $16.50 (3 vol. set).

This multivolume set consists of: volume 1 - Awareness Papers, volume 2 - Final Report, volume 3 - Implementation Plan. Volume 1 contains the papers which participants read in preparation for the conference. They cover health, social, education, economic, and special concerns and are intended to be readable and thought provoking. Volume 2 contains conference history, recommendations and resolutions, transcripts of speeches, statistical data, the list of official delegates, and a guide to resolutions. Volume 3 has very specific statements on implementing the resolutions. Each plan is identified as to government level (federal, state or administrative), type (administrative or legislative), and target completion date. The conference brought together 3700 people for the period May 23-27, 1977. The business they accomplished gives encouragement and support to all disabled individuals, because of the importance of their findings and their effective implementation plan. This landmark document is a must for any reference collection which includes materials on disabilities.

Y 3.T22/2:2T22/6. Technology and Handicapped People. Washington, D.C.: Congress of the U.S., Office of Technology Assessment, 1982. 214 pp. For sale by: the Supt. of Docs. U.S. G.P.O. $7.50.

FEDERAL GOVERNMENT PUBLICATIONS

The Senate Committee on Labor and Human Resources requested the Office of Technology Assessment to conduct a study of technologies for handicapped individuals. The study examines factors that affect research and development, evaluation, marketing, delivery, use, and financing of technologies related to disabled people. Chapters in the report cover disability, technology, resource allocation and policy options. Also included is a legislative overview, a glossary of acronyms and terms, and a list of references. This is an excellent summary of the state of the art, and provides a basis for deciding where we go from here.

14 JOURNALS

PHYLLIS C. SELF/Health Sciences Librarian, Library of
the Health Sciences, University of Illinois, Urbana, Illinois

INTRODUCTION

The importance of journal literature to the information world is well-documented. Journal literature is more timely than other forms of publication. It provides both research and practical articles, and in many professions, particularly the sciences, the research literature is published in serials rather than in books. However, the spiralling costs of serials due to inflation has been devastating and libraries have been forced to cancel peripheral titles with current budgets superimposing restrictions on the selection and acquisition of these materials. Therefore, it becomes essential for selectors to become knowledgeable about current serials before initiating a purchase request. For a comparison of average prices and price indexes, 1978-1981 see Piper 1982.(1)

Because of the differences in selection, acquisition, control and inflation associated with journals and the interdisciplinary nature of subjects in the field of rehabilitation a separate chapter is devoted to the journal literature. Subscription prices quoted have been included and should be used for the purpose of obtaining estimates as journal prices are constantly changing.

The average cost of journals listed in this chapter is approximately $38.00.

One journal which may have been more appropriately placed in the Independent Living chapter under the Aids and Devices section is the Bulletin of Prosthetic Research. This is an exceptionally fine publication for researchers in bioengineering and orthopedics, and is a must for any library supporting research in these areas.

The purpose of this chapter is to identify, provide bibliographic information, and describe the various serials available to professionals working in the field of rehabilitation. The journals listed within this chapter for the most part are aimed at professionals in the fields of speech-hearing-language, medicine, occupational and physical therapy, bioengineering, and rehabilitation. However, many of these serials would also be useful to laypersons providing such persons with information on new therapies, aids and devices, and new publications. Just as the layperson should be made aware of the professional literature, the literature written for or by laypersons should not be overlooked by the rehabilitation professional. As Bopp (1981) states "... periodicals offer information not found elsewhere about publications and services for the disabled. More importantly, they can educate librarians, rehabilitation professionals, and the general public about the needs and abilities of those Americans who are physically disabled."(2)

A few general publications which are not strictly aimed at professionals but would be useful in terms of providing background information about disabled persons have been included. Examples of such serials are: Disabled USA, Ostomy Quarterly, and The Deaf American. Such publications as the Deaf American would be useful to the general audience providing information about the deaf community which many in the hearing world know little to nothing about.

Most serials included in this chapter are published by professional organizations and/or societies working in the various fields of rehabilitation with only three titles being produced by the U.S. Government. The greatest concentration of the journal literature is directed toward the broad subjects of Speech-language/hearing/and deafness, and rehabilitation. Few professional publications are solely devoted to visual and mobility impairments. Disciplines which are represented by at least one serial in the field of rehabilitation are: art, counseling, medicine, music, nursing, psychiatry, and sports.

A survey of the literature demonstrates that many professional organizations have begun to devote time, energy, and money to the development of serials dealing specifically with rehabilitation but greater attempts need to be made to coordinate efforts to disseminate information in this multi-disciplinary subject area.

In an examination of indexes to the serial literature (those serials cited in this chapter) the following indexes were found to be the major indexes and abstracts in the field of rehabilitation:

    Exceptional Child Education Resources
    dsh Abstracts
    Social Science Citation Index
    Index Medicus
    Sociology Abstracts
    National Institute of Mental Health
    Psychological Abstracts
    ERIC

Today, all of these except dsh Abstracts are available through online database vendor such as BRS, SDC, and Lockheed. Those journals which are indexed by a variety of indexing and abstracting services are:

    American Annals of the Deaf
    American Speech and Hearing Association (ASHA)

Exceptional Children
Journal of Learning Disabilities
Journal of Speech and Hearing Disorders
Journal of Speech and Hearing Research.

Because of the interdisciplinary nature of rehabilitation and the scattering of the literature, a number of journals have made attempts to aid their readers by providing citations of recent articles appearing in journals which the reader might not normally scan. An example of this feature can be found in Developmental Medicine and Child Neurology's "Current Articles" section.

A number of journals appear in this chapter even though their major focus is not rehabilitation including such journals as Behavior Research and Therapy. Because adjustment to disability is the primary step in the rehabilitation process these interdisciplinary journals have been included and they may be useful to a variety of professionals working with behavioral problems associated with individuals having physical disabilities.

Other useful features employed by several journals are the inclusion of summaries or abstracts and key word lists. These two features are extremely useful for individuals maintaining personal reference files. These features can generally be found in those journals which claim to be international in scope such as International Journal of Artificial Organs, Developmental Medicine and Child Neurology, International Rehabilitation Medicine, and Paraplegia.

The primary purpose of journals published by professional associations is to extend information to their membership about current events, publications effecting the profession, current research techniques or methodologies, and controversies within the profession. An organization may publish a variety of publications to cover the variety of interests of its membership. Such an organization is the American Speech-Language Hearing Association. It publishes three journals to address the clinical, research, and professional activities of the Association. They are, respectively; The Journal of Speech and Hearing Disorders, Journal of Speech and Hearing Research, and ASHA.

One serial which holds a very prominent position in the field of rehabilitation for both the consumer and the professional is Rehabilitation Literature. Although published by the National Easter Seal Society, it in no manner serves as the newsletter for that society. Rather it is both a reviewing and an abstracting journal attempting to bring all interested persons and rehabilitation information together and is more comparable to an index for the field of rehabilitation. It is an excellent current awareness source for both professionals and laypersons.

Because of the interdisciplinary nature of the fields of physical disability and rehabilitation and the expense involved in purchasing and processing journals, this chapter was written as a guide to journals available in todays professional rehabilitation literature. No attempt has been made to identify retrospective materials. Two other chapters which include journal and serial titles are: "Legal Rights: Advocacy, Legislation, Litigation, and Programs" and "Federal Publications." Readers are encouraged to use all three chapters to obtain a more comprehensive list of those publications published on a serial basis.

NOTES

1. Nelson A. Piper, "Prices of U.S. and Foreign Published Materials" in The Bowker Annual of Library and Book Trade Information (New York: R.R. Bowker Company, 1982), pp. 396-413.
2. Richard E. Bopp, "Periodicals for the Disabled: Their Importance as Information Sources," The Serials Librarian, Vol. 5 (2), Winter 1980: 61-70.

ANNOTATED BIBLIOGRAPHY

ASHA. Rockville, Md.: The American Speech-Language-Hearing Association, Monthly. $50.00.

This journal serves as the "house organ" of the American Speech-Language-Hearing Association and as such focuses its attention to the "professional and administrative activities of speech-language pathology, audiology, and the Association." Articles are of a "broad professional interest and may be philosophical, conceptual, historical or synthesizing." Like other association publications it includes a listing of available employment positions, a calendar of upcoming events, and book reviews. It is written for practitioners and educators. Indexed in Biological Abstracts, Index Medicus, and Psychological Abstracts. Recommended for medical and social science libraries as well as those libraries serving speech, language, and hearing professionals.

American Annals of the Deaf. Silver Spring, Md.: Conference of Educational Administrators Serving the Deaf/Convention of American Instructors of the Deaf. Bimonthly. $27.50.

This is the official organ of the Conference of Educational Administrators Serving the Deaf/Convention of American Instructors of the Deaf. It is "a national professional journal for teachers, specialists and school administrators working for education of the deaf." Articles include abstracts and extensive bibliographies. As the official organ this publication carries convention announcements, symposia, committees, roster of members, and classified ads. Indexed in Biological Abstracts, Education Index, Index Medicus, P.A.I.S., Psychological Abstracts, and Social Science Citation Index. Recommended for education and medical libraries.

American Archives of Rehabilitation Therapy. North Little Rock, Ark.: Association for Rehabilitation Therapy, Three times a year. $17.00.

This publication is directed toward rehabilitation practitioners in schools, colleges and community agencies and covers the broad field of rehabilitation including learning disabilities, schizophrenia, and others. Published three times a year it attempts to present "current professional issues, innovative practices and programs and scientific research of benefit and interests to practitioners..." The publishers do not require the reader to seek permission to reproduce complete articles in the Archives, a valuable feature for any educator. Indexed in Index Medicus. This publication is not a must for a research collection but would be useful to practitioners to keep abreast of happenings in related areas within the broad field of rehabilitation. Recommended for medical and social science libraries.

American Corrective Therapy Journal. San Diego, Calif.: American Corrective Therapy Association, Inc., Bimonthly. $27.00.

Appears to serve as the "House Organ" for the American Corrective Therapy Association by providing a calendar of events,

Association business items, certification information, and book reviews. Formerly the Association for Physical and Mental Rehabilitation Journal, this publication attempts to publish "Research studies, theoretical articles and systematic reviews of special areas relating to corrective or adaptive physical education, psychology, physiology and special education..." Indexed in Biological Abstracts, Index Medicus, Psychological Abstracts, and Hospital Literature Index. Useful publication for practitioners and educators. Recommended for medical libraries and rehabilitation and physical education collections.

American Journal of Art Therapy. Washington, D.C.: Elinor Ulman in affiliation with the American Art Therapy Association, Quarterly. $20.00.

Art therapy plays a vital role in the rehabilitation of both the mentally and physically disabled. This journal, published in association with the American Art Therapy Association, contains many of the same features as other professional journals, namely: news, job information exchange, signed book reviews and citations to recent literature of interest to the membership. The articles are written from a practical point of view in the areas of education, rehabilitation, and psychotherapy. Indexed in Index Medicus, Psychological Abstracts, Social Science Citation Index, Exceptional Child Education Abstracts, Hospital Literature Index, and Mental Retardation Abstracts. Recommended for medical libraries and art and rehabilitation collections.

The American Journal of Occupational Therapy. Rockville, Md.: American Occupational Therapy Association, 13 times a year. $30.00.

This is the official publication of the American Occupational Therapy Association and as such includes featured articles, news items, letters to the editor, book reviews and classified ads. It is the primary publication for educators and practitioners in occupational therapy because it contains "new approaches and techniques of practice, development, theory, research and educational activities, and professional trends." It is another journal whose publishers have lifted copyright restrictions for educational purposes. Indexed in Index Medicus, Cumulative Index to Nursing Literature, Current Index to Journals in Education; Mental Health Index, and Current Contents in Educational and the Behavioral, Social, and Management Sciences. A must for all medical libraries and rehabilitation collections.

American Journal of Physical Medicine. Baltimore, Md.: Williams and Wilkins Company, Bimonthly. $28.00.

This journal is directed toward researchers and clinicians in the field of physical medicine and rehabilitation, primarily, rehabilitation of long-term conditions of amputation, stroke, arthritis, and brain damage. The "New Equipment and New Products" section while useful as a means for the reader to keep abreast of new equipment on the market is prepared from the material submitted by the manufacturers and provides no evaluation for the reader. The journal does include a useful "New Notes" section which provides information on advanced courses, symposia, workshops, association meetings, new journals, governmental agencies announcements, and many other items which cover the broad field of physical and/or rehabilitation medicine. Indexed in Index Medicus and Currents Contents/Clinical Medicine. A must for all medical libraries and rehabilitation and physical education collections.

American Rehabilitation. Washington, D.C.: Rehabilitation Services Administration, Bimonthly. $9.00.

This is the official publication of the Rehabilitation Services Administration. It includes short invited articles, publication announcements, short book reviews, and descriptions of new aids and devices. It includes little new information but would be useful to the layperson or perhaps to librarians as an acquisition source. This publication is available from the U.S. Government Printing Office. Recommended for public libraries.

Amicus. Notre Dame, Ind.: National Center for Law and the Handicapped, Bimonthly. Ceased.

An excellent, authoritative, well-written legal journal for the handicapped which ceased publication in 1980 as a result of Federal funding cuts to support the National Center for Law and the Handicapped. Its regular features included legal news, legislation, cases in the courts and special reports. There is no other publication which attempts to cover the legal field as well as this one did. The loss of this publication is a great loss to all professionals working with physically and mentally disabled individuals.

Archives of Physical Medicine and Rehabilitation. Chicago: American Congress of Rehabilitation Medicine, Monthly. $35.00.

This journal is the official journal of and is published jointly by the American Congress of Rehabilitation Medicine and the American Academy of Physical Medicine and Rehabilitation. Although it is the official journal of these organizations, it contains less association business and many more scientific articles than most journals of its kind. All articles contain an abstract and many references. The journal does contain classified ads and signed book reviews and articles are written for rehabilitation medicine professionals both researchers and clinicians. Indexed in Index Medicus, Current Contents/Clinical Practice, Physical Education Index, and Cumulative Index to Nursing and Allied Health Literature. This is a must for medical libraries and rehabilitation and physical education collections.

Artificial Organs. Cleveland, Ohio: International Society for Artificial Organs, Quarterly. $80.00

This journal is the official publication of the International Society for Artificial Organs and claims to publish articles of original research and clinical application. Articles are reviewed by an editorial board of international scholars and "includes the design of studies, the performance and evaluation of biomaterials and devices, physiological effects of various artificial organs, innovative concepts and approaches and case reports." The journal does carry a few membership items and a section for international news but basically it is a research journal. Indexed in Index Medicus, Biological Abstracts, Chemical Abstracts, Current Contents and Science Citation Index. Recommended for medical and academic libraries and bioengineering collections.

Audecibel. Livonia, Mich.: National Hearing Aid Society, Quarterly. $10.00.

This journal is written for otologists, clinical audiologists, and other professionals interested in the field of hearing and audiology. As the official journal of the National Hearing Aid Society it contains research, clinical, and educational articles; association business; book reviews; educational opportunities; and other items for professionals to assist the hard-of-hearing. Because it is not indexed in any major indexing service this journal has limited usefulness to the researcher. Included with the journal, as a separate, is an annual "Directory of Members."

Audiology: Journal of Auditory Communication. Switzerland: S. Karger Medical and Scientific Publishers, Bimonthly. $132.00.

This is the official organ of the International Society of Audiology. Articles may appear in French as well as English, but all articles include a "Resume" in French, an abstract, and key words. They are research oreinted and would be useful for the audiologist and otolaryngologist. The Journal contains signed book reviews and a minimal amount of association business. Recommended for medical libraries and professional audiology collections.

Behavior Therapy. New York: Association for Advancement of Behavior Therapy, Five times a year. $80.00.

"Interdisciplinary journal primarily for publication of original research of an experimental and clinical nature which contributes to the theories, practices, and evaluation of behavior therapy or behavior modification." It covers any aspect of living in which behavior can be modified from nailbiting to obesity and to encouraging women to seek cervical cytology. Articles include brief reports, case reports and book reviews. Indexed in Biological Abstracts, Physchological Abstracts, and Social

Science Citation Index. Recommended for social sciences libraries and rehabilitation collections.

Behaviour Research and Therapy: An International Multi-Disciplinary Journal. New York: Pergamon Press, Bimonthly. $130.00.

Although not specifically oriented toward the physically disabled, this interdiscipline journal would be useful to any professional working with behavioral problems associated with individuals having a physical disability. Articles appear in English and include an abstract and many references. It is not a journal for laypersons but for professionals in behavioral medicine and medical psychology. Indexed in Biological Abstracts, Index Medicus, Psychological Abstracts, and Social Science Citation Index. Recommended for medical and academic libraries.

Bulletin of Prosthetics Research. Washington, D.C.: Veterans Administration. Dept. of Medicine and Surgery, Semiannual. Price varies per issue. For sale by: Supt. of Docs., U.S. G.P.O.

A federal document which publishes Veterans Administration funded research and development projects. The R&D articles cover all aspects of living from specific limb prosthetics to driving, writing, automated retrieval of information on assistive devices, wheelchair cushions, and many other such topics. Other sections include: technical notes, which are not formally refereed, progress reports, recent patents, abstracts of recent articles appearing in journals from around the world, publications of interest, and a calendar of events. Articles contain an abstract, references, and many illustrations. This is an extremely valuable source for bioengineers, mechanical engineers, and orthopedic surgeons working in the area of prosthetics and sensory aids development. Indexed in Engineering Index, Excerpta Medica, Index Medicus, and Current Contents/Clinical Practice. Recommended for medical, engineering, and academic libraries.

The Canadian Journal of Occupational Therapy. Toronto: Canadian Association of Occupational Therapists, Five times a year. $15.30.

This journal contains many of the same features as do other official journals of an association: announcements, book reviews, job announcements, and does include clinical, theroretical, educational and research articles of interest to occupational therapists. General announcements appear in both French and English whereas full length articles appear in either French or English determined by the author and include an abstract in the other language. Indexed in Index Medicus and Hospital Literature Index. A must for medical libraries and most rehabilitation collections.

Cleft Palate Journal; an International Journal of Craniofacial anomalies. Baltimore, Md.: American Cleft Palate Association printed by Waverly Press, Inc., Quarterly $35.00.

"....an international publication designed to reflect research and clinical activities in the...study and treatment of cleft lip and cleft palate, other craniofacial anomalies, and related problems." It is the official organ of the American Cleft Palate Association and as such includes association business, letters to the editor, announcements, and book reviews. The articles contain abstracts and key words which are useful to readers who maintain reprint files. Articles appear in English, are illustrated, and contain many references. It is another publication which has lifted copyright restrictions for educational purposes. Indexed in Index Medicus, and Index to Dental Literature. This publication is a must for anyone working in the field of craniofacial anomalies including dentistry, otolaryngology, and plastic surgery and is recommended for most medical libraries.

The Deaf American. Silver Spring, Md.: National Association for the Deaf, Eight times a year. $10.00.

As the official publication of the National Association for the Deaf this journal provides general and organizational information to and about the deaf community and is neither research nor clinical in nature. A useful publication for public libraries primarily for individuals of or serving the deaf community and should be useful to local community planners. Appears not to be indexed in any major indexing service.

Developmental Medicine and Child Neurology. Philadelphia: J. B. Lipincott, Bimonthly. $50.00.

This is the official journal of the American Academy for Cerebral Palsy and Developmental Medicine, and of the British Paediatric Neurology Association. It is an international and professional journal covering the medical aspects of child neurology, cerebral palsy, and developmental medicine. Articles appear in English but include summaries in French, German, and Italian. The section "Current Articles" lists articles which appear in other journals and which would be of interest to its readers. The journal includes editorials, original articles, case reports, annotations, and news items of interest to its members. Indexed in biological Abstracts, Index Medicus, Psychological Abstracts, dsh Abstracts, Science Citation Index, Index to Dental Literature, and Mental Retardation Abstracts. Recommended for all medical and social sciences libraries.

Education of the Visually Handicapped. Washington, D.C.: Heldref Publications, Quarterly. $15.00.

Articles cover a very broad range of topics in the area of educating the visually impaired. They include an abstract, and are well-written and referenced. The journal contains lengthy and signed book reviews, editorials, and conference announcements. Because it contains both practical and research oriented articles and is indexed in most all of the major indexes in the field of education, this journal is a must for education libraries and for professionals working with the visually handicapped and/or their parents.

Epilepsia: Journal of the International League Against Epilepsy. New York: Raven Press, Bimonthly. $94.00.

A scholarly research publication which contains original manuscripts "on any aspect of epilepsy (clinical, experimental, biochemical, etc.)" Articles must follow a very structured format and include summaries in French, German, and Spanish when possible, a very valuable feature for a publication which claims to be international. In addition, the journal includes excellent book reviews and announcements of meetings and awards. Indexed in Biological Abstracts, Chemical Abstracts, Index Medicus and Psychological Abstracts. This journal is a must for life science, medical, and social science libraries.

Exceptional Children. Reston, Va.: The Council for Exceptional Children, Bimonthly. $25.00.

This journal contains many excellent articles covering the clinical, research, and educational areas for professionals working with exceptional children. Articles are well-written and include an abstract and many references. The journal includes full-length articles; brief communications; media reviews; and "ERIC's Newsfront;" which lists news items, ERIC acquisitions, and computer search reprints of interest to "Exceptional Children's" readership. Indexed in Psychological Abstracts, Exceptional Child Education Resources, Language and Language Behavior Abstracts, Abstracts for Social Workers, and Current Index to Journals in Education. A must for education, social science and psychology collections.

Handicapped Americans Report. Arlington, Va.: Capitol Publishers, Semimonthly. $127.00.

A semimonthly newsletter published to keep readers abreast of current proposals, legislation, programs, and grants which effect handicapped Americans. This is a very useful publication for those professionals involved with federal funding and legislation affecting employment or services and for laypersons. It is not indexed by any of the major indexing services. Recommended for public, law, and academic libraries.

Hearing Rehabilitation Quarterly. New York: League for the Hard of Hearing, Quarterly, $4.00.

This publication lies somewhere between a newsletter and a journal. It is the official publication of the New York League for the Hard-of-Hearing, licensed as an out-of-hospital health facility. It contains a "News in Brief" section and signed book reviews and would be of interest to otolaryngologists, audiologists and other communication therapy professionals. Indexed in dsh Abstracts. Recommended for speech, language, hearing, and rehabilitation collections.

Hearing Research. North-Holland: Elsevier Biomedical Press, Bimonthly. $153.60.

As the title implies this journal is research oriented with emphasis on experimental studies although there are some theoretical papers. The journal aims to publish articles on "auditory neurophysiology, ultrastructure, psychoacoustics and behavioral studies of hearing in animals and models of auditory functions." Articles are in English and include an abstract, key words, and many references. Besides research articles the journal includes short communications, review articles, announcements, and book reviews. Indexed in Biological Abstracts, Chemical Abstracts, Current Contents/Life Sciences, Excerpta Medica, and Psych INFO. Recommended for research oriented life science and medical libraries and professional hearing collections.

International Journal of Artificial Organs. Milano, Italy: Wichtig Editore. Bimonthly. $93.00.

This international journal contains both clinical and experimental articles about the use of artificial organs. The editors have divided it into eleven sections which may or may not appear in every issue of the journal. The sections are: Artifical Kidney and Dialysis, Gas Exchange and Artificial Lung, Artificial Heart and Related Topics, Liver Assist Devices, Detoxification, Bio-artificial Devices, Biomaterials, Hemapheresis, New Trends, Editorials, and Letter to the Editor. Articles appear in English and contain an abstract and list of key words which assist the reader in maintaining personal reference files. Indexed in Current Contents and Index Medicus. Recommended for all medical libraries and biological research collections.

International Journal of Rehabilitation Research. Heidelberg, Germany: G. Schindele Verlag, Quarterly. $42.50.

A quarterly publication which publishes international research in all areas of rehabilitation. Articles appear in English but include summaries in English, German, French, and Spanish. Indexed in Current Contents/Social and Behavioral Resources, Excerpta Medica, Psychological Abstracts, Social Science Citation Index, Rehabilitation Literature, and many other indexing services. Recommended for academic and medical libraries.

International Rehabilitation Medicine. Basel, Switzerland: EULAR Publishers, Quarterly. $56.00.

This international journal attempts to publish "...clinical studies directed towards rehabilitation medicine, communications concerned with physical therapy, occupational therapy, speech therapy, the psychosocial aspects of disablement, rehabilitation engineering, and resettlement and the vocational training of disabled people..." It represents the broadest range of information published within a single journal. Although it is the official journal of the International Rehabilitation Medicine Association, it contains very few items directed only toward its membership. Its primary emphasis is the publishing of clinical studies and communications of rehabilitation information. Articles appear in English but include summaries in both French and German and a list of key words. Indexed in Index Medicus. This journal is recommended for all medical libraries.

International Rehabilitation Review. New York: Rehabilitation International, Quarterly. $10.00.

A truely international newsletter written for laypersons and professionals in all fields of rehabilitation. It includes short articles of developments in various countries around the world discussing laws, transportation, employment, education, housing, and others. It is a superficial but very informative newsletter. It is not indexed by any of the major indexing services. Recommended for public and academic libraries and rehabilitation collections.

Journal of Applied Rehabilitation Counseling. Falls Church, Va.: National Rehabilitation Counseling Association, Quarterly. $30.00.

Articles in this journal are relevant to practitioners, educators, and students in the field of rehabilitation counseling. The journal includes both theoretical and practical issues, a few book reviews, and Letters to the Editor. Indexed in Psychological Abstracts. Recommended for social sciences and medical libraries and rehabilitation and counseling collections.

Journal of Auditory Research. Croton, Conn.: C. W. Shilling Auditory Research Center, Inc., Quarterly. $12.00.

This is an interdisciplinary journal covering the fields of "otology, audiology, psycho-acoustics, musicology, speech and communications, neurophysiology of audition, instrumentation for hearing research, and auditory aspects of human engineering." It is a highly research oriented publication and would be useful primarily to those involved in the scientific study of hearing. Therefore, it is recommended to only those libraries supporting such studies. The journal contains no book or media reviews or any supplementary sections other than the original articles it publishes. Indexed in Index Medicus.

Journal of Learning Disabilities. Glassboro, N.J.: Educational Press Association of America, Monthly. $27.00.

"A multidisciplinary publication containing articles on theory and practice related to learning disabilities. It includes reports of research, program and curriculum evaluation, case reports, and discussion of issues which are the concern of all discipline engaged in the field." This is a refereed journal. It contains an annual index and arranged by author, subject, and title. It is useful for the educator but not necessarily for health practitioners. Subjects covered include eye movement patterns, reading comprehension, psychotropic drugs, peer tutoring, foods and hyperactivity. Indexed in Biological Abstracts, Education Index, Excerpta Medica, Psychological Abstracts, and many others. Recommended for education, medical and academic libraries.

Journal of Music Therapy. Lawrence, Kan.: National Association for Music Therapy, Quarterly. $12.00.

As the official publication of the National Association for Music Therapy this journal contains few of the features found in most membership journals. It is basically composed of articles and signed book reviews which would interest the researcher, clinician and educator in Music Therapy. A small but useful publication. Indexed in Exceptional Child Education Resources, Psychological Abstracts, Hospital Literature Index, dsh Abstracts, and Music Therapy Index. Recommended for academic libraries and rehabilitation collections.

Journal of Occupation Medicine. Chicago: The American Occupational Medical Association and American Academy of Occupational Medicine, Monthly. $25.00.

Another professional association journal containing many of the same features and emphasis as others of this type of journal. A very useful feature for individuals working in this multidisciplinary field is "Selected Reviews from the Literature" which covers international journals as well. Indexed in Biological Abstracts, Chemical Abstracts, Index Medicus, and Social Science Citation Index. Recommended for Medical and Social Science Libraries, for physicians in occupation medicine and/or Family Practice, and Sociologists.

Journal of Orthopaedic and Sports Physical Therapy. Baltimore, Md.: Orthopaedic and Sports Physical Therapy Sections of the American Physical Therapy Association, Quarterly. $30.00.

The primary audience for this manual is professionals in orthopaedics and sports physical medicine. Articles are reviewed by an Editorial Board representing the fields of: medicine, psychology, biomechanics, basic science, neurology, dentistry, sports medicine, and others. It contains book reviews, educational opportunities, abstracts of current literature, classified ads, and many advertisements. It does not appear to be indexed in any of the major indexing and abstracting services. Recommended for orthopaedic, osteopathic, physical therapy, other sports medicine professionals; medical libraries; and physical education collections.

Journal of Rehabilitation. Alexandria, Va.: National Rehabilitation Association, Quarterly. $20.00.

This is the official publication of the National Rehabilitation Association and as such attempts to publish articles of interest to rehabilitation professionals across the broad field of rehabilitation. It is not a research publication, but is a publication by, for, and about the membership and as such includes signed book reviews, association news, and educational opportunities. Indexed in Index Medicus, Psychological Abstracts, Social Science Citation Index and Hospital Literature Index. Recommended for all rehabilitation professionals regardless of disability specialization for its broad overview to the field of rehabilitation and for social science and medical libraries.

Journal of Rehabilitation of the Deaf. Silver Spring, Md.: American Deafness and Rehabilitation Association, Quarterly. $25.00.

Although this journal is the official organ of the American Deafness and Rehabilitation Association, it contains more research and education articles than do other comparable association journals. It is published quarterly and would be useful to all professionals working with the deaf. Indexed in Psychological Abstracts and Social Sciences Citation Index. Recommended for social science and education libraries and rehabilitation collections.

Journal of Speech and Hearing Disorders. Rockville, Md.: The American Speech-Language-Hearing Association, Quarterly. $50.00.

This journal "pertains to the nature and treatment of disordered speech, hearing, and language and to the clinical and supervisory processes by which this treatment is provided." Articles included are based on their clinical significance and contain an abstract and generally extensive bibliographies. The Journal is directed toward the clinician and is a very professional type journal. It contains no advertisements and literally no association news. Indexed in Biological Abstracts, Education Index, Index Medicus, Psychological Abstracts, Social Science Citation Index and dsh Abstracts. Recommended for all professionals and libraries in the areas of speech, language, and hearing.

Journal of Speech and Hearing Research. Rockville, Md.: The American Speech-Language-Hearing Association, Quarter. $50.00.

A highly research oriented journal which "pertains broadly to studies of the processes and disorders of speech, hearing, and language." Articles are included which are experimental reports -- theoretical, tutorial or review papers. Indexed in

Biological Abstracts, Chemical Abstracts, Education Index, Index Medicus, Social Science Citation Index and dsh Abstracts. Recommended for academic libraries and those medical libraries supporting speech and hearing research.

Journal of Visual Impairment & Blindness. New York: American Foundation for the Blind, Monthly. $20.00.

An interdisciplinary journal which will appeal to researchers and practitioners working with the blind and visually impaired. Articles cover a broad range of topics including libraries, attitudes, technology and education. Indexed in Chicorel Abstracts to Reading and Learning Disabilities, Current Contents. Exceptional Child Education Abstracts, Excerpta Medica, Psychological Abstracts, and many others. Recommended for public, and social science libraries and education collections.

Ostomy Quarterly. Los Angeles, Calif.: United Ostomy Association, Quarterly. $10.00.

A publication for and about ostomates. It contains many articles written from the personal perspective and a variety of helpful articles written by health professionals. It includes organizational news and events, product and equipment information, and publication announcements. Written for the layperson, this publication would be useful for nurses, doctors, and therapists working with ostomates to help better understand the complexities and difficulties of living with an ostomy. It is not indexed by any of the major indexing services. Recommended for medical and public libraries.

Paraplegia. Edinburgh, Scotland: International Medical Society of Paraplegia, Bimonthly. $69.00.

This publication is written for clinical and research oriented physicians working with paraplegics and is not a publication for the layperson. Articles appear in English, but include summaries in both French and German. They also contain abstracts and key words which are useful for those physicians maintaining personal reference files. The journal does include a few signed book reviews and conference announcements. Indexed in Index Medicus. Recommended for medical libraries.

Paraplegia News. Bethesda, Md.: Paralyzed Veterans of America, Monthly. $5.00.

As the offical organ of the Paralyzed Veterans of America "it is published in the interest of and for the benefit of paraplegics, civilians and veterans all over the world." It is primarily useful to keep abreast of current legislation but covers all aspects of life such as employment, recreation, travel, and education affecting physically disabled individuals. As an association journal it includes announcements, calendars, and "chapter briefs." The many advertisements for aids and devices make this a useful publication for the layperson and vocational rehabilitation counselors. It is not indexed in any of the major indexing services. Recommended for public libraries and rehabilitation collections.

Physical & Occupational Therapy in Pediatrics: The Quarterly Journal of Developmental Therapy. New York: Haworth Press, Quarterly. $66.50.

This is a relatively new journal which began in 1980 and publishes research reports, reviews, and case studies. It is written for both physical and occupational therapists in practice or in education and is concerned with the application to children. The editors and the contributing authors represent the fields of psychology, physical and occupational therapy, orthopedics, neurology, nursing, and special education. It contains signed book reviews, annotated bibliographies, and news items of interest to its readers. Indexed in Cumulative Index to Nursing and Allied Health Literature. Recommended for medical and social sciences libraries.

Physical Therapy. Washington, D.C.: American Physical Therapy Association, Monthly. $22.00.

As the official journal of the Association it includes articles and sections aimed at both the science and practice of physical therapy. The regular features: "Continuing Education," "Abstracts of Theses and Dissertation," "Abstracts of Current Literature," "Book Reviews," "Products News," and "Positions Available" make this a valuable publication for the practicing therapist. Indexed in Index Medicus, Current Contents/Clinical Practice, and Exceptional Child Education Resources. This is a must for all medical libraries and rehabilitation collections.

Psysiotherapy. London: Chartered Society of Physiotherapy, Monthly. $25.00.

As the "Journal of the Chartered Society of Physiotherapy" the major portion of the journal is devoted to the dissemination of professional information to its membership by its regular features of newsletters, educational opportunities, society news and elections, book reviews, audiovisual programs, and many more. The articles are clinical in nature and would appeal to physical therapists, occupational therapists and nurses. Its classified ad section makes this publication extremely useful for finding a position as a physiotherapist. Indexed in Index Medicus. Recommended for medical libraries.

Physiotherapy Canada/Physiotherapie Canada. Toronto, Ontario: Canadian Physiotherapy Association, Bimonthly. $12.00.

As the official journal of the Canadian Physiotherapy Association it contains many features of interest to its membership: educational opportunites, classified ads, international news, calendar of events, and book reviews. The journal would be useful to clinicians, educators, and researchers. The articles appear in English and include abstracts in both English and French and key words which are useful for personal indexing files. Indexed in Cumulative Index to Nursing and Allied Health Literature, Hospital Literature Index, and Rehabilitation Literature. Recommended for all medical libraries and rehabilitation collections.

Prosthetics and Orthotics International. Copenhagen: International Society for Prosthetics and Orthotics, Three times a year. $38.00.

Referred to as the Journal of the International Society for Prosthetics and Orthotics, it publishes articles which would appeal to individuals in occupational and physical therapy, orthopaedic surgery, rehabilitation engineering, biomechanics, orthotics, and prosthetics. Articles may be clinical or research oriented and appear in English. Abstracts appear in German, French, and Italian in the journal issue following the actual publication of the article. This is a definite flaw in the journal format. Readers would be better served if the foreign abstracts appeared with the publication of the article rather than three months later. The journal includes a calendar of educational opportunities at the National Centre for Training and Education in Prosthetics and Orthotics and often signed book reviews. Indexed in Exerpta Medica and Index Medicus. Recommended for all medical libraries and those libraries supporting bioengineering and biomechanic research.

Rehabilitation Counseling Bulletin. Falls Church, Va.: American Rehabilitation Counseling Association, Five times a year. $12.50.

Published as the Journal of the American Rehabilitation Counseling Association it is directed toward both clinicians and educators in the field of rehabilitation counseling and not toward laypersons. It is a very professional publication. The January 1982 issue contains the "1980 Annual Dissertation Review: An Annotated Bibliography" in Rehabilitation Counseling. Indexed in Social Science Citation Index and Social Work Research & Abstracts. Recommended for academic libraries and for rehabilitation counselors/social workers.

Rehabilitation Digest. Toronto, Ontario: Canadian Rehabilitation Council for the Disabled, Quarterly. $6.40.

An informative newsletter type of publication which reprints articles from other journals of interest to physically disabled individuals. It is a Canadian publication but would be useful for comparative purposes and for the announcements and reviews of books and audiovisual materials. Indexed in Excerpta Medica and

Exceptional Child Education Abstracts. This publication is written for laypersons and is recommended for public libraries.

Rehabilitation in Australia. Deakin, Australia: Australian Council for Rehabilitation of Disabled, Quarterly. $17.50

This is the official publication of the Australian Council for Rehabilitation of Disabled and as such contains organization news and conference announcements. It contains more features and more international news than does its American counterparts and carries no advertising. Some useful features are: the "Rehab Reading," which provides current awareness to other professional journals in the rehabilitation field; Book Reviews; "Newly Cataloged Titles"; and "Rehab Viewing" section which describes audio-visual materials available for use from the Film & Information Service; and an international calendar of "Coming Events." It is not indexed by any of the major indexing services. Recommended for academic libraries.

Rehabilitation Literataure. Chicago: National Easter Seal Society, Bimonthly. $18.00.

This is an interdisciplinary journal "published for professional and students concerned with the rehabilitation of the handicapped." It is intended to keep the professional up to date not only in his field but also in other related fields. Although it is published by the National Easter Seal Society, it in no way serves as the official journal of that association. Articles are extremely easy to read and are written by people outstanding in their fields. It contains an "Article of the Month," a "Special Article," "Events and Comments", book reviews, and abstracts. This publication serves as both a reviewing and an abstracting journal. It is an extremely valuable publication which would be useful to any professional expecially to librarians as a current awareness and selection tool. As an educational service the publishers have given permission to reproduce up to 100 copies of an article for an organization or classroom use or the Editor can supply at cost reprints of the Article of the Month or the Special Article. Indexed selectively in Index Medicus, Psychological Abstracts, Hospital Literature Index, dsh Abstracts, Exceptional Child Education Resources, Current Index to Journals in Education and Cumulative Index to Nursing & Allied Health Literature. Recommended for all medical, academic, and public libraries.

Rehabilitation Nursing. Evanston, Ill.: Association of Rehabilitation Nurses, Bimonthly. $20.00.

This is the official publication of the Association of Rehabilitation Nurses and as such includes news items for the membership. It is "Designed to reflect thought, trends, policies, and research in rehabilitation nursing care." Indexed in Cumulative Index to Nursing and Allied Health Literature. Recommended for medical and nursing libraries.

Rehabilitation Psychology. Washington, D.C.: American Psychological Association, Quarterly.

The publication of this journal has been delayed. An announcement by Springer claims "the emphasis will be on reporting the results of sound empirical research in rehabilitation settings and issues relevant to clinical practice." Recommended for academic and medical libraries.

Rehabilitation World: The U.S. Journal of International Rehabilitation News and Information. New York: Rehabilitation/World, Quarterly. $10.00.

This publication is written to keep Americans abreast of international events affecting physically disabled individuals. It is definitely written for the laypersons but would be useful to librarians because of the "International Calendar" and list of "Books Recently Received." Indexed in Excerpta Medica and Exceptional Child Education Abstracts. Recommended for academic and public libraries and rehabilitation collections.

Rheumatology and Rehabilitation. London: Bailliere Tendall, Quarterly. $55.00.

Formerly known as Annals of Physical Medicine and Rheumatology and Physical Medicine this publication serves as the official journal of the British Association for Rheumatology and Rehabilitation. An international clinically oriented journal which would be useful to anyone studying or working with patients suffering from rheumatoid disease. Articles appear in English and include a short summary/abstract and cover such topics as assessment, repair and reconstruction, monitoring movement, anti-inflammatory drugs, and many other related topics. The journal contains excellent, and well-written, and signed reviews of books and media. Indexed in Biological Abstracts, Chemical Abstracts and Index Medicus. Highly recommended for medical libraries and rehabilitation collections.

Scandinavian Journal of Rehabilitation Medicine. Stockholm: Almqvist & Wiksell Periodical Company, Quarterly. $47.00.

A very professionally oriented medical journal which "publishes original articles, editorials and invited reviews, and case reports." Articles are formatted to be very concise, appear in English, and include an abstract and three to twelve key words from Medical Subject Headings which the author believes suitably describes the article. Indexed in Biological Abstracts and Index Medicus. Recommended for medical libraries.

Sexuality and Disability: A Journal Devoted to the Study of Sex in Physical and Mental Illness. New York: Human Sciences Press, Quarterly. $58.00.

An excellent journal for both clinicians and researchers involved in the study of sex and physical and mental illnesses and various disabling conditions including geriatric problems, endocrinologic diseases, and drug addiction. Articles may appear as clinical practice reports, case studies, research and survey data reports, state-of-the-art papers, guidelines for clinical practice, contemporary developments in special programs in sex education and counseling for the disabled, and the like. Three very useful sections in this journal are "Q & A Answering your Questions about Sexual Medicine," "Book Reviews", and "Media Reviews". It is indexed in "Sociological Abstracts, Human Sexuality Update, Excerpta Medica, Pastoral Care and Counseling Abstracts, Current Contents/Social and Behavioral Sciences, Social Sciences Citation Index, and Social Service Abstracts. Articles are well-written for both professionals and laypersons and include an abstract and many references. Recommended for all medical and social sciences libraries.

Spina Bifida Therapy: an International Journal. Oak Brook, Ill.: Eterna Press, Quarterly. $30.00.

"...multidisciplinary professional publication addressing physicians, nurses, therapists, counselors, educators, and social workers involved in the treatment and care of people with Spina Bifida." The journal includes a section entitled "Previews and Reviews" which summarizes a variety of articles about spina bifida which have appeared in professional medical journals. It is not indexed by any of the major indexing services. Recommended for all medical libraries and anyone involved in the work or study of Spina Bifida.

Volta Review. Washington, D.C.: Alexander Graham Bell Association for the Deaf, Inc., Seven times a year. $35.00.

This is the official journal of the Alexander Graham Bell Association for the Deaf. The organization was established in 1890 to encourage the teaching of speech, speechreading, and the use of residual hearing to deaf persons. It is one of the best indexed journals in the field; it is indexed by at least 10 indexing and abstracting sources. Articles are of a practical nature and include an abstract and lengthy bibliographies. The journal contains book reviews, association news, calendar of events, and a Directory of Services. Recommended for academic and education libraries and speech-language-hearing collections.

15 AUDIOVISUAL REFERENCE SOURCES

FRANCESCA ALLEGRI/Assistant Health Sciences Librarian,
University of Illinois, Urbana, Illinois

INTRODUCTION

The usefulness of audiovisual materials in various settings has been testified to by various persons, primarily educators. As Dwyer states in his preface to <u>Strategies for Improving Visual Learning:</u>

> "The use of visualized materials (drawings, photographs, films, television, transparencies, charts, computer assisted instruction, etc.) to complement regular classroom instruction has become a common instructional technique at all levels of education - extending from pre-school activities through graduate school and also into in-service training and development programs."(1)

The widespread use of audiovisuals in these various settings and others has stimulated much discussion as to their effectiveness and Dwyer continues by stating that a great deal of research is needed in this area. However, the fact that audiovisuals have an important role in the presentation of information and instruction now and in the future is confirmed. In a report issued by the Carnegie Commission on Higher Education, the special role instructional technology will have for the disabled is also noted:

> "...by the year 2000 it now appears that a significant proportion of instruction in higher education on campus may be carried on through informational technology - perhaps in a range of 10 to 20 percent. It certainly will penetrate much farther than this into off-campus instruction at all levels

beyond the secondary school - in fact it may become dominant there at a level of 80 percent or more.

Better than ever before, it can bring education to the sick, the handicapped, the aged, the prisoners, the members of the armed forces, persons in remote areas, and to many adults who could attend classes on campus but who will find instruction at home more convenient. It can create new uses for leisure time, can facilitate job-to-job movement through new training, and can improve community participation by imparting greater skill and knowledge to citizens."(2)

One of the most significant contributing factors to the revolution in instructional technology has been techniques of mass communication, primarily television. Peterson in The Learning Center: A Sphere for Nontraditional Approaches to Education describes this development and how television has given rise to new expectations in our audiences, particularly those of school-age today.(3)

There are many potential values of the use of visuals, some of which are listed by Dwyer.(4) Relevant to the disabled audience, some media have become standards of communication. Examples are captioned or signed visuals for the deaf and audiorecordings for the blind. The popularity of captioned film centers and the Library of Congress Talking Book Service have established these modes as major channels of communication with these two populations.

In addition to these uses of audiovisuals by the disabled, audiovisuals have been successfully used as consciousness-raising devices and stimulants for discussion on physical disabilities and societal and individual attitudes toward the disabled. One film typically used for this purpose is "What Do You Do When You See a Blind Person?" produced by the American Foundation for the Blind in 1971.

Due to the wide variety of audiences and potential applications for audiovisuals there will be many groups for which materials listed in this chapter will be useful. In addition to public libraries which may be primarily interested in films similar to "What Do You Do When You See a Blind Person?", patient educators, and consumer or advocacy groups may find audiovisuals valuable. Recently, more instructors in medical and other health professions programs are making use of materials on rehabilitation topics in order to expand student awareness in these areas. The same materials are being used in continuing education programs for practicing professionals whose curricula did not offer these topics several years ago. The National Library of Medicine Literature Search, <u>Audiovisual Aids, Computer Assisted Instruction, and Programmed Instruction in Education for the Health Professions</u>, lists numerous articles discussing the advantages of audiovisuals in the context of health professions education.(5)

All types of libraries, whether public, special, school or academic, will find reference tools listed in this chapter which would help in acquiring audiovisuals on rehabilitation topics. This chapter covers audiovisual catalogs which list nonprint media about the disabled for either professional or general audiences. These catalogs may be used for the purposes of selection or reference in the area of rehabilitation. In this chapter, specialized tools are examined, as well as a few general catalogs which contain good coverage of physical disability or provide unique information in this subject area. Catalogs of materials for the disabled themselves, for example the catalog of the Captioned Films for the Deaf Distribution Center, are not included.

As is common in other subject areas, reviews or evaluative information on nonprint media are not frequently provided. A rare exception is <u>Looking Ahead: Filmstrips for the Hearing Impaired</u>, compiled by Rouleau, which lists only programs which meet specified criteria. Reviews, if available, are more likely to be found in organizational newsletters or professional journals. Some of these journals feature regular columns on audiovisuals, such as "Valuable Viewing" in <u>Rehabilitation Digest</u> (Toronto: Canadian Rehabilitation Council for the Disabled). This publication is a definite must for keeping abreast of newly produced media in the area of rehabilitation.

The sources of information for audiovisual programs is extremely varied. They include commercial producers, professional organizations, newsletters and specialized subject catalogs. Several examples of each of these are included. There are also, in addition to general catalogs in the health area, related specialized tools such as About Aging: A Catalog of Films with a Special Section on Videocassettes.(6) Rental catalogs, such as the Rehabfilm Rental Catalogue, are useful for program planning or preview purposes if not for collection development. Schools for the deaf or blind, although they tend to collect materials for use by their students, are also sources of audiovisuals for the professional or general audience about these particular disabilities.

Professional organizations and national associations or societies often include nonprint media in their publications lists or may issue a separate catalog for these materials. As these lists are very abundant and usually ephemeral in nature only a few have been annotated in this chapter. Examples of those which are available but not annotated in this chapter are Illinois Heart Association Public Health Education Catalog of Films and Slides, National Association of the Deaf Catalog of Publications, A.G. Bell Publications by Alexander Graham Bell Association for the Deaf and the Educational Multimedia-CME Catalog by the American Academy of Orthopaedic Surgeons.

Some of the general sources included in the annotations for this chapter are the catalogs produced by the Veterans Administration. Other governmental agencies, both state and federal, may also be sources of nonprint media in the area of rehabilitation. A noted general selection tool, due to its concentration on inexpensive programs, is the Educator's International Guide to Free & Low-Cost Health Audio-Visual Teaching Aids by Nolan. Another general tool, which provides access to materials which have gained increasing importance recently, is Human Sexuality Methods and

AUDIOVISUAL REFERENCE SOURCES   425

Materials for the Education, Family Life and Health Professions: An Annotated Guide to the Audiovisuals by Daniel.

Several catalogs of rehabilitation research institutes have been included as they are excellent sources of audiovisuals for professionals. The Rehabilitation Institute of Chicago's catalog is a good example of this type. Related to these are the catalogs of the nineteen Rehabilitation Research and Training Centers. Although a union catalog is annotated in this chapter, Publications and Audio-Visual Aids Directory of the Rehabilitation Research and Training Centers, most of the centers issue individual materials catalogs which tend to be more current than this general one. Selectors interested in materials for professionals in the rehabilitation field would want to be on the training centers' mailing lists in order to receive, for example, the eight-page Research and Training Materials Catalogue, 1979-80 of the Rehabilitation Research and Training Center No. 9 at George Washington University. This catalog lists four videotapes in addition to books and journal articles.

Another category of selection/reference tools are aimed at particular aspects of rehabilitation, for example, independent living or physical education. One of several examples included here is Instructional Materials in Independent Living by Smith and Fry. Two of this type which are not annotated due to their ephemeral nature are "Selected Resources for Accessibility" issued by the Architectural and Transportation Barriers Compliance Board, Washington, D.C. and "Tools for Accessibility: A Selected List of Resources for Barrier Free Design" by the National Center for a Barrier Free Environment. Between the two, they list eight audiovisual programs with no overlap between the brochures examined. Another type of specialized catalog covers a particular disability, such as Saltzman's Guide to Films about Blindness.

Commercial catalogs may list audiovisuals on rehabilitation or disabilities but due to the lack of a centralized source of subject access to these, they are difficult to discover. An example of such a catalog is "Films, Video Filmstrips, Slides" by Focus International. This company specializes in audiovisuals on sexuality and includes a section on disability which usually lists three to four titles. The catalog is aimed at health professionals but the titles under disability would be valuable consciousness-raisers for general audiences and the disabled themselves.

As can be seen by these examples and the materials annotated, there are a variety of information sources for rehabilitation audiovisuals and no centralized dissemination source at this time. In addition to these printed tools there are computerized databases incorporating audiovisual programs such as AVLINE, ERIC (Educational Resources Information Center), NARIC (National Rehabilitation Information Center) and NICSEM/NIMIS (National Information Center for Special Education Materials).

The AVLINE database, prepared by the National Library of Medicine, does contain hard-to-find reviews as well as availability information on health science audiovisuals. Searching the database for rehabilitation topics has been described briefly in another publication.(7) The audiovisuals in AVLINE, due to the educational purposes for which the database was constructed, are primarily intended for students and practicing health professionals rather than the lay public. However, it is often possible to identify producers who may also distribute materials for the nonprofessional.

Content and tips for searching audiovisuals in all of the above-mentioned databases have been described by Van Camp in a series of articles.(8,9) In "Health Science Audiovisuals in On-line Databases: Part 2", Van Camp describes how to locate catalogs or directories of audiovisual materials similar to those listed in this chapter through the various computerized systems. A hint for increasing the retrieval of the sample search shown in the article is to utilize other synonyms for audiovisuals such as "film(s)", "media", "video(s)", and "multimedia". The following retrieval resulted from such an expansion: GPOM (GPO Monthly Catalog), 50; MDOC (Medoc), 19; NRIC (National Rehabilitation Information Center), 23; NIMI (National Information Center for Special Education Materials), 3; and ECER (Exceptional Child Education Resources), 50. In two databases in which the initial retrieval was large, ERIC (Educational Resources Information Center), 394, and NTIS (National Technical Information Service), 88, several rehabilitation terms were added to focus the search results. This retrieved 38 references on ERIC and 7 on NTIS. In this manner, readers may keep updated on new audiovisual productions as well as new catalogs of materials on rehabilitation topics.

NOTES

1. Francis M. Dwyer, Strategies for Improving Visual Learning: A Handbook for the Effective Selection, Design, and Use of Visualized Materials (State College, Pa.: Learning Services, 1978), p. xiii.
2. Carnegie Commission on Higher Education, The Fourth Revolution: Instructional Technology in Higher Education (New York: McGraw-Hill, 1972), pp. 1-2.
3. Gary T. Peterson, The Learning Center: A Sphere for Nontraditional Approaches to Education (Hamden, Conn.: Linnet Books, 1975), p. 13.
4. Dwyer, Stategies for Improving Visual Learning, p. 12.
5. National Library of Medicine, Audiovisual Aids, Computer Assisted Instruction, and Programmed Instruction in Education for the Health Professions, Literature Search No. 81-27, (Bethesda, Md.: National Library of Medicine, 1981).
6. Mildred V. Allyn, comp., About Aging: A Catalog of Films with a Special Section on Videocassettes, 4th ed. (Los Angeles: The Ethel Percy Andrus Gerontology Center, University of Southern California, 1979).
7. Richard E. Bopp, and Francesca A. Anstine, "Rehabilitation Literature: A Guide to Selection Materials," Library Resources and Technical Services 25, no. 3 (July/September 1981): 232-233.
8. Ann Van Camp, "Health Science Audiovisuals in Online Databases," Database 3, no. 3 (September 1980): 17-27.
9. Ann Van Camp, "Health Science Audiovisuals in Online Databases: Part 2," Database 5, no. 3 (August 1982): 23-29.

ANNOTATED BIBLIOGRAPHY

Arthritis Information Clearinghouse. <u>Arthritis Information Clearinghouse: Audiovisual Materials Catalog</u>. Bethesda, Md.: Arthritis Information Clearinghouse and National Institute of Arthritis, Metabolism and Digestive Diseases, 1981. 95 pp.

Lists various audiovisuals under nearly 150 subject headings. Unique feature is excellent indexing and organization: provides format, primary audience, title, subject and source indexes which list citation number and title of audiovisual. Full citation is listed in separate section. Some producers' annotations are included. Availability information provided as items are not available from Clearinghouse. List is nonevaluative. Includes some items for continuing education credit. Nine related print items are also listed; these are referenced by document number where appropriate. Very useful for selection purposes.

Daniel, Ronald S. <u>Human Sexuality Methods and Materials for the Education, Family Life and Health Professions: An Annotated Guide to the Audiovisuals</u>. Brea, Calif.: Heuristicus Publishing Co., 1979. 509 pp.

Includes the topic, "Mentally/Physically Compromised," which lists approximately sixty titles primarily for college or general audiences. Fourteen titles are marked for senior high and younger; seven are suitable for professionals. Majority of titles are dated 1977 and earlier. An alphabetical listing by title includes annotations and distributor. Entries under topic list title, format, date and other topics referenced. Some of the titles are not listed elsewhere. Text also includes references to sexuality of cancer and cardiac patients which makes this general index useful to other rehabilitation personnel.

<u>Disability Attitudes: A Film Index</u>. Portland, Maine: Human Services Development Institute, University of Southern Maine, 1978. 40 pp.

Lists approximately seventy films that may be effective in changing attitudes toward persons with disabilities by presenting accurate information about the disabled. Lists title only in alphabetic and subject indexes. Broad subject divisions are by disability. Gives descriptive annotations. Provides rental/purchase information in most cases. Includes various formats.

<u>Educational Materials</u>. Minneapolis: Sister Kenny Institute, 1980. 17 pp.

Table of contents divides fourteen subject areas into print and nonprint materials. Approximately 45 audiovisual titles listed, most under three headings, "Neuroaugmentation-Neurostimulation Training Series," "Care of the Handicapped" and "Stroke". The neuroaugmentation series is unique and includes detailed programs for professionals plus shorter more general presentations for the patients. Most materials in this guide however, are aimed at health professionals. Includes summaries of all programs plus content notes. June 1981 supplement to this catalog contains new programs.

Filmakers Library, Inc. <u>Films for Nursing, Rehabilitation and Special Education</u>. New York: Filmakers Library, Inc., n.d. 19 pp.

Lists twenty-one 16mm films on varied rehabilitation topics including breast cancer, Down's Syndrome, cerebral palsy, stroke and deafness. Also describes a film on language development and normal infant development. Several paragraph summaries are listed as well as reviewers' comments. One drawback is that no dates are listed. These films are useful for both professionals and laypersons.

<u>Guide to Audiovisual Resources for the Health Care Field</u>. Pittsburgh, Pa.: Medical Media Publishers, 1981. 198 pp.

Most items listed under 56 subject categories are for the professional; one subject heading is Health/Patient Education but it is not subdivided. Information is supplied by producer or distributor and not reviewed. Includes many titles in area of physical disability under various subject headings e.g., amputations, genetics, neurology and rehabilitation. Includes advertisements of AV producers, list of AV producers' address, phone and contact person (if available), and services and equipment manufacturers listed under type of service and equipment. Has list of lending libraries and distributors for other production companies. Gives information on two publications which list programs not in this guide: <u>Health Education Resource Catalogue, Inc.</u> and <u>Medical Catalogue of Selected, Audiovisual Materials</u>. Complete entry for items in this guide is under subject heading. Gives audience, purchase/rental price, availability of non-English versions and brief summary. Dates not always provided. This guide contains much useful information.

Information and Research Utilization Center in Physical Education and Recreation for the Handicapped. <u>Annotated Listing of Films, Physical Education and Recreation for Impaired, Disabled, and Handicapped Persons</u>. 2d ed. Washington, D.C.: American Alliance for Health, Physical Education and Recreation, 1976. 118 pp.

Contains 314 references to 16mm films and other media. Unique feature is inclusion of materials for or about the able-bodied which can be used with the disabled. Reviews include summary, possible uses, or audiences. Has index of key descriptors and list of additional sources of audiovisuals. One flaw: entries from first edition listed separately from second edition entries.

<u>International Rehabilitation Film Review Catalogue</u>. New York: Rehabilitation International, U.S.A., 1977. 65 pp.

Lists seventy-one 16mm films in English on mental and physical rehabilitation. Includes sales distributor list, alphabetic title index, list of subject categories, and index by subject. Evaluative reviews state potential usefulness and audiences. Many foreign producers are included. Most of the titles are recommended for both professionals and the disabled or their families.

Looking Ahead: Filmstrips for the Hearing Impaired: An Annotated Bibliography Featuring...Living Skills, Community Involvement, Vocational Options. Compiled by Ruth O. Rouleau. Pittsburgh, Pa.: Western Pennsylvania School for the Deaf, 1980. 254 pp.

Introduction describes the value of filmstrips for hearing and language impaired. Includes only those filmstrips which have met specified evaluative criteria. Lists series titles and individual titles under subject headings. Arrangement is alphabetical by title. Includes annotations and list of resource materials and distributors and producers. This is a valuable bibliography because it is evaluative but its indices could have been consolidated better, e.g., integrated series and individual title list, using "captioned" vs "noncaptioned" as subheadings of the subjects rather than the reverse. Materials listed would be useful for both professional and general audiences.

National Catalog of Films in Special Education. 2d ed. Compiled by National Center on Educational Media and Materials for the Handicapped and the New York State Education Department, Area Learning Resource Center. Columbus, Ohio: National Center, Educational Media and Materials for the Handicapped, 1978. 89 pp.

This catalog uses over two hundred descriptors to categorize audiovisuals primarily intended to instruct teachers and parents. A list of descriptors includes scope notes for each heading. Multiple descriptors are assigned and the title appears under each descriptor. An alphabetic arrangement is used to list the complete entries; the latter include a brief annotation. Intended to supplement the National Instructional Materials Information System (NIMIS) catalog. Also intended to be a more comprehensive list of special education films than is currently available; however, selection criteria are not clearly stated, therefore the latter is difficult to determine. Includes many audiovisuals in areas of behavior modification, mental retardation and learning disabilities but also areas of physical disability such as architectural barriers, blindness, mobility aids, and hearing impairment. Lists producers/distributors' addresses. Includes bibliography of catalogs consulted and lists first edition titles which are out of print. Unique feature is quite extensive list of titles being considered for next edition of this catalog. This catalog shows a lot of planning which makes it a very useful purchase for professionals or laypersons.

The 1980-1981 Rehabfilm Rental Catalogue. New York: Rehabfilm, 1980. 29 pp.

Lists ninety-one titles of films and videotapes for rental; several titles listed for sale. All items have summary and review. Forty-seven subject categories used. Catalog also has an alphabetic index by title with reviews listed alphabetically by title. Films tend to be directed more toward general audiences than professionals but professionals would find many of the titles useful for counseling, patient education and other work with the disabled.

Nolan, Maureen A., Educator's International Guide to Free and Low-Cost Health Audio-Visual Teaching Aids, 2d ed. Long Island City, N.Y.: Pharmaceutical Communications, Inc., 1979. 312 pp.

Divided into two sections: (1) Materials of Professional Interest and (2) Materials of Interest to Allied Medical Personnel and the General Public. Lists approximately 100 titles under subsection, "Disabilities, Rehabilitation, and the Disabled." Titles of interest to professionals in area of rehabilitation are listed in subsections of the catalog for example "Spinal Disorders" and "Physical Medicine, Disabilities, and Rehabilitation." Provides the source, audience and rental or purchase price as well as ordering instructions. Excellent as selection tool for inexpensive or free rehabilitation audiovisuals.

Publications and Audio-Visual Aids Directory of the Rehabilitation Research and Training Centers. Washington, D.C.: Rehabilittation Services Administration, 1978. 542 pp.

Lists 287 audiovisuals for professionals developed by and/or currently available through the nineteen research and training centers. Formats grouped under each research and training center are (1) audiotape or disc; (2) film, slide, overhead transparency, or filmstrip; (3) videotape; and (4) other. Includes brief description of content, recommended audience, and availability information. "Recommended follow-up" is also provided but most items are listed as self-contained units. Subject headings are fairly specific. Includes index of lecturers.

Rehabilitation Institute of Chicago. 1981 Publications and Visual Aids. Chicago: Research Dissemination, Rehabilitation Institute of Chicago, 1981. 36 pp.

Materials primarily for the health professional listed under "Educational and Instructional Training Packages" and "Other Audiovisuals." Most deal with spinal cord injuries and neurologic disabilities. Each entry contains summary, rental/purchase information, and audience. Very detailed programs dealing with management of physical disability. Includes several lectures by staff of Rehabilitation Institute.

Rehabfilm Newsletter. New York: Rehabfilm, Rehabilitation International U.S.A., Quarterly. $10.

An inexpensive quarterly. Contains reviews of films in one or two subject areas in each issue and feature articles on new audiovisuals. Includes articles on new technical developments, upcoming events, interviews, and bibliographies. Reviews other selection tools plus provides an extensive review of one film per issue. Reviews contain availability information and usually purchase recommendations. Valuable selection aid.

Saltzman, Joel, ed. Guide to Films about Blindness. New York: American Foundation for the Blind, Inc., 1978. 93 pp.

Not limited to this organization's films. Lists about eighty audiovisuals; most are available for a minimal rental fee or free. Provides summary, information on multiple formats, multiple distributors, and long/short versions. Indexed by twenty-nine broad subject categories. Drawbacks include an agency index which only lists names, not addresses; symbol N/A is used for several purposes. Lists other free film catalogs of materials not in this guide.

Smith, Bradley C., and Fry, Ronald R. Instructional Materials in Independent Living. Menomonie, Wis.: Stout Vocational Rehabilitation Institute, University of Wisconsin, 1978. 30 pp.

Lists 103 items, mostly print, which can be used by professionals to teach daily living skills to either the physically or mentally disabled. Provides availability, loan or purchase information for all items. Subject index has fourteen broad headings which are subdivided. Annotated list is not organized in a discernable way and subject index lists only the number of the annotated entry rather than the title. Despite these drawbacks in organization, the list is usefully annotated and the types of materials indexed may be difficult to locate elsewhere.

Stuckey, K. A., Deaf-Blind Bibliography. Rev. ed. Watertown, Mass.: Perkins School for the Blind, 1977. 186 pp.

Chapter, "Films, Videotapes, and Slides," (pp. 152-62) lists approximately ninety audiovisual titles dealing with this dual-sensory disability. Contains brief summary as well as format and availability information. Suggests audience in some cases. Most of items are available on free loan but a good number have a pre-1976 production date. Materials are geared toward professionals, parents of deaf-blind and advocates for deaf-blind individuals. Valuable as one of few selection tools devoted to deaf-blind materials, but list needs updating.

Veterans Administration. VA Film Catalog. Washington, D.C.: Veterans Administration, 1978. 98 pp.

This general film catalog lists twenty titles under heading, "Rehabilitation". Most of other materials are not geared specifically to physical disability but VA services and techniques in general. Materials listed are available on "free loan" from the Veterans Administration Central Office Film Library. Some entries marked for VA use only. Primarily 16mm format but also lists audiocassettes, videocassettes, filmstrips, and 35mm slides.

Veterans Administration. Union List of Audiovisuals in the Library Network of the Veterans Administration. Washington, D.C.: Veterans Administration, 1976. 595 pp.

Most of the materials are geared to the professional and discuss treatment aspects; occasionally lists audience and some have summaries. Complete information is provided under title. Many of the subject headings deal with physical disability. Lists holdings of the Library Network of the Veterans Administration, VALNET. Contains 3500 items in four formats: 16mm, audiocassette, videocassette, and 2"X2" slides. Has author, title, and subject indices. Also has name and subject heading authority lists. Unfortunately, no indication is given in the catalog as to whether these materials are available to persons outside the Veterans Administration Library Network. Needs updating.

The Videolog: Programs for the Health Sciences, 1979. New York: Esselte Video, Inc., 1979. 399 pp.

Formerly the Health Sciences Video Directory. Lists only videocassette/videotape programs. For health professions students or practitioners but does have approximately 800 programs under "Patient Education". There is a subheading, "Handicaps", under "Patient Education". Has at least forty specific subject headings which list over 350 programs of interest to rehabilitation personnel. Title only is listed under up to three Medical Subject Headings; full entry under title includes pricing, distribution information, producer's summary, audience, and video formats. Program was not included if summary was not provided. Has list of producers' addresses and phone numbers. Lists four video subscription services.

West Virginia Rehabilitation Research and Training Center. Products from the West Virginia Research and Training Center. Dunbar, W. Va.: West Virginia Rehabilitation Research and Training Center, n.d. 23 pp.

Briefly summarizes eleven film and sound/slide programs on vocational rehabilitation and affirmative action. No dates given for programs or catalog. Supplies rental/purchase information. Materials are intended for counselor or employer. Good example of materials available from specialized rehabilitation centers. Programs are aimed at professionals.

AUTHOR INDEX

Abeson, A., 248, 251, 252, 268
Abramson, A. S., 342
Abreu, B. C., 207, 213
Adams, J. M., 277
Adams, R. C., 326
Aiello, J., 387
Albrecht, G. L., 7, 84
Allan, B., 4, 26
Allen, A., 326
Allen, K. E., 350
Allen, W. A., 316
Allyn, M. V., 427
Alonso, L., 386
Alpiner, J. G., 164
Alvin, J., 327
American Alliance for Health Physical Education and Recreation, 337, 338, 342, 365, 366
American Art Therapy Association, 405
American Automobile Association, 126
American Deafness and Rehabilitation Association, 147
American Foundation for the Blind, 32, 34, 35, 36, 109, 114, 115, 126, 309, 422
American Hospital Association, 277
American Institute of Architects Potomac Valley Chapter, 7
American Medical Association, 207, 213
American National Standards Institute, 4, 7, 386, 387

American Speech-Language-Hearing Association, 160, 164, 402, 403, 404, 414
Ancona, G., 169
Ancona, M. B., 169
Andersen, V. W., 115
Anderson, E. M., 351
Anderson, F., 301
Anderson, H., 115
Anderson, M. H., 214
Anderson, W., 327
Andrews, B. G., 240
Annand, D. R., 324, 327, 345
ANSI, 386
Anstine, A., 427
Anthony, L. K., 133
Architectural and Transportation Barriers Compliance Board, 396, 425
Arkansas Rehabilitation and Training Center, 126
Arnheim, D. D., 323, 327
Aronson, S. M., 237
Arthritis Foundation, 116
Arthritis Information Clearinghouse, 428
Asbell, B., 40
Asenjo, J. A., 36
Association of Occupational Therapists, 408
Atkinson, J., 277
Atwater, M. H., 324, 328
Aurelia, J. C., 212, 214
Austin, R. L., 323, 328
Auxter, D., 323, 327
Avedon, E. M., 329
AVLINE, 426

Bachner, J. P., 384
Baer, W. P., 278
Baker, B. L., 116, 140, 141
Baker, C., 162, 164, 165, 175, 176
Bailey, D., 146
Ballantyne, J., 55, 60
Ballard, J., 252
Ballison, R., 164
Bamford, J., 157, 165
Banks, J., 118
Bardach, J., 301
Barley, M., 158, 182, 183
Barnerjee, S. N., 214
Barnes, E., 85
Baron, H., 116
Barraga, N. C., 36
Barrett, J., 28
Barrier Free Environments, 8
Barrow, R. L., 249, 252
Basmajian, J. V., 207, 214
Bass, M., 301
Batelaan, J., 139
Batelle Institute, 388
Batson, T. W., 56, 60
Bauer, H. J., 2, 8, 21, 215
Bauman, M. K., 37
Bautch, J. C., 240
Baxter, R. T., 313
Bean, B., 250, 253
Beasley, M. C., 117, 302
Beasley, R. W., 215
Becker, E. F., 295, 313
Becker, G., 61
Bednar, M. J., 9
Behrmann, M. M., 258
Belgum, D. R., 274, 278
Bellugi, U., 162, 184
Bench, J., 157, 165
Bender, R. E., 61
Benderly, B. L., 56, 61
Bennet, J. L., 221
Benton, A. L., 2, 9
Berg, F. S., 159, 166
Bergen, A., 111, 127
Berger, G., 85
Berger, K. W., 157, 167
Bergman, E., 56, 60
Bergman, M., 163, 167
Bergsma, D., 351
Berkowitz, E. D., 253
Berkowitz, M., 253

Berlin, A. J., 287
Berrigan, C., 85
Beryl, L., 60
Bess, F. H., 167, 179
Biehl, G. R., 247, 253
Bielfelt, S. W., 46
Biklen, D., 85, 254
Binder, D. P., 313
Birnbaum, S., 325
Bishop, D. S., 81, 85
Bishop, M., 386
Bishop, S., 386
Bitter, J. A., 78, 86
Blackwell, P. M., 160, 168
Blakeslee, M. E., 117
Bland, J. H., 278
Blasch, B. B., 34, 50
Blaxter, M., 83, 86
Blea, W. A., 37
Bleck, E. E., 208, 215, 277
Block, J. R., 105
Blount, W. P., 210, 215
Bluestone, C. D., 179
Blum, Barry, 302
Blum, G. T., 302
Blumenfeld, J., 279
Board, M. A., 141, 142, 144
Boblitz, M. H., 243
Bolick, N., 252, 254
Boller, F., 302
Bolles, M. M., 307
Bolton, B., 6, 57, 62, 80, 100
Bopp, R. E., 400, 403, 427
Bornstein, H., 163, 168
Boswell, D. M., 86, 88
Boucher, R. T., 235
Bowar, M. T., 110, 117
Bowe, F., 79, 82, 87, 249, 254
Bowker, T. H., 216
Bowley, A. H., 348, 351
Braddock, D. L., 268
Bradford, L. J., 55, 62, 64
Braille, L., 34
Brattstrom, M., 117
Bray, J. J., 214
Brechin, A., 83, 88
Breen, J. E., 324, 331
Bregman, S., 314
Brehm, H. P., 259
Brewer, G. A., 350
Bricker, D. D., 352
Brickner, R. P., 3, 9

Brightman, A. J., 116, 140, 141
Brodsky, C. M., 142
Bromley, I., 216
Brooks, H., 329
Brown A., 3, 9, 209, 216
Brown, C., 10
Brown, S. L., 352
Browne, J. A., 88
Browning, P., 256
Bruck, L., 249, 255, 275, 279
Bruckner, R., 39
Buell, C. E., 324, 329
Bullard, D. G., 295, 303, 318
Bunch, W. H., 210, 216
Bunin, N., 10
Burgdorf, R. L., Jr., 249, 255
Burke, D. C., 299
Burke, E. A. S., 217
Burn, G., 349, 360
Burns, D., 117, 302
Buscaglia, L., 82, 88, 350, 353

Cailliet, R., 217
Caldwell, B. M., 353
Calhoun, M. L., 349, 353
Califia, P., 296, 300
California Department of Public Health, 118
Calvert, D. R., 161, 169, 186
Campling, J., 89
Canadian Rehabilitation Council for the Disabled, 423
Carmen, R., 135
Carnegie Commission on Higher Education, 421, 427
Carnell, C. M., 114, 142
Carnes, G. D., 83, 89
Carrell, J. A., 200
Carroll, T. J., 30, 37
Carter, Goble, Robert, Inc., 393
Carver, V., 90
Cary, C., 5, 99
Cary, J. R., 10
Cassatt-Dunn, 152
Casterline, D. C., 200
Casto, G., 366

Casto, M. D., 143
Chadwick, D. M., 330
Chapey, R., 213, 217
Chapman, E. K., 349, 353, 354
Charlip, R., 169
Chartered Society of Physiotherapy, 127, 416
Chasin, J., 5, 11, 12
Children, R. A., 317
Children's Bureau, 383
Chipouras, S., 303
Christian, W. P., 354
Christopher, D. A., 161, 169
Clark, C. A., 330
Clark, L. L., 127
Clearfield, D., 112, 128
Clellan, R., 247, 255
Clifford, K., 319
Clowers, M. A., 238
Clymes, E. W., 176
Cobb, A. B., 3, 90
Cohan, H., 167
Cohen, L. K., 170, 179
Cohen, O., 44
Cohen, S., 79, 90
Cokely, D., 162, 165, 175, 176
Cole, J. A., 113, 141, 142, 143, 144, 146
Cole, S. S., 300
Cole, T. M., 300, 317
Collins, W., 394
Colson, J. H. C., 330
Comfort, A., 303
Committee on Sexual Problems of the Disabled, 300
Comoss, P. M., 211, 217
Constantian, M. B., 209, 218
Consumers' Association, 118
Convention of American Instructors of the Deaf, 404
Coons, M., 11
Cooper, I. S., 279
Cooper, S., 10
Copeland, K., 128
Corbet, B., 12
Cordellos, H. C., 330, 331
Cornelius, D. A., 91, 294, 299, 303

Council for Exceptional
  Children, 246
Council of Organizations
  Serving the Deaf, 63
Courtial, D., 234
Cox-Gedmark, J., 274, 279
Cozad, R. L., 171
Craft, A., 300
Craft M., 300
Craig, H. B., 157, 171
Craig Hospital. Family Service Department, 12
Craik, R., 241
Cratty, B. J., 324, 331, 354
Creer, T. L., 354
Crewe, N. M., 145
Croneberg, C. G., 200
Crosson, A., 256
Croucher, N., 331
Crowe, W. C., 323, 327
Crowell, W. M., 289
Cruickshank, W. M., 2, 12, 348, 354
Cull, J. G., 30, 40, 65, 91, 94, 208, 218
Curtis, B., 145
Curtis, S., 33, 38, 355

Dahlberg, C. C., 4, 13
Dale, D. M. C., 160, 172
Danhauer, J. L., 157, 172
Daniel, A. N., 326
Daniel, R. S., 425, 428
Daniels, S. M., 293, 299, 300, 303, 304
Danzig, A., 118
Dardier, E. L., 212, 219
Dardig, J. C., 358
Darley, F. L., 226
Davidson, R., 145
Davis, H., 62, 156, 173
Davis, J. A., 280
Davis, M. Z., 13
Davis, W. M., 129
Day, S. S., 143
Dean, R. J. N., 21
DeGraff, A. H., 275, 280
De Jong, G., 84, 145, 146, 256
Delk, J. H., 157, 173
Delk, M. J., 73

Dell Orto, A. E., 3, 6, 81, 82, 83, 96, 98, 99
DeLoach, C., 80, 92, 298
Demarco, B., 341
Des Jardins, C., 256
Dibner, A. S., 349, 355
Dibner, S. S., 349, 355
Dicker, L., 163, 174
Dickman, I., 314
Dickman, I. R., 32, 38, 249, 256, 304
Dietz, J. H., 210, 219
Dinsmore, A. B., 163, 174
Dinsmore, J., 268
DiQuizio, D., 265
Disabled Living Foundation, 344
Dittmar, S. S., 235
Dixon, A., 284
Dixon, J. T., 331
Dong, C. H., 118
Donlon, E. T., 33, 38, 355
Doose, H., 305
Dorros, S., 280
Downey, J. A., 348, 355
Downie, P. A., 210, 219
Doyle, P. B., 280
Drouillard, R., 355
Dubow, S., 257
Duckworth, B., 119
Duffy, Y., 295, 314
Duncan, J. L., 248, 257
Duval, R. J., 92
Dwyer, F. M., 421, 422, 427

Eareckson, J., 13
ECER, 427
Edgar, B. J., 14
Edington, D., 349, 356
Educational Resources Information Center, 426
Edwards, E. M., 332
Egolf, D. P., 186
Eisenberg, M. G., 92, 208, 220, 297, 304, 314
Eldridge, P. B., 220, 280
Elson, R., 223
Enby, G., 307, 315
Engen, E., 168
England, E. J., 233

AUTHOR INDEX

Engleman, E. P., 275, 281
Epilepsy Foundation of America, 249, 257
ERIC, 426
Esselte Video, Inc., 433
Evans, C. D., 220
Evans, J., 281
Evans, L., 197
Exceptional Child Education Resources, 427

Fabing, H. D., 249, 252
Fait, H. F., 343
Falconer, J. A., 220
Falk, M. L., 287, 291
Fallon, B., 272, 281
Fant, L. J., 174
Fant, L. J., Jr., 162, 175
Farber, S. D., 220
Fardy, P. S., 211, 221
Favors, A., Jr., 386
Feathersone, H., 356
Feingold, S. N., 273, 282
Fellendorf, G. W., 63
Feller, I., 207, 221
Ferron, D. T., 378
Fiedler, M. F., 175
Field, E. J., 221
Filmakers Library, Inc., 429
Fine, P. J., 176, 356
Firing, M., 93
Fischgrund, J. E., 168
Fishler, A. L., 114, 146
Fishman, D., 14
Fitch, W. J., 200
Flaherty, P. T., 222
Fletcher, S. G., 159, 166
Focus International, 426
Fodor, E., 325
Foott, S., 119
Ford, J. R., 119
Fortunate-Schwandt, W., 25
Foulds, R. A., 137, 190
Frank, E., 302
Frankman, J. P., 158, 192
Fraser, B. A., 282
Fredrickson, A., 326
Freedman, C. R., 277
Freeman, P., 33, 38, 349, 357
Freiberger, H., 132

Freud, S., 364
Frieden, L., 113, 141, 144, 146
Friedman, L. A., 162, 176
Friedmann, L. W., 2, 208, 209, 222
Fries, J. F., 282
Frisna, R., 63
Fry, R. R., 425, 432
Fuller, J. L., 46
Funk, D., 332
Furse, A., 222
Furth, H. G., 64

Gallaudet College, 56, 71
Gallender, D., 119, 120
Gambrell, E., 315, 318
Gannon, J. R., 64
Garcia, R. M., 211, 223
Gardner, L., 348, 351
Garee, B., 15, 132
Garrett, J. F., 3, 93
Gauger, J. S., 158, 176
Gault, E., 333
Gebhard, P. H., 300
Geddes, D., 324, 333
George Washington University, 299
Gerben, D., 84
Gerber, S. E., 159, 176, 177, 189
Gerwin, K. S., 159, 178
Giffiths, C., 178
Gilbert, A. E., 133
Gilbertson, K., 333
Gill, D., 50
Ginsburg, B. E., 46
Giolas, T. G., 159, 196
Gitler, D., 357
Gliedman, J., 348, 357
Gloor, B., 39
Glorig, A., 159, 178
Goble, R. E. A., 15
Goldberg, M. H., 39
Goldenson, R. M., 6, 35, 78, 93, 299
Goldfinger, G. H., 282
Goldsmith, S., 16
Goldstein, H., 39
Goltz, D. L., 258

Goodgold, J., 301
Goodman, J. F., 280
Gordon, S., 274, 283, 300, 315
Gould, E., 334
Gould, L., 334
GPO (Monthly Catalog), 427
GPOM, 427
Grabb, W. C., 221
Grayson, D., 35, 52
Greengross, W., 315, 316
Greer, B. G., 80, 92, 298
Greer, P. S., 34, 41
Gregory, M. F., 294, 300, 305
Gregory, S., 64
Greif, E., 81, 94, 223
Griesse, R., 16
Griffith, E. R., 305
Griffith, V. E., 283
Griggins, C., 92
Grilley, K., 140
Grofs-Selbeck, G., 305
Groom, J. N., Jr., 17
Gross, L., 283
Grotsky, J. N., 280
Groves, L., 324, 334
Groves, P. A., 34, 51
Gugerty, J., 133
Gugerty, J. J., 379
Gunn, S. L., 334
Gustason, G., 163, 178
Guttman, L., 335

Hackler, E. N., 16
Hale, G., 133
Halliday, C., 349, 358
Hamill, C. M., 335
Hamilton, L. B., 168
Hampton, D., 394
Hanak, M. A., 282
Hardy, A. G., 212, 223
Hardy, R. E., 30, 40, 65, 91, 94, 209, 218, 224
Hardy, W. G., 55, 62, 64
Harford, E. R., 159, 179
Harkness, S. P., 17
Harris, E., 240
Harris, G. M., 160, 179
Hart, B. O., 160, 179
Hart, V., 358

Hartbauer, R. E., 94, 180
Hartman, D., 33, 40
Hartman, E. C., 237
Haskins, J., 95
Hass, J., 252
Hastings, K., 306
Hawisher, M. F., 349, 353
Hawk, B., 266
Haynes, W. D., 213, 224
Hedgecock, L. D., 200
Hedley, E., 335
Heifetz, L. J., 116, 140
Heisler, V., 284
Heiss, M., 240
Hellenberg, M., 158, 180
Hellerstein, H. K., 242
Helms, T., 17
Henderson, P., 348, 358
Hennessy, C. A., 214
Hensinger, R. N., 282
Hermann, A. M. C., 247, 258
Heron, P. A., 291
Heslinga, K., 306
Hess, G. H., 284
Heward, W., 358
Hicks, D., 229
Higgins, P. C., 59, 65
High, E. C., 134
Hill, K., 335
Hinshaw, S. P., 141
Hippolitus, M. L., 392
Hirsch, E. A., 17
Hirsch, L. M., 185
Hockberg, I., 201
Hodgins, E., 18
Hodgson, W. R., 157, 180
Hoehne, C. W., 30, 40
Hoemann, H. W., 162, 175, 181
Hoffman, A. M., 120
Hoffman, S. J., 147
Hoffman, R. B., 111, 134
Holcomb, R. K., 56, 66
Holm, V. A., 350
Holt, N. B., 229
Hooley, A. M., 323, 345
Hopper, C. E., 316
Horr, K., 361
Hotte, E. B., 120, 123
Hourihan, J. P., 378
Howards, I., 259
Huffman, J., 182
Hughes, J., 226

AUTHOR INDEX

Hull, K., 249, 259
Human Resources Center, 132, 134, 139, 335, 336
Human Services Development Institute, 428
Humm, W., 224
Hurvitz, J., 135
Husted, J., 183
Hutchinson, P., 322, 336

ICTA Information Centre, 126, 139
Illinois Department of Children and Family Services, 121
Illinois Governor's Council on Developmental Disabilities, 144
Illinois State Office of Education. Bureau of Education for the Handicapped, 359
INA Mend Institute, 284
Information and Research Utilization Center in Physical Education and Recreation for the Handicapped, 342, 429
Ingenito, R., 224
Institute for Information Studies, 95, 260
Institute on Rehabilitation Issues, 147, 259
Intermed Communications, 234
International Symposium on Interpretation of Sign Languages, 163, 182

Jackson, R. W., 326
Jacobs, L. M., 56, 66
Jaffe, B. F., 55, 67, 159, 182
Jaffe, J., 4, 13
James, J. I. P., 225
Janz, Dieter, 298, 306
Jasperse, D., 10

Jastrzembska, Z. S., 41
Jay, P. E., 121
Jayson, M., 284
Jeffers, J., 158, 182, 183
Jenkins, W. M., 18
Jeter, K. F., 285
Johnson, M., 163, 183
Johnson, W. G., 253
Johnson, W. R., 316
Johnstone, M., 212, 225
Joint Commission on Accreditation of Hospitals, 277
Jones, B. W., 194
Jones, M. A., 18
Jurgens, M. R., 41

Kaarlela, R., 51, 125
Kakalik, J. S., 350
Kamenetz, H. L., 19
Kaplan, P. E., 226
Karnes, M. B., 359
Karp, A., 158, 198
Katz, I., 95
Katz, J., 156, 183
Katz, L., 273, 285
Kay, J. G., 337
Kay, L., 41
Keagy, R. D., 210, 216
Keith, R. L., 226
Keith, R. W., 184
Kelly, J. D., 337
Kenedi, R. M., 207, 226
Kernaleguen, A., 110, 121
Kerns, E., 250, 260
Kidwell, A. M., 34, 41
Kijek, J. C., 231
Kiley, A., 260
Kinney, R., 33, 42
Kirlin, B. A., 88
Kirlin, R. L., 186
Kirtley, D. D., 31, 42
Klein, J. O., 179
Kleinfield, S., 79, 96
Klemz, A., 43
Klima, E. S., 162, 184
Klinger, J. L., 121, 136
Knight, S. E., 295, 303
Koestler, F. A., 33, 43
Kolodny, R. L., 359

Kostuik, T. P., 226
Kottke, F. T., 227
Kowle, C. P., 379
Krambs, R. E., 256
Kramer, L. C., 163, 185
Kreisler, N., 135
Kreisler, T., 135
Krenzel, J. R., 212, 227
Kretschmer, L. W., 160, 179, 185, 200
Kretschmer, R. E., 60, 160, 194
Kretschmer, R. R., Jr., 179, 185, 200
Krusen, F. H., 227
Kubler-Ross, E., 274, 277
Kunder, L. H., 19
Kurzhals, I. W., 349, 358
Kwatny, E., 135

Labanowich, S., 19
Lagos, J. C., 286
Laker, M., 148
Lancaster-Gaye, D., 83, 96, 295, 306
Landis, C., 307
Lang, J., 301
LaRocca, J., 112, 136
Larson, C. W., 222
Larson, D., 286
Larson, M. R., 148
Larson, V. D., 186
Lash, J. P., 33, 43
Lasky, R. G., 81, 96
Lassen, P. L., 297, 300
Lauri, G., 148
Lawrence, E. D., 56, 67
Lawton, E. B., 122
Lear, R., 360
Leavitt, G. S., 163, 186
Lee, R. C., 359
Lees, D., 97
Leggett, J. M., 385
Lehman, W. B., 208, 227
Lehmann, T. F., 227
Lehr, S. T., 310
Lenneberg, E., 286
Leshin, G., 186
Levering, C., 265

Levine, E. S., 3, 57, 58, 59, 67, 68, 71, 93, 160, 186, 222
Liben, L. S., 68
Licht, S., 210, 228
Liddiard, P., 83, 88
Liebergott, J., 386
Lieberman, G., 109, 122
Lifchez, R., 5, 20
Lindemann, J. E., 97
Ling, A. H., 159, 187
Ling, D., 159, 161, 187
Liskey, N., 317
Lloyd, G. T., 71, 377
Logigian, M. K., 228
Longacre, J. J., 207, 208, 228
Lord, J., 322, 336
Loring, J., 349, 360
Low, M. L., 348, 355
Lowell, E. L., 187
Lowenfeld, B., 31, 44
Lowman, E. W., 136
Lowthian, P., 136
Lukoff, I. F., 32, 44
Lynch, J., 157, 198

McCartney, J., 308
Macartney, P., 110, 123
McDaniel, J. W., 98, 298
McDevitt, G. M., 98
McDonald, E. T., 286, 287
McGarney, B. D., 261
McKay, E., 167
McKinney, L. A., 379
McMichael, J. K., 360
McNamara, J., 274, 287
McNarmar, B., 287
McPherson, D. L., 188
Mace, R. L., 20
Madsen, W. J., 162, 188
Makas, E., 303
Malick, M. H., 210, 229
Malles, I., 167
Manley, M. S., 318
Mann, L., 280
Marinelli, R. P., 3, 82, 83, 98
Marquit, S., 20

AUTHOR INDEX

Martin, F. N., 188
Martin, N., 211, 229
Martin, R., 246, 260, 261
Mastro, B. A., 210, 229
Mastro, R. T., 229
Matarazzo, R. G., 81, 94, 223
Materson, R. S., 226
Mathews, B., 21
Mathis, S. L., 69
Mathis, S. L., III, 285
May, E. E., 123
MDOC, 427
Meade, J. G., 261
Meadow, K. P., 58, 59, 69, 73
Means, B. L., 31, 35, 47, 100, 149
Medical Media Publishers, 429
Meece, A. R., 243
Meighan, T., 45
Mencher, G. T., 159, 177, 189
Mendelssohn, A. N., 286
Menelaus, M. B., 208, 230
Mental Health Law Project, 261
Merrill, E. C., Jr., 285
Meyer, C. M. H., 229
Midwest Symposium on Therapeutic Recreation, 339
Miller, A. G., 339
Miller, A. L., 159, 189, 287
Miller, D., 199
Miller, J. B., 190
Miller, J. D., 137
Miller, M. H., 157, 190,
Miller, N. R., 273, 282
Miller, T. R., 209, 230
Milner, M., 11, 21
Mindel, E., 360
Mindel, E. D., 58, 69
Minkin, M., 183
Moakley, T. J., 261
Moberg, E., 208, 230
Moe, J. H., 215
Moersch, M. S., 352
Monbeck, M., 31, 45
Monteiro, L. A., 209, 230
Montgomery, G., 70
Mooney, T. O., 317
Moore, C. B., 383
Moores, D. F., 55, 70, 160, 190

Morrison, A. W., 207, 231
Morrison, D., 361
Morton, K. G., 383
Moses, H. A., 361
Mossman, P. L., 231
Mueller, J., 5, 21
Mulder, D. W., 207, 231
Muller, H., 339
Mullins, J. B., 361
Murphy, D. M., 116, 140
Murphy, E. H., 253
Murray, D. D., 299
Murray, J. N., 362
Murray, R., 211, 231
Musselwhite, C. R., 232
Myklebust, H. R., 57, 70

Nagel, D. A., 277
Nagi, S. Z., 259
Namir, L., 162, 197
NARIC, 426, 427
Nathanson, I., 388
National Arthritis Advisory Board, 380
National Association of State Directors of Special Education, 262
National Center for a Barrier Free Environment, 5, 22, 425
National Center for Health Statistics, 374
National Center for the Law and the Deaf, 251, 263
National Center for Law and the Handicapped, 144, 250, 252, 262, 266
National Center on Educational Media and Materials for the Handicapped, 430
National Conference on Program Development for and with Deaf People, 71
National Easter Seal Society, 170, 276
National Federation of the Blind, 45, 263
National Information Center for Special Education Materials, 426, 427

AUTHOR INDEX

National Institute for Advanced Studies, 385
Nationoal Library of Medicine, 423, 427
National Paraplegia Foundation, 301, 309
National Public Law Training Center, 250, 263
National Rehabilitation Information Center, 426, 427
National Technical Information Service, 427
National Workshop on Rehabilitation Centers, 149
Neff, W. S., 99
Nelson, J. G., 325, 340
Nerbonne, M. A., 158, 197
New Jersey. Department of the Treasury. Division of Building and Construction, 22
New York University Medical Center, 137
Newby, H. A., 190
Newman, J., 340
Nichols, P. J. R., 15, 207, 232
Nickel, V. H., 233
NICSEM/NIMIS, 426, 427, 430
Nielsen, D. W., 204
Nix, G. W., 249, 264
Nolan, M. A., 424, 431
Noland, R. L., 350, 362
Nordqvist, I., 317
Norris, C., 318
Norris, C. M., 272, 277, 288
Northern, J. L., 159, 190
NTIS, 427
Nursing Clinics of North America, 211, 235

O'Brien, M. T., 212, 232
O'Connor, E., 341
Ohio. Governor's Committee on Employment of the Handicapped, 23
Oliver, R. C., 335
Oppelt, K., 341
Oppenheim, C. J., 329

O'Rourke, T. J., 161, 191, 192
O'Shea, B. J., 139
Ovellette, S. E., 71
Overbeck, D., 199
Overs, R. P., 341
Owen, E. S., 342
Oyer, H. J., 158, 183, 191, 192

Padden, C., 165
Pahz, C. S., 163, 193
Pahz, J. A., 163, 193
Palkes, H. S., 290, 363
Pallett, P. J., 232
Palver, A. E., 351
Parker, C. A., 362
Parks, A. L., 264
Parrott, C. A., 390
Paterson, G. W., 274, 288
Paul, J. P., 226
Pearman, J. W., 209, 233
Pentz, C. M., 72
People's Housing, Inc., 23
Perlman, L. G., 32, 45
Perlmutter, A. D., 289
Petal, M., 72, 149
Peterson, A., 366
Peterson, G. T., 422, 427
Peterson, Y., 23, 296, 307
Pfaffenberger, C. J., 46
Pfetzing, D., 178
Pflueger, S. S., 113, 150
Phillips, J. W., 200
Phillips, W. R. F., 265
Pieper, B., 289
Pieper, E., 289
Pierce, D., 208, 233
Pilling, D., 289
Piper, N. A., 399, 403
Platt, R. T., 142
Podair, S., 102
Poling, D. A., 301
Pollack, M. C., 193
Pollack, M. L., 233
Pothier, P., 361
Potok, A., 46
Power, D. J., 194
Power, P. W., 68, 81, 99

AUTHOR INDEX 445

Prensky, A. L., 290, 363
Prescod, S. V., 193
President's Committee on Employment of the Handicapped, 111
Preston, R. P., 211, 234
Priestley, L., 224
Pritham, C., 243
Progressive Architecture, 387
Public Technology, Inc., 394

Quigley, S. P., 160, 194

Rabin, B. J., 293, 299, 308
Rainey, C., 125
Rantz, M. F., 212, 234
Raynor, S., 355
Read, R., 123
Reamy, L., 324, 342
Redden, M. R., 24, 25, 265
Redford, J. B., 137, 210, 235
Reed, M., 246
Rehab Group, Incorporated, 384
Rehabfilm, 431, 432
Rehabilitation Engineering Center, 210, 228 229
Rehabilitation Institute of Chicago, 326, 431
Rehabilitation International, 429, 432
Rehabilitation Research and Training Center, 425
Rehabilitation Services Administration, 431
Reitz, N. L., 221
Rice, B. D., 150, 265
Richards, L., 146
Riekehof, L. L., 161, 194
Riffle, K. L., 211, 236
Rintelmann, W. F., 157, 195
Roberts, A., 31, 46
Roberts, G. A., 308
Roberts, J., 266
Robinault, I. P., 99, 138, 308

Robinson, F. M., 343
Robinson, K. P., 240
Robinson, R. L., 47
Rodda, M., 90
Rodriquez, D. B., 312
Roessler, R., 80, 100
Roessler, R. T., 6, 31, 35, 47, 100, 149, 150
Rogers, M. A., 290
Rohman, B. F., 189
Rohrer, L. M., 227
Rolen, G., 339
Rose, D. E., 195
Rosenbaum, E. H., 318
Rosenbaum, I. R., 318
Rosenberg, A. L., 272, 290
Rosenberg, J., 265
Rosenstein, S. N., 208, 236
Roshal, A. F., 133
Ross, D., 212, 236
Ross, M., 157, 159, 195, 196
Rossett, A., 358
Rossi, P., 210, 237
Rossi, S. L., 171
Roth, W., 348, 357
Rouleau, R. O., 423, 430
Rousseau, M. K., 264
Routh, T., 47
Routledge, L., 363
Royal National Institute for the Deaf, 189
Royse, R. E., 150
Rubin, M., 157, 196
Rullman, L., 326
Rusalem, J., 167
Russell, W. R., 237
Russo, A., 72
Rustad, L. C., 314
Ryan, M., 123
Safilios-Rothschild, C., 81, 84, 100
Sahs, A. L., 237
Salmon, F. C., 48
Saltman, J., 11
Saltzman, J., 425, 432
Sams, T. A., 354
San Francisco Cancer Symposium, 311
Sanders, D. A., 158, 196
Saulnier, K. L., 168
Saunders, F. A., 137, 138, 190

Savage, J. F., 197
Savage, R. D., 163, 197
Savitz, H. M., 101, 343
Scadden, L., 132
Scarlett, S., 308
Schapiro, S., 250, 253
Schein, J. D., 73
Schellen, A. M., 306
Schiefelbusch, R. L., 350
Schiller, V., 167
Schlesinger, H. S., 58, 59, 73
Schlesinger, I. M., 162, 197
Schmidt, C., 246, 266
Schmidt, D. H., 233
Schnur, R., 31, 48
School of Art, University of Michigan, 8
Schow, R. L., 158, 197
Schowe, B. M., 54, 59, 74
Schroedel, J. G., 101
Schroeder, S. A., 386, 387
Schroeder, S. L., 125
Schubert, E. D., 198
Schwab, L. O., 151, 152, 392
Schweikert, H. A., Jr., 25
Scott, J. P., 46
Scott, R. A., 48
Scholl, G., 31, 48
Seay, D. M., 379
Seligman, M., 102, 350, 364
Selim, G., 4, 25
Sensory Aids Foundation, 49
Sha'ked, A., 294, 299, 310
Shaw, S., 97
Shearer, A., 301
Shedd, D. P., 237
Sherrick, E. E., 132
Sherrill, C., 343
Shinnick, M. D., 147
Shipes, E. A., 310
Shivers, J. S., 343
Shontz, F. C., 81, 102
Siedar, G., 260
Silver, R. A., 74
Silverman, M., 275, 281
Silverman, S. R., 62, 156, 161, 169, 173, 186
Silverstein, A., 291
Silverstein, V. B., 291
Simkins, J., 151

Singh, S., 157, 172, 198
Sins, V. A., 157, 171
Sioux Vocational School, 151
Sister Kenny Institute 16, 124, 428
Skinner, P. H., 157, 180
Sloan, L. L., 49, 138
Small, R. E., 4, 26
Smith, B. C., 425, 432
Smith, C. R., 158, 198
Smith, F. T., Jr., 266
Smith, J., 266
Smith, L. M., 392
Snobl, D. E., 148
Solnit, A. J., 348, 364
Sorensen, R. J., 26
Sosne, M., 324, 344
Sourcebook Publications, 133
Soyka, P. W., 364
Spastic Society and SPOD, 301
Spencer, S., 236
Sperry, J. C., 141, 142, 143, 144
Spiegel, A. D., 102
Spillman, S. J., 280
Splaver, S., 291
Staab, W. J., 158, 199
Stark, R. E., 157, 199
Stedman, D. J., 353
Steinfeld, E., 386, 387
Steinkamp, M. W., 194
Stephens, P., 317
Stewart, J., 365
Stewart, L., 160, 199
Stewart, L. G., 58, 74
Stewart, W. F. R., 295, 301, 310
Stile, S. W., 186
Stills, M., 243
Stillwell, G. K., 227
St. Louis, K. W., 232
Stocker, C. S., 49
Stoklosa, J. M., 297, 318
Stokoe, W. C., 162, 165, 200
Stolov, W. C., 238
Stoner, M., 187
Stratton, J., 365
Strebel, M. B., 124
Streng, A. F., 160, 200

AUTHOR INDEX

Streng, A. H., 160, 200
Stryker, R., 211, 238
Stryker, S., 212, 238
Stubbins, J., 3, 82, 83, 102
Stuckey, K. A., 37, 50, 432
Studebaker, G. A., 201
Sullivan, T. V., 339
Sullivan, R. F., 185
Sullivan, T., 50
Sussman, A. E., 58, 74
Swails, S. H., 217
Swain, J., 83, 88
Swinyard, C. A., 291
Switzer, L., 267
Sykes, S., 333
Symington, D. C., 139

Taggie, J. M., 318
Task Force on Concerns of Physically Disabled Women, 296, 311, 319
Templer, J. A., 394
Thain, W. S., 366
Thatcher, J. W., 188
Thomas, D., 103, 366
Thomason, B., 309, 319
Thompson, F. V., 189
Thompson, P. E., 279
Thury, C. 308
Thvedt, J. E., 152
Timms, R. J., 305
Tindall, L. W., 379
Tomko, M. A., 305
Townsend, P., 82, 104
Tradewell, M. D. J., 133
Trela, J. E., 152
Trieschmann, R. B., 2, 6, 27, 209, 239, 299
Turem, J. S., 112, 136
Tymchuk, A. J., 350, 366

Ullman, M., 3, 27
United Cerebral Palsy Associations, 311
United Ostomy Association, 276, 277, 288
U.S. Congress. Office of Technology Assessment, 396, 397

U.S. Department of Education. Office for Handicapped Individuals, 375, 376
U.S. Department of Education. Office of Special Education and Rehabilitatative Services Clearinghouse on the Handicapped, 375, 376
U.S. Department of Health and Human Services. Bureau of Community Health Services, 383
U.S. Department of Health and Human Services. Public Health Service, 374, 381, 382
U.S. Department of Health, Education and Welfare. Maternal and Child Health Services, 380
U.S. Department of Health, Education and Welfare. Office of Human Development Services. Administration for Children, Youth and Families, 385, 386
U.S. Department of Health, Education and Welfare. Office of Human Development Service. Office for Handicapped Individuals, 378, 385
U.S. Department of Health, Education and Welfare. Office of Resources for the Handicapped, 377
U.S. Department of Health, Education and Welfare. Public Health Service. National Institutes of Health, 381, 382, 384
U.S. Department of Health, Education and Welfare. Social Security Administration. Office of Research and Statistics, 378
U.S. Department of Housing and Urban Development. Office of Housing, 388, 390
U.S. Department of Housing and Urban Development. Office of Policy

[ment. Office of Policy] Development and Research, 387, 388, 389
U.S. Department of the Interior. National Park Service, 390
U.S. Department of Transportation Transportation Systems Center, Technology Sharing Program Office, 392, 393
U.S. Department of Transportation. Urban Mass Transportation Administration, 394
U.S. Employment and Training Administration, 390
U.S. Government Printing Office., 369, 374, 375, 377
U.S. Library of Congress. Copyright Office, 384, 391
U.S. National Institute of Arthritis, Metabolism and Digestive Diseases, 381
U.S. National Institute of Mental Health. Saint Elizabeths Hospital, 384
U.S. National Institute of Neurological and Communicative Disorders and Stroke, 382
U.S. National Library Service for the Blind and Physically Handicapped, 391
U.S. Office of Personnel Management, 391
U.S. President's Committee on Employment of the Handicapped, 391, 392
U.S. Rehabilitation Services Administration, 377, 406
U.S. Superintendent of Documents, 374, 377
U.S. Veterans Administration, 395
U.S. Veterans Administration. Central Office Library, 395

U.S. Veterans Administration. Department of Medicine and Surgery, 395
University of Maryland Law School, Developmental Disabilities Law Project, 248, 251, 267
University of Wisconsin-Madison. Wiscconsin Vocational Studies Center, 375
Utrup, R. G., 110, 124

Vaeth, J. M., 311
Van Camp, A., 426, 427
Vanderheiden, G. C., 140
Varela, R. A., 103
Varma, V. P., 366
Vash, C., 6, 80, 84, 140, 239
Velleman, R. A., 277
Verkeryl, A., 306
Verlag, G. S., 411
Vernon, M., 58, 69
Veterans Administration, 432, 433
Veterans Administration Hospital, 297, 312
Vigliarolo, D., 357
Vitali, M., 210, 240
Vogel, B. S., 279
Volle, F. O., 291
Von Eschenbach, A. C., 312
Vorce, E., 201
Voysey, M., 367

Waggoner, N. R., 123
Wagner, E., 33, 38, 355
Walberg, F., 344
Walker, A., 82, 104
Walker, F. C., 240
Walker, J. M., 268
Walker, L., 250, 258
Wallace, R., 212, 240
Walls, R. T., 152
Walsh, A., 211, 241
Walter, F., 323, 344
Walton, K. M., 114, 152

AUTHOR INDEX

Wannstedt, G., 210, 241
Ward, J., 201
Watson, D., 56, 75
Watt, S., 88
Webster, E. J., 350, 367
Wehrum, M. E., 125
Weinberg, B., 237, 241
Weiner, W., 51
Weintraub, F. J., 268
Weiss, J., 117
Weiss, J. M., 302
Weiss, L., 324, 345
Weiss, M., 208
Welsh, J., 25
Welsh, R. L., 34, 50, 51
Wenger, N., 242
West Virginia Rehabilitation Research, and Training Center, 433
Wheeler, R. H., 323, 345
White, D. A., 139
White House Conference on Handicapped Individuals, 396
Whitehurst, M. W., 160, 202
Whiteman, M., 32, 44
Wicka, D. K., 287, 291
Widerberg, L., 51
Widerberg, L. C., 125
Wiedel, J., 34, 51
Wilbur, R. B., 162, 176, 202
Williams, J., 254
Williams, M. A., 221, 239
Williams, M. C., 246, 266
Willoughby, D. M., 275, 292
Willoughby, M., 147
Wilshere, E. R., 129, 130, 131

Wilson, A. B., 210, 211
Wilson, A. B., Jr., 242, 243
Wilson, D., 301
Wineman, J. D., 394
Wingrove, J., 86, 88
Winslow, B., 5, 20
Witt, P. A., 322, 345
Wittmeyer, M., 28
Woods, N. F., 312
Woodward, J., 161, 203, 313
Woolever, L. D., 176
Wright, B. A., 80, 104
Wright, D., 56, 75
Wright, G. N., 78, 105
Wright, V. K., 152

Yanick, P., Jr., 203
Yeadon, A., 30, 35, 52, 109, 125
Yohalem, D., 268
Yoken, C., 33, 52, 163, 204
Yost, A. C., 125
Yost, W. A., 204
Young, M., 176
Yount, W. R., 58, 75
Yuker, H. E., 105

Zane, T., 152
Zarcadoolas, C., 168
Zawolkow, E., 178
Zimmer, A. B., 268
Zola, I. K., 145
Zuckerman, R., 135
Zupan, I., 308

TITLE INDEX

About Aging, 424, 427
Accent on Living, 325, 326
Access, 249, 255, 275, 279
Access Chicago, 326
Access for All, 4, 23
Access National Parks, 371, 390
Access to Historic Buildings for the Disabled, 390
Access to the Built Environment, 387
Access to the World, 324, 345
Access Travel, 325
Accessibility Assistance, 22
Accessibility Modifications, 20
Accessibility Standards Illustrated, 4, 18
Accessible Buildings for People with Severe Visual Impairment, 387
Accessible Buildings for People with Walking and Reaching Limitations, 386
Accessible Housing, 7
Accreditation Manual for Hospitals, 277
Acoustical Factors Affecting Hearing Aid Performance, 201
Activities Coordinator's Guide, 384
Activities of Daily Living for Physical Rehabilitation, 122
Adapt Your Own, 117

Adaptations and Techniques for the Disabled Homemaker, 124
Adapting Activities for Therapetic Recreation Service, 331
Adapting Historic Campus Structures for Accessibility, 21
Adaptive Housing for the Physically Handicapped, 143
Adjustment to Severe Physical Disability, 80, 92, 298
A.D.L. Activities of Daily Living Test, 122
Adult Rehabilitation, 228
Advancing Your Citizenship, 256
Advice to Parents of a Cleft Palate Child, 287, 291
Advocacy for/with the Mentally Ill and Handicapped, 250, 263
Against All Odds, 17
Aids for Children, 111, 125
Aids for the Severely Handicapped, 128
Aids to Independent Living, 136
Aids to Make You Able, 129
Airlines and Disabled Travellers, 339
All about Jimmy and his Friend, 288
...All Things are Possible, 295, 314

American Annals of the Deaf, 332, 401, 404
American Archives of Rehabilitation Therapy, 404
American Corrective Therapy Journal, 404
American Journal of Art Therapy, 405
American Journal of Nursing, 277
American Journal of Occupational Therapy, 405
American Journal of Physical Medicine, 405
American Journal of Sports Medicine, 326
American National Standard Specifications for Making Buildings and Facilities Accessible to and Usable by Physically Handicapped People, 4, 7
American Rehabilitation, 406
American Sign Language, 175, 179, 181
American Sign Language: a Look at its History, Structure, and Community, 165
American Sign Language: a Teacher's Resource Text on Grammer and Culture, 162, 165
American Sign Language and Sign Systems, 162, 202
American Speech and Hearing Association (ASHA), 401, 403
American Statistics Index, 373, 375
Ameslan, 162, 175
Amicus, 251, 252, 406
Amplification for the Hearing Impaired, 293
Amputation Surgery and Rehabilitation, 226
Amputations and Prostheses, 210, 240
Amyotrophic Lateral Sclerosis, 381
Annotated Bibliography: the Exceptional Child and the Law, 266

Annotated Listing of Films, Physical Education and Recreation for Impaired, Disabled, and Handicapped Persons, 429
Annual Report of the Rehabilitation Services Administration to the President and the Congress on Federal Activities Related to the Administration of the Rehabilitation Act of 1973, as Amended, 377
Annual Report of the U.S. Dept. of Health, Education, and Welfare to the Congress of the United States on Services Provided to Handicapped Children in Project Head Start, 385
Aphasia Rehabilitation, 212, 236
Aphasia Therapy Manual, 212, 214
Aphasic Patient, 278
The Application of Technological Developments to Physically Disabled People, 112, 136
Applied Audiology for Children, 172
Aquatic Recreation for the Blind, 330
Architectural Accessibility for the Disabled on College Campuses, 396
Architectural Barriers Removal, 375
Archives of Physical Medicine and Rehabilitation, 406
The Arthritic's Cookbook. 118
Arthritis: A Comprehensive Guide, 282
Arthritis: Medical Treatment and Home Care, 278
The Arthritis Book, 275, 281
Arthritis Information Clearinghouse, 428
The Arthritis Program, 381

TITLE INDEX

Arthritis Research and Education in Nursing and Allied Health, 380
Artificial Organs, 407
Arts and Crafts for Physically and Mentally Disabled, 334
Arts and the Handicapped,, 322, 328
ASHA, 401, 403
Assistive Devices and Equipment for Rehabilitation, 126, 127
Assuring Access for the Handicapped, 24
Attendant Care Manual, 148
Attendees and Attendants, 275, 280
Attitudes Toward Blind Persons, 44
Attitudes Toward Persons with Disabilities 101
Audecibel, 407
Audiological Assessment, 195
Audiological Evaluation and Aural Rehabilitation of the Deaf-Blind Adult, 163, 185
Audiological Handbook of Hearing Disorders, 193
Audiology, 190
Audiology: Journal of Auditory Communication, 407
Audiology for the Physician, 184
Audiometry in Infancy, 159, 176
Auditory and Hearing Prosthetics Research, 186
Auditory Dysfunction, 177
Auditory Management of Hearing Impaired Children, 159, 196
Auditory Rehabilitation for Hearing Impaired Blind Persons, 163, 167
Audiovisual Aids, Computer Assisted Instruction, and Programmed Instruction in Education for the Health Professions, 423, 427
Audiovisual Materials Catalog, 381

Aural Habilitation, 159, 180, 187
Aural Rehabilitation, 158, 196
Aural Rehabilitation Process, 158, 192
Avocational Activities for the Handicapped, 341

Barrier Awareness, 91
Barrier Free Design, 25
Barrier Free Design: The Law, 248, 261
Barrier Free Design for Providing Facilities for the Physically Handicapped in Public Buildings, 22
Barrier-Free Environments, 9
Barrier-Free Meetings, 25
Barrier Free Rapid Transit, 7
Barrier Free School Facilities for Handicapped Students, 19
Basic Components of Orientation and Movement Techniques, 51
A Basic Course in Manual Communication, 161, 170, 191
Basic Terminology for Therapeutic Recreation and Other Action Therapies, 334
A Basic Vocabulary, 192
Basic Vocabulary: American Sign Language for Parents and Children, 161, 192
Bathroom Facilities Accommodating the Physically Disabled and the Aged, 8
Be Opened! 58, 75
Beginning with the Handicapped, 358
Behavior Therapy, 407
Behavioral Approaches to Rehabilitation, 81, 94, 223
Behavioral Change in Cerebrovascular Disease, 2, 9
Behavioral Changes in Patients Following Strokes, 3, 27

Behavioral Problems and the Disabled, 81, 85
Behaviour Research and Theraphy, 402, 407
Bibliography on Deafness, 63
A Bicentennial Monograph on Hearing Impairment, 63
Black's Law Dictionary, 251
The Blind and Physically Handicapped in Competitive Employment, 263
The Blind Child in the Regular Kindergarten, 365
The Blind Monitor, 263
Blinded Veterans of the Vietnam Era, 47
Blindness, 373
Blindness: What It Is, What It Does, and How to Live with It, 30, 37
Blindness and Disorders of the Eye, 45
Blindness and Partial Sight, 43
Blindness Research, 39
Blindness, Visual Impairment, Deaf-Blindness, 37
Boating for the Handicapped, 335
The Body-Image of Blind Children, 354
Bowker Annual of Library and Book Trade Information, 403
Braille Monitor, 263
Brief Consumer's Guide to Sexuality and the Disabled Woman, 299, 304
Bright Promise for Your Child with Cleft Lip and Cleft Palate, 287
Building without Barriers for the Disabled, 17
Bulletin of Prosthetics Research, 400, 408
By, For and With... Young Adults with Spina Bifida, 289

The Canadian Journal of Occupational Therapy, 408
Cancer Rehabilitation, 210, 219
Cardiac Patient Rehabilitation, 209, 230
Cardiac Rehabilitation: a Comprehensive Nursing Approach, 211, 217
Cardiac Rehabilitation: Implications for the Nurse and Other Allied Health Professionals, 211, 221
Cardiac Rehabilitation for the Patient and Family, 280
Care of the Neurologically Handicapped Child, 290, 363
Caring for the Disabled Patient, 220, 280
Case Reporter, 248, 251, 267
Catalog of Aids for the Disabled, 135
Catalog of Federal Domestic Assistance, 258, 261, 375, 376, 385
Catalog of the Captioned Films for the Deaf Distribution Center, 423
Central Auditory and Language Disorders in Children, 184
Cerebral Palsy, 2, 12
Cerebral Palsy and Sexuality, 317
C.F.R., 251
Challenging Barriers to Change, 105
Changing Patterns of Law, 265
The Changing Status of the Blind, 31, 44
Child with Disabling Illness, 348, 355
The Child with Spina Bifida, 289, 291
Childhood Deafness, 167
The Childhood Story of Christy Brown, 10
Children with Hearing Impairment, 385
Children with Orthopedic Handicaps, 386

TITLE INDEX 455

Children with Speech and Language Impairments, 386
Children with Visual Handicaps, 386
Chronically Ill and Handicapped Children, 354
The CIL, 150
CIS/Index, 375
Cleft Palate Journal, 408
Clinically Adapted Instruments for the Multiply Handicapped, 330
Clothes Sense, 110, 123
Clothing Designs for the Handicapped 110, 121
Clothing for the Handicapped, 110, 117
Clothing for the Handicapped, the Aged, and other People with Special Needs, 120
The Clubfoot, 208, 227
Coalition Building, 254
Code of Federal Regulations, 251
The College Student with a Disability, 392
Colostomies, 286
Combatting Exclusionary Zoning, 261
Comeback, 79, 87
Communicating with Deaf People, 162, 181
Communication, 170
Communication Aids for the Brain Damaged Adult, 170
Communication for the Hearing Handicapped, 192
Communication Programming for the Severely Handicapped Vocal and Non-Vocal Strategies, 232
Communicative Skills Program, 170
Community Leisure Services and Disabled Individuals, 322, 345
Community Living Alternatives for Persons with Developmental Disabilities, 144

Community Living for the Disabled, 144
Community Resources for the Social Adjustment of Severely Disabled Persons, 99
A Comprehensive Cardiac Rehabilitation Program, 209, 218
A Comprehensive Dictionary of Audiology, 157, 173
Comprehensive Guide to Employment Discrimination of the Handicapped, 262
Comprehensive Rehabilitation Nursing, 211, 229
Conceptual Study of Handicapped Facilities for New Subway Station Designs, 372, 394
Confrontation Between the Young Deaf-Blind Child and the Outer World, 41
Congressional Information Service's Index, 373, 375
The Conquest of Deafness, 61
Consider... Understanding Disability as a Way of Life, 101
A Constant Burden, 367
Consumer Involvement/Policy Development Consultation, 265
Consumer Warranty Law, 250, 253
A Continuing Summary of Pending and Completed Litigation Regarding the Education of Handicapped Children, 251
Conversational Sign Language II, 162, 188
Coping with Disablement, 118
Coping with Physical Disability, 274, 279
Counseling and Rehabilitating the Cancer Patient, 209, 224
Counseling in Communicative Disorders, 94
Counseling Parents of Exceptional Children, 365

Counseling Parents of the Ill and the Handicapped, 350, 362
Counseling the Person with Spinal Cord Injury on Sex and Sexuality, 301
Counseling with Deaf People, 58, 74
Counseling with Parents of Handicapped Children, 367
Counseling with Physically Handicapped High School Student, 361
Crafts for the Disabled, 333
Crafts for the Very Disabled and Handicpped, 337
Creating an Accessible Campus, 11
Creative Arts for the Severely Handicapped, 343
Crooked Shall be Made Straight, 16
Current Perspectives in Rehabilitation Nursing, 211, 231

Daily Living Skills, 109, 122
Dance for Physically Disabled Persons, 335
Dancing to Learn, 344
Dancing Without Music, 56, 60, 61
Database, 427
A Deaf Adult Speaks Out, 56, 66
The Deaf American, 400, 409
Deaf-Blind Bibliography, 50, 432
Deaf Blind Children, 33, 38, 355
The Deaf Child and His Family, 64, 371, 377
The Deaf Child in the Public Schools, 273, 285
Deaf Children, 68
The Deaf Experience, 56, 60
Deaf Heritage, 64
The Deaf Man and the World, 63
The Deaf Population of the United States, 73

Deafness, 55, 56, 60, 75
Deafness and Child Development, 58, 69
Deafness in Infancy and Early Childhood, 176, 356
The Demography of Blindness Throughout the World, 39
The Denial of Death, 234
Dentistry in Cerebral Palsy and Related Handicapping Conditions, 208, 236
Design Competition Program, 389
Design for Accessibility, 26
Design for Independent Living, 5, 20
Designing for Everyone...Access America, 396
Designing for Functional Limitations, 5, 21
Designing for the Disabled, 16
Detection of Hearing Loss and Ear Disease in Children, 159, 178
Developing Assessment Programs for the Multihandicapped Child, 362
Development, Management, and Evaluation of Community Speech and Hearing Centers, 114, 142
The Development of a Sex Education Curriculum for a State Residential School for the Deaf and Social Hygiene Guides, 300
Development of Individualized Education Programs (IEPS) for the Handicapped in Vocational Education, 371, 379
Development of Interpretation as a Profession, 163, 182
Development of Work Programs for the Multihandicapped, 114, 146
Developmental Disabilities, 351
Developmental Medicine and Child Neurology, 402, 409
Developmental Studies of Deaf Children, 175

TITLE INDEX 457

Devices and Systems for the Disabled, 135
The Diagnosis and Treatment of Amyotrophic Lateral Sclerosis, 207, 231
Diagnostic Procedures in Hearing, Language and Speech, 157, 198
A Dictionary of American Sign Language on Linguistic Principles, 162, 200
Dictionary of Occupational Titles, 49
A Difference in the Family, 356
Digest of Data on Persons with Disabilities, 370, 384
Digest of State and Federal Laws, 254
The Dilemmas of Care, 211, 234
Directory of Agencies Serving the Visually Handicapped in the U.S., 35
Directory of National Information Sources on Handicapping Conditions and Related Services, 376
Disability, 207, 226
Disability: Our Challenge, 378
Disability and Rehabilitation Handbook, 6, 35, 78, 93, 299
Disability and the Environment, 90
Disability Attitudes, 428
Disability, from Social Problem to Federal Program, 259
Disability, Home Care, and Relative Responsibility, 256
Disability in Britain, 82, 104
Disability in Childhood and Youth, 348, 349, 358
Disability Policies and Government Programs, 253
Disability Survey 72, 370, 378
The Disabled and Their Parents, 82, 88, 350, 353
The Disabled Homemaker, 115
Disabled People as Second-Class Citizens, 92

The Disabled Person and Family Dynamics, 309, 319
The Disabled Schoolchild, 351
Disabled USA, 400
Down All the Days, 10

Early Childhood, 359
Early Diagnosis of Hearing Loss, 159, 177
Early Intervention, 350
Early Management of Hearing Loss, 159, 189
The Early Stroke Patient, 212, 219
Early Therapeutic, Social and Vocational Problems in the Rehabilitation of Persons with Spinal Cord Injuries, 208, 242
Easy Path to Gardening, 332
Eating Handicaps, 119
Ecology of Deafness, 160
The Ecology of Early Deafness, 57, 58, 67, 68, 71, 186
Educating Handicapped Children, 246, 260
Educating the Deaf, 55, 70, 160, 190
Education, 429
Education and Rehabilitation of Deaf Persons with Other Disabilities, 73
The Education for all Handicapped Children, 262
Education for Children with Epilepsy, 257
Education for the Handicapped Law Report, 247, 257
The Education of Deaf Children, 160, 194
Education of the Visually Handicapped, 409
Educational and Psychosocial Aspects of Deafness, 65
Educational Audiology, 166
Educational Games for Physically Handicapped Children, 324, 331

Educational Materials, 428
Educational Multimedia-CME Catalog, 424
Educator's International Guide to Free & Low-Cost Health Audio-Visual Teaching Aids, 424, 431
The Effects of Blindness and other Impairments on Early Development, 41
Elderly and Handicapped Transportation, 394
Employing the Handicapped, 268
Encyclopedia of Associations, 36
Entitled to Love, 315
Environmental Control Systems and Vocational Aids for Persons with High Level Quadriplegia, 137
Epilepsia, 410
Epilepsy, 291
Epilepsy and the Law, 249, 252
Epilepsy and You, 291
Epilepsy, Pregnancy, and the Child, 298, 306
Epilepsy-Problems of Marriage, Pregnancy, Genetic Counseling, 305
Episode, 18
Equipment for the Disabled
  Vol. 1 Communication, 112, 129
  Vol. 2 Clothing and Dressing for Adults, 112, 129
  Vol. 3 Home Management, 112, 130
  Vol. 4 Outdoor Transport, 112, 130
  Vol. 5 Wheelchairs, 112, 130
  Vol. 6 Leisure and Gardening, 112, 130
  Vol. 8 Personal Care, 112, 131
  Vol. 9 Housing and Furniture, 112, 131
  Vol. 10 Hoists Walking Aids, 112, 131
  Vol. 11 Disabled Child, 111, 131
Escape from Evil, 234

The Estimated Cost of Accessible Buildings, 387
European Rehabilitation, 83, 89
Evaluating Driving Potential of Persons with Physical Disabilities, 132
Evaluating Orthopedic Disability, 209, 230
Evaluation of a Disabled Living Unit, 15
An Evaluation of Making Rail Transit Systems Accessible to Handicapped Persons, 370, 394
Evaluation of the Limb-Load Monitor, 210, 241
Everybody can Cook, 116
Exceptional Children, 402, 410
Exercises and Self-care Activities for Quadriplegic People, 115
The Expanded Role of the Rehabilitation Nurse, 211, 241
Expanding Horizons in Therapeutic Recreation, 339
The Experience of Handicap, 103

Facilitating Manual Communication for Interpreters, Students, and Teachers, 163, 174
Fact Book - National Institute of Neurological and Communicative Disorders and Stroke, 382
Facts about Sex, 300
Facts about Sex for Exceptional Youth, 300
Family Planning Services for Disabled People, 370, 383
The Feasibility of Accommodating Physically Handicapped Individuals on Pedestrian Over and Undercrossing Structures, 394
Federal Assistance for Programs Serving the Handicapped, 385

TITLE INDEX

Federal Assistance for Programs Serving the Visually Handicapped, 261
Federal Personnel Manual, 391
Feeding can be Fun, 123
Feeding the Child with a Handicap, 380
Feeling Good About Yourself, 302
Female Sexuality following Spinal Cord Injury, 295, 313
Films for Nursing, Rehabilitation and Special Films, Video Filmstrips, Slides, 426
Focus on Deafness, 56, 67
Food, Nutrition and the Disabled; An Annotated Bibliography, 222
Foundations of Orientation and Mobility, 34, 50
The Fourth Revolution, 427
Frontiers of Radiation Therapy and Oncololgy (Vol. 14) Body Image, Self-Esteem, and Sexuality in Cancer Patients, 311
Functional Aids for the Multiply Handicapped, 138
Functional Evaluation and Rehabilitation of Cardiac Patients, 210, 237
Fundamentals of Hearing, 204

Games, Sports, and Exercises for the Physically Handicapped, 326
General Information to Help the Recently Disabled, 284
Getting the Buck to Stop Here, 258
Getting There, 15
The God of the Deaf Adolescent, 72
Government Reports Announcements and Index, 373, 374, 375
Green Pages Rehab Sourcebook, 133

Group Counseling and Group Psychotherapy with Rehabilitation Clients, 102
Group Counseling and Physical Disability, 81, 96
Growing Old in Silence, 61
Guide Dogs for the Blind, 46
A Guide for Trainers, 300
Guide to Audiovisual Resources for the Health Care Field, 429
A Guide to Clinical Services in Speech-Language Pathology and Audiology, 160, 164
A Guide to College/Career Programs for Deaf Students, 65
A Guide to Designing Accessible Outdoor Recreation Facilities, 10
A Guide to Expanding Social Services to the Blind Under Title XX of the Social Security Act, 248, 257
Guide to Films about Blindness, 425, 432
A Guide to Organizations, Agencies, and Federal Programs for Handicapped Americans: Report I, 250, 268
Guide to the Section 504 Self-Evaluation for Colleges and Universities, 247, 253
Guide to the Selection and Use of the Teaching Aids of the Signed English System, 163, 168
Guidelines for Planning Travel for the Physically Handicapped, 332
Guides to the Evaluation of Permanent Impairment, 207, 213

Hand Controls and Assistive Devices for the Physically Disabled Driver, 134
Handbook for One-Handers, 118
Handbook of Adapted Physical Education Equipment and Its Use, 324, 344

Handbook of Adult Rehabilitative Audiology, 164
Handbook of Clinical Audiology, 156, 183
Handbook of Employment Rights of the Handicapped, 247, 248, 258
Handbook of Hearing Aid Measurement, 395
Handbook of Selective Placement of Persons with Physical and Mental Handicaps in Federal Civil Service Employment, 391
Handbook of Severe Disability, 238
Handbook of Spinal Cord Medicine, 294, 299
Handbook on Sexuality after Spinal Cord Injury, 318
Handicap, 360
Handicap in a Social World, 83, 87, 88
The Handicapped, 373, 377
Handicapped Americans' Report, 410
The Handicapped Child, 348 351
The Handicapped Child and His Family, 357
The Handicapped Child in the Family, 284
Handicapped Children, 350
The Handicapped Driver's Mobility Guide, 126
The Handicapped Experience, 98
The Handicapped Forum, 300
Handicapped Married Couples, 296, 300
The Handicapped Person in the Community, 86
Handicapped Requirements Handbook, 247, 250, 258
Handicapping America, 79, 87
Handling the Handicapped. 127
Handtalk, 169
The Hard of Hearing Child, 159, 166
Hazards of Deafness, 56, 66
Health Education Resource Catalogue Inc., 429

Health Science Audiovisuals in Online Data Bases, 426, 427
Health Sciences Video Directory, 433
Hearing, 198
The Hearing Aid, 157, 167
Hearing Aid Assessment and Use in Audiologic Habilitation, 157, 180
Hearing Aid Handbook, 158, 199
Hearing Aids, 157, 190
Hearing Aids: Current Developments and Concepts, 157, 196
Hearing Aids and You, 157, 171
Hearing and Deafness, 55, 62, 156, 173
Hearing and Hearing Disability, 373, 377
Hearing and Hearing Impairment, 55, 62, 64
Hearing Assessment, 157, 195
Hearing Disorders, 159, 190
Hearing Loss, Hearing Aids and Your Child: A Guide for Parents, 287
Hearing Loss in Children. 55 67, 159, 182
Hearing Rehabilitation Quarterly, 410
Hearing Research, 411
Hearing Therapy for Children, 160, 200
Heart Disease and Rehabilitation, 233
Helen and Teacher, 33, 43
Help Them Grow!, 279
Help Yourselves, 121
Helping the Severely Handicapped Child, 280, 355
Helping Your Handicapped Child, 274, 288
Hemiplegia, Current Approaches to Patient Positioning, 224
The Hidden Minority, 79, 96
Highway Rest Areas for Handicapped Travelers, Access Amtrak, National Parks, 325, 391
Holidays for the Physically Handicapped, 336

TITLE INDEX

Home Economics Rehabilitation, 125
Home in a Wheelchair, 5, 11, 12
Home Mechanics for the Visually Impaired, 110, 124
Homemaking Manual, 121
Horticulture as a Therapeutic Aid, 329
Housing Adaptability Guidelines, 23
Housing and Home Services for the Disabled, 148
Housing for the Handicapped, 373
Housing Needs of the Rural Elderly and Handicapped, 388
How to Build Special Furniture and Equipment for Handicapped Children, 111, 134
How to Cope with Arthritis, 371, 381
How to Create Interiors for the Disabled, 5, 10
How to Integrate Aging Persons who are Visually Handicapped into Community Senior Programs, 32, 35
How to Organize an Effective Parent/Advocacy Group and Move Bureaucracies, 249, 256
How to Set Up an Independent Living Program, 145
HUD Challenge: 390
Human Sex Behavior Research, 300
Human Sexuality, 311
Human Sexuality: The Handicapped, the Aging, 302
Human Sexuality and Rehabilitation Medicine, 299, 310
Human Sexuality in Health and Illness, 312
Human Sexuality in Physical and Mental Illnesses and Disabilities, 310
Human Sexuality Methods and Materials for the Education, Family Life and Health Professions, 425, 428

Ideas for Making Your Home Accessible, 15
Identity Crisis in Deafness, 54, 59, 74
If You Could See What I Hear, 50
Ileostomy, 283
Illinois Heart Association Public Health Education Catalog of Films and Slides, 424
An Illustrated Handbook for Barrier Free Design, 26
ILRU Source Book, 113, 146
Images of Ourselves, 89
Impairment, Disability, and Handicap, 97
Impedence Screening for Middle Ear Disease in Children, 159, 179
Implementation of Independent Living Programs in Rehabilitation, 147
In the Mainstream, 251, 259
Independence through Environmental Control Systems, 139
Independent Living (Hoffman), 147
Independent Living (Pflueger), 113, 150
Independnet Living and Deafness, 72, 149
Independent Living Assessments for Persons with Disabilities, 151
The Independent Living Behavior Checklist, 152
Independent Living Evaluation-Training Program, 151
Independent Living for Physically Disabled People, 145
Independent Living for the Handicapped and the Elderly, 123
Independent Living Skills for the Severely Handicapped Deaf Person Preparing to Enter Gainful Employment, 71, 147

Independent Living Techniques and Concepts, 114, 152
Independent Living with Attendant Care, 141, 142
Independent Living Without Sight and Hearing, 33, 42
Index Medicus, 373, 374, 375
Infant Education, 353
Instructional Materials in Independent Living, 425, 432
Instrumentation in the Hearing Sciences, 188
Integration of Handicapped Children in Society, 349, 360
Integration or Segregation for the Physically Handicapped Child, 349, 355
Intermediate Sign Language, 162, 175
International Directory of Services for the Deaf, 69
International Guide to Aids and Appliances for Blind and Visually Impaired Persons, 126
International Journal of Artificial Organs, 402, 411
International Journal of Rehabilitation Research, 411
International Rehabilitation Film Review Catalogue, 429
International Rehabilitation Medicine, 402, 411
International Rehabilitation Review, 412
International Symposium on Interpretation of Sign Languages, 163
Interpreter Training, 163, 204
Intervention with At-Risk and Handicapped Infants, 352
Interviewing Guides for Specific Disabilities, 390
Introduction to Audiology, 188
Introduction to Aural Rehabilitation, 158, 197
Introduction to Independent Living Rehabilitation Services, 150
Introduction to Rehabilitation, 78, 86
An Introduction to Working with the Aging Person who is Visually Handicapped, 32, 36
An Investigation of the Self Concept of Blind and Visually Handicapped Adolescents, 45
Involving Impaired, Disabled, and Handicapped Persons in Regular Camp Programs, 337

Job Placement and Adjustment of the Handicapped, 379
Joint HEW-UMTA Evaluation of Elderly and Handicapped Transportation Services in Region IV, 393
Joni, 13
Journal of Applied Rehabilitation Counseling, 412
Journal of Auditory Research, 412
Journal of Learning Disabilities, 402, 412
Journal of Leisurability, 345
Journal of Occupation Medicine, 413
Journal of Music Therapy, 413
Journal of Orthopaedic and Sports Physical Therapy, 413
Journal of Rehabilitation, 414
Journal of Rehabilitation of the Deaf, 414
Journal of Speech and Hearing Disorders, 402, 403, 414
Journal of Speech and Hearing Research, 402, 403, 414
Journal of Visual Impairment & Blindness, 415
The Joy of Signing, 161, 194

Kitchen Sense for Disabled People of all Ages, 119
Krusen's Handbook of Physical Medical and Rehabilitation, 227

TITLE INDEX

Language Development and Intervention with the Hearing Impaired, 160, 185
Language Development in Deaf and Partially Hearing Children, 160, 172
Language for the Preschool Deaf Child, 160, 179
Language Intervention Strategies in Adult Aphasia, 213, 217
Language, Learning, and Deafness, 160, 200
Laryngectomee Rehabilitation, 226
Law and the Handicapped Child, 246, 266
The Learning Center, 422, 427
Learning to Live with Disability, 95
Least Restrictive Alternative for Handicapped Students, 371, 379
Legal Change for the Handicapped through Litigation, 248, 252
The Legal Rights of Handicapped Persons, 248, 249, 255
The Legal Rights of Persons with Epilepsy, 249, 257
Legal Rights Primer for the Handicapped, 266
Leisure Time Activities for Deaf-Blind Children, 118
Let Our Children Go, 249, 254
Let there be Love, 307, 315
Library Resources and Technical Services, 427
Life Together, 317
Lifting, Moving, and Transfering Patients, 212, 234
Limb Prosthetics, 211, 242, 243
Limb Prostetics for Vocational Rehabilitaion Workers, 211, 243
Listening for the Visually Impaired, 49
Literature on the Deaf-Blind, 37
Living at Your Best with Multiple Sclerosis, 284
Living Comfortably with your Ilestomy, 286
Living Fully, 273, 283
Living Independently, 113, 143
Living with a Hearing Impairment, 60
Living with Chronic Neuroligic Disease, 279
Living with Deaf-Blindness, 33, 52
Living with Impaired Vision, 30, 35, 52
Living with Multiple Sclerosis, 13
Living with Your Arthritis, 272, 290
Lobbying for the Rights of Disabled People, 260
Look, Now Hear This, 182
Looking Ahead, 423, 430
Love Matters, 301
Lower-Limb Orthotics, 210, 228

Mainstreaming Preschoolers: Children with Hearing Impairment, 371, 385
Mainstreaming Preschoolers: Children with Orthopedics Handicaps, 386
Mainstreaming Preschoolers: Children with Speech and Language Impairments, 386
Mainstreaming Preschoolers: Children with Visual Handicaps, 386
Making Buildings and Facilities Accessible to and Usable by the Physically Handicapped, 386
The Making of Blind Men, 48
Making Physical Education and Recreation Facilities Accessible to All, 322, 338
Management of Housing for Handicapped and Disabled Persons, 389
Management of Sensorineural Deafness, 207, 231
Managing Physical Handicaps, 282

Manual Communication, 161, 169
Manual for an Ultralight Below-Knee Prosthesis, 210, 243
Manual of Above-Knee Socket Prosthetics, 214
Manual on Legal Rights and Responsibilities of Developmentally Disabled Persons in Illinois, 250, 260
Manual on Management of the Quadriplegic Upper Extremity, 210, 229
A Manual on Multiple Sclerosis, 2, 8, 21, 215
Marital Adjustments in Couples of which one Spouse is Physically Handicapped, 23, 296, 307
Marriage, Sex, and Arthritis, 316
Materials on Creative Arts (Arts, Crafts, Dance, Drama, Music and Bibliotherapy) for Persons with Handicapping Conditions, 338
Mealtime Manual for People With Disabilities and the Aging, 121
Mealtime Manual for the Aged and Handicapped, 119
The Meaning of Blindness, 31, 45
The Meaning of Disability, 83, 86
Measures of Psychological, Vocational, and Educational Functioning in the Blind and Visually Handicapped, 31, 48
Medical and Psychological Aspects of Disability, 3, 90
Medical Catalogue of Selected Audiovisual Materials, 429
Medical Devices and Equipment for the Disabled, 112, 128
Mental Health in Deafness, 384
The Metamorphosis, 234
Methods of Communication Currently Used in the Education of Deaf Children, 189
Methods of Communication with Deaf-Blind People, 163, 174
Midwest Symposium on Therapeutic Recreation. St. Louis, 1975, 339
The Milwaukee Brace, 210, 215
Ministering to the Silent Majority, 67
Ministry to the Deaf, 72
Mobile Homes, 372, 388
Mobility in the Wheelchair Home, 12
Modern Stoma Care, 240
Monograph on Sexual Function and Paraplegia, 300
Monthly Catalog of Government Publications, 370, 372, 374, 376
Move it!, 355
The Movement for Independent Living, 84, 145
Multidimensional Speech Perception by the Hearing Impaired, 157, 172
Multiple Sclerosis, 21, 237, 277
Multiple Sclerosis in Childhood, 221
Multiple Sclerosis Scars of Childhood, 277
Music Education for the Deaf, 332
Music for the Handicapped Child, 327
My Left Foot, 10
My Second Twenty Years, 3, 9

National Association of the Deaf Catalog of Publications, 424
National Catalog of Films in Special Education, 430
National Center for Law and the Deaf: Final Report, 257
National Recreational Boating for the Physically Handicapped, 335, 336

TITLE INDEX

National Research Strategy for Neurological and Communicative Disorders, 382
The Need for Personal Care Services by Severly Physically Disabled Citizens of Massachusetts, 146
Neurorehabilitation: A Multisensory Approach, 220
New Life for Millions, 91
New Options, 113, 143, 144
New Options Training Manual, 113, 144
New Outlook for the Blind, 45
Newsletter, 251, 263
NIMIS Catalog, 430
The NINCDS Program. Spinal Cord Injury and Nervous System Trauma, 382
The NINCDS Research Program. Epilepsy, 382
The NINCDS Research Program. Multiple Sclerosis, 382
The NINCDS Research Program. Spina Bifida and Neural Tube Defects, 382
The NINCDS Research Program. Stroke, 382
94-142 and 504: Numbers that Add up to Educational Rights for Handicapped Children, 268
Non-Vocal Communication Techniques and Aids for the Severely Physically Handicapped, 140
Normal and Handicapped Children, 366
Not Made of Stone, 306
Nursing Home Activities for the Handicapped, 148

Of Sound and Mind, 70
On Being the Parent of a Handicapped Youth, 300
On Death and Dying, 274, 277
On the Other Hand, 162, 176
Only Child's Play, 363
Opening Doors, 5, 22

Ophthalmological Considerations in the Rehabilitation of the Blind, 30, 40
Oppelt Standard Method of Therapeutic and Recreational Ice Skating, 341
Options, 12
Oral-Aural Communications (OAC), 163, 186
Ordinary Daylight, 46
An Orientation to Deafness for Social Workers, 56, 71
Orientation to Hearing Aids, 158, 176
Orthopaedic Management of Cerebral Palsy, 208, 215
The Orthopaedic Management of Spina Bifida Cystica, 208, 230
Orthotics and Prosthetics, 230
Orthotics Etcetera, 137, 210, 235
The Ostomy Handbook, 275, 288
The Ostomy Library, 277, 288
Ostomyt Quarterly, 288, 400, 415
Ostomy Review II, 288
Outdoor Pursuits for Disabled People, 331
Outreach to the Aging Blind, 32, 38
Outsiders in a Hearing World, 59, 65
Overdue Process, 264

Paraplegia, 290, 402, 415
Paraplegia News, 325, 326, 415
Paraplegic and Quadraplegic Individuals, 212, 227
Paraplegics Discuss Their Sexual Problems, 301
Parent & Family Therapy, 350, 366
Parents on the Team, 352
Parkinson's, 280
A Patient's Bill of Rights, 277

Peer-Oriented Group Work for the Physically Handicapped Child, 359
Personal Achievement Skills; An Introduction, 35, 100
Personal Achievement Skills Training for the Visually Handicapped, 31, 47
Personal Achievement Skills Training Package, 149
Personal Relationships, the Handicapped and the Community, 83, 96, 295, 306
Personality and Sexuality of the Physically Handicapped Woman, 307
Perspectives in Reproduction and Sexual Behavior, 300
Physical Activities for Individuals with Handicapping Conditions, 324, 333
Physical & Occupational Therapy in Pediatrics, 416
Physical Disabilities, 85
Physical Disabilities Manual, 207, 213
Physical Disabilty- A Psychological Approach, 80, 104
Physical Disability and Human Behavior, 98, 298
Physical Education and Recreation for Impaired, Disabled and Handicapped Individuals...Past, Present and Future, 342
Physical Education and Recreation for the Visually Handicapped, 329
Physical Education for Blind Children, 324
Physical Education for Special Needs, 323, 324, 334
Physical Education for the Handicapped, 323, 345
Physical Education for the Visually Handicapped, 324
Physical Education, Recreation and Sports for Individuals with Hearing Impairments, 333
Physical Illness and Handicap in Childhood, 348, 364
Physical Management for the Quadriplegic Patient, 119
Physical Medicine and Rehabilitation Approaches in Spinal Cord Injury, 208, 218
Physical Rehabilitation for Daily Living, 122
Physical Therapy, 416
The Physically Handicapped Child in Your Classroom, 349, 356
Physically Handicapped Children, 274, 277
Physically Impaired Population of the United States, 93
Physiological and Psychological Considerations in the Management of Stroke, 3, 9, 209, 216
Physiotherapy, 416
Physiotherapy Canada/Physiotherapie Canada, 416
The Planner's Guide to Barrier Free Meetings, 5, 24, 25
Planning Barrier Free Libraries, 391
Planning Effective Advocacy Programs, 249, 254
Play Helps, 360
Play It By Ear, 187
A Playground for all Children, 389
Playgrounds and Playspaces for the Handicapped, 323, 328
Playing and Coaching Wheelchair Basketball, 342
Pocket Guide to Federal Help for the Disabled Person, 377
Portable Urinals and Related Appliances, 136
Practical Management of Spinal Injuries, 212, 223
The Practice of Rehabilitation Medicine, 226
Preparation of Orientation and Mobility Maps for the

TITLE INDEX

[and Mobility Maps for the] Visually and Physically Handicapped, 48
Preschool Learning Activities for the Physically Disabled, 359
Pressure Ulcers, 209, 218
A Primer on Due Process, 246, 252
Principles and Methods of Adapted Physical Education and Recreation, 323, 327
Principles of Aural Rehabilitation, 159, 195
Principles of Joint Protection in Chronic Rheumatic Disease, 117
Principles of Orthotic Treatment, 210, 216
A Problem-Oriented Approach to Stroke Rehabilitation, 231
Proceedings of the National Conference for and with Deaf People, 71
Proceedings of the International Conference on Auditory Techniques, 178
Proceedings of the International Congress on Technology and Blindness, 127
Proceedings of the Supreme Court (Davis) Decision, 247, 265
Proceedings of the Third Biennial Registry of Interpreters for the Deaf, 163, 183
Products from the West Virginia Research and Training Center, 433
Professional Approaches with Parents of Handicapped Children, 350, 367
Progressive Exercise Therapy in Rehabilitation and Physical Education, 330
Prosthetics and Orthotics International, 417
Providing Early Mobility, 212, 234

Psychological and Behavioral Aspects of Physical Disability, 97
The Psychological and Social Impact of Physical Disability, 3, 82, 98
The Psychological Aspects of Physical Illness and Disability, 81, 102
Psychological Consultation, 362
Psychological Factors in the Management of Parkinson's Disease, 20
Psychological Practice with the Physically Disabled, 3
The Psychological Rehabilitation of the Amputee, 2, 14, 209, 222
Psychological, Sexual, Social and Vocational Aspects of Spinal Cord Injury, 308
Psychology and Communication in Deaf Children, 163, 197
The Psychology of Blindness, 31, 42
Psychology of Deafness, 187
Psychology of Deafness: Sensory Deprivation, 57, 70
The Psychology of Deafness: Techniques of Appraisal for Rehabilitation, 57, 68
Psychology of Deafness for Rehabilitation Conselors, 57, 62
The Psychology of Disability, 80, 84, 104, 239
Psychology of Exceptional Children and Youth, 348, 354
Psychosocial Adjustment to Disability, 80, 100
Psychosocial Rehabilitation of the Blind, 31, 46
Public Law 94-142 and Section 504, 252
The Public Law Supporting Mainstreaming, 264
Public Policy Toward Disability, 253

Publications and Audio-Visual Aids Directory of the Rehabilitation Research and Training Centers, 425, 431
Publications Reference File, 373, 374

Range of Motion Exercise, 222
A Reader's Guide for Parents of Children with Mental, Physical or Emotional Disabilities, 383
Reading Aids for the Partially Sighted, 49, 138
Readings in Speech Following Total Laryngectomy, 241
Readings on Deafness, 56, 75
Recommended Aids for the Partially Sighted, 138
Reconstruction and Rehabilitation of the Burned Patient, 207, 208, 221
Recreation and Leisure for Handicapped Individuals, 371, 376
Recreation for Disabled Persons Recreation Integration, 322, 336
Recreation Programming for Visually Impaired Children and Youth, 337
Recruitment, Admissions, and Handicapped Students, 265
Reducing Public Barriers of the Severely Handicapped, 7
Regional Directory of Services for Deaf Persons, 72
Rehabfilm Newsletter, 432
Rehabfilm Rental Catalogue, 424
Rehabilitating America, 79, 87
Rehabilitating People with Disabilities into the Mainstream of Society, 102
Rehabilitation Administrative Procedures for Extended Care Facilities, 145

Rehabilitation after Myocardial Infarction, 211, 223
Rehabilitation after Severe Head Injury, 220
Rehabilitation Centers for the Blind and Visually Impaired, 114, 149
Rehabilitation Counseling Bulletin, 417
Rehabilitation Counseling of the Blind, 47
Rehabilitation Digest, 417, 423
Rehabilitation Engineering Aids and Devices for Persons with Impaired Hearing, 138
Rehabilitation Engineering and Product Information, 376
Rehabilitation Engineering Sourcebook and Supplement, 140
Rehabilitation Environment, 142
Rehabilitation for Independent Living, 110, 151, 392
Rehabilitation for Independent Living, A Selected Bibliography, 1982, 110, 392
Rehabilitation in Australia, 418
Rehabilitation Literature, 403, 297, 418
Rehabilitation Literature: A Guide to Selection Materials, 427
Rehabilitation Management of Amputees, 214
Rehabilitation Medicine, 207, 232
Rehabilitation Nursing, 418
Rehabilitation Nursing, 211, 235
Rehabilitation Nursing and Related Readings, 211, 235
Rehabilitation of the Coronary Patient, 242
Rehabilitation of the Facially Disfigured, 207, 228

TITLE INDEX

Rehabilitation of the Lower Limb Amputee, 224
Rehabilitation of the Older Blind Person, 32, 45
Rehabilitation of the Physically Handicapped, 374
Rehabilitation of the Severely Disabled, 18
Rehabilitation of the Visually Disabled and the Blind at Different Ages, 39
Rehabilitation Oncology, 210, 219
Rehabilitation Practices with the Physically Disabled, 93
Rehabilitation Psychology, 99, 309, 419
Rehabilitation Services and the Social Work Role, 88
Rehabilitation Strategies for Sensorineural Hearing Loss, 203
Rehabilitation Teaching for the Blind and Visually Disabled, 36
Rehabilitation Techniques in Severe Disability, 91
Rehabilitation World, 419
Rehabilitative Aspects of Acute and Chronic Nursing Care, 211, 238
Rehabilitative Nursing, Case Studies, 211, 236
Report from the Study Group on Legal Concerns of the Rehabilitation Counselor, 259
Report of the Workshop on Communication Systems for Persons with Impaired Hearing or Speech, 137
Report of the Workshop on Sensory Deficits and Sensory Aids, 132
Reproduction of Copyrighted Works for the Blind and Physically Handicapped, 391
Research and Training Materials Catalogue, 1979-80, 425
Residential Facility Programs for the Hearing Impaired Developmentally Disabled, 160, 199
Resource Guide for Parents and Educators of Blind Children, 275, 292
Resource Guide to Habilitative Techniques and Aids for Cerebral Palsied Persons of all Ages, 134
Resources Book, 389
Resources for the Vocational Preparation of Disabled Youth, 392
Resources in Education, 373, 374, 375
Restoration of Motor Function in the Stroke Patient, 212, 225
Rheumatology and Rehabilitation, 419
A Right to Love, 301
The Rights of Hearing-Impaired Children, 249, 264
Rights of Parent and the Responsibilities of Schools, 261
The Rights of Physically Handicapped People, 249, 259
Rights of Special Education and Handicapped Students in School Disciplinary Procedures, 262
The Role of Facilitites in Training Rehabilitation Personnel, 152
Role of the Family in the Rehabilitation of the Physically Disabled, 81, 99
Roll'on, 324, 328

Salvaging our Sexuality, 313
Sapphistry: The Book of Lesbian Sexuality, 296, 300
Scandinavian Journal of Rehabilitation Medicine, 419
School Nurses Working with Handicapped Children, 363

Scoliosis, 217, 225
Section 504: Civil Rights for the Handicapped, 247, 255
Section 504 and Blind Employees, 263
SEICUS Report, 297
Seizures, Epilepsy, and your Child, 286
Selected Equipment for Pediatric Rehabilitation, 110, 127
Selected Litigation and Legislation Affecting the Handicapped, 263
Selected Reading Suggestion for Parents of Mentally Retarded Children, 383
Selected Readings, 210, 229
Selected Resources for Accessibility, 425
A Selective Listing of Legal Resources for the Handicapped, 250, 266, 268
Self Care for the Hemiplegic, 124
Self-Help Clothing for Children who have Physical Disabilities, 120
Self-Help Groups in Rehabilitation, 103
Self-Help Manual for Patients with Arthritis, 116
Sensory Aids for Employment of Blind and Visually Impaired Persons, 49
Sensory Capabilities of Hearing Impaired Children, 157, 199
Sensory-Motor Dysfunction and Therapy in Infancy and Early Childhood, 361
The Sensuous Wheeler, 299, 308
Sentences and Other Systems, 160, 168
Serving Physically Disabled People, 174, 277
Severe Disabilities, 91, 94
Sex: Rehabilitation's Stepchild, 309
Sex and Disability, 297, 304

Sex and Spina Bifida, 301
Sex and the Handicapped, 297 312, 395
Sex and the Male Ostomate, 315
Sex and the Physically Handicapped, 300
Sex and the Spinal Cord Injured, 297, 300, 314
Sex, Courtship and the Single Ostomate, 313, 318
Sex Education and Counseling of Special Groups, 316
Sex Education and Family Life for Visually Handicapped Children and Youth, 304
Sex Education for Disabled Persons, 314
Sex Education for Physically Handicapped Youth, 316
Sex Education for the Handicapped and an Annotated Bibliography of Selected Resources, 301
Sex Education for the Visually Handicapped in Schools and Agencies...Selected Papers, 309
Sex, Pregnancy and the Female Ostomate, 315, 318
Sex, Society, and the Disabled, 308
Sexual Adjustment, 194, 195, 300, 305
Sexual Consequences of Disability, 303
Sexual Counseling for Ostomates, 310
Sexual Dysfunction in Neurological Disorders, 302
Sexual Health Care, 300
Sexual Health Care Services for the Disabled, 399, 304
Sexual Options for Paraplegics and Quadriplegics, 317
Sexual Problems of Patients with Spinal Injuries, 305
Sexual Rehabilitation of the Urologic Cancer Patient, 312

TITLE INDEX

Sexual Rights for the People...Who Happen to be Handicapped, 315
The Sexual Side of Handicap, 295, 310
Sexuality and Cancer, 197, 318
Sexuality and Disability, 197, 303
Sexuality and Disability, 419
Sexuality and Neuromuscular Disease, 301
Sexuality and Physical Disability, 295, 300, 303
Sexuality and the Disabled, 308
Sexuality and the Spinal Cord Injured Woman, 314
Sexuality Article Packet, 299, 300
Shopping Centers and the Accessibility Codes, 14
Shout in Silence, 74
Sign Language, 162, 174, 175
Sign Language of the Deaf, 162, 197
Sign Language and the Deaf Community, 164
Signing Exact English, 163, 178
Signs of Drug Use, 161, 203
Signs of Language, 162, 184
Signs of Sexual Behavior, 161, 203, 313
Single-Handed, 132
Sites Perception and the Nonvisual Experience, 34, 41
So You're Paralyzed... , 272, 281
Social and Psychological Aspects of Disability, 3, 82, 102
Social and Rehabilitation Services for the Blind, 40
Social Psychology of Childhood Disability, 366
The Social Sources of Adjustment to Blindness, 32, 44
The Sociology and Social Psychology of Disability and Rehabilitation, 81, 100

The Sociology of Physical Disability and Rehabilitation, 84
Socio-Sexual Distance, 301
Sound and Sign, 58, 73
A Source Book: Rehabilitating the Persons with Spinal Cord Injury, 395
Source Book for the Disabled, 133
The Special Child Handbook, 274, 287
Special Devices for Hard of Hearing, Deaf, and Deaf-Blind Persons, 135
Special People, 79, 90
Speech After Stroke, 212, 238
Speech and Deafness, 161, 169
Speech and the Hearing-Impaired Child, 161, 187
Speech Clinician and the Hearing Impaired Child, 171
Speech for the Hearing Impaired Child, 186
Speech-Hearing Test and the Spoken Language of Hearing Impaired Children, 157, 165
Speechreading (Lip reading), 158, 183
Spinal Bifida and Neural Tube Defects, 382
Spina Bifida Therapy, 420
Spinal Cord Injuries, 2, 27, 209, 239, 299
Spinal Cord Injury, 395
Spinal Cord Injury: A Guide for Care, 282
Spinal Cord Injury and Nervous System Trauma, 382
Sport and Physical Recreation for the Disabled, 344
Sports Centers & Swimming Pools, 323, 344
Sports for the Handicapped, 326
Sports 'n Spokes, 343
Staff Manual for Teaching Patients About Rheumatoid Arthitis, 212, 240
Starting Over, 17

State Law and Education of Handicapped Childen, 247, 268
State of the Art, 342
Statistical Abstract of the United States, 372, 374
The Status of Handicapped Children in Head Start Progams, 371
Status Report of Interagency Linkages at the State Level, 375
A Step-by-Step Guide to Personal Management for Blind Persons, 109, 115
Steps to Independence, 140
Sticks and Stones, 289
Stigma, 95
Stimulating Environments for Children Who are Visually Impaired, 349, 358
Strategies for Helping Parents of Exceptional Children, 350, 364
Strategies for Improving Visual Learning, 421, 427
Stresses in Children, 366
Stroke, 4, 13, 237
Stroke and Its Rehabilitation, 210, 228
A Stroke in the Family, 283
Stroke Patient, 212, 225
Stroke Rehabilitation and Re-Socialization, 16
Study and Evaluation of Integrating and Handicapped in HUD Housing, 370, 388
Subject Bibliographies, 373
A Summary of Selected Legislation Relating to the Handicapped 1975-1976, 267
The Supplemental Security Income Program for the Aged, Blind and Disabled, 378
Surgical and Prosthetic Approaches to Speech Rehabilitation, 237
The Surgical Rehabilitation of the Amputee, 108, 222
Swimming for Children with Physical and Sensory Impairments, 340
Symposium of Management of Upper Limb Amputations, 215
Symposium on "Dental Management of the Handicapped Child," Iowa City, Iowa, 1973, 208, 239
Symposium on Special Problems in Orthopedic Rehabilitation, 216

Tactual Mapping, 34, 51
Talk with Me, 182
Talking Book Topics, 45
A Teacher's Guide to Management of Physically Handicapped Students, 361
Teaching and Learning Strategies for Physically Handicapped Students, 249, 353
Teaching Communication Skills to the Preschool Hearing Impaired Child, 160, 202
Teaching Driver Education to The Physically Disabled, 139
Teaching Eating and Toileting Skills to the Multi-handicapped in the School Setting, 120
Teaching Patients, 277
Teaching Physical Activities to Impaired Youth, 339
Teaching Reading to Deaf Children, 160, 179
Teaching Speech to Deaf Children, 201
Teaching the Physically Handicapped to Swim, 327
Technical Aids for the Speech-Impaired, 139
Techniques for Eating, 125
Techniques of Daily Living, 125
Technology and Handicapped People, 396
Test of Syntactic Abilities, 194
Testing for Impaired, Disabled, and Handicapped Individuals, 365

TITLE INDEX 473

Tetraplegia and Paraplegia, 216
Textbook of Sport for the Disabled, 335
Therapeutic Activities for the Handicapped Elderly, 335
Therapeutic and Adapted Recreational Services, 343
Therapeutic Exercise, 207, 214
Therapeutic Re-Creation, 343
Therapeutic Recreation, 340
Therapeutic Recreation Service, 329
These Special Children, 285
They Grow in Silence, 58, 69, 360
Thinking/Learning/Doing, 249, 256
Thinking Without Language, 64
Thru the Arthritis Maze, 380
Thursday's Child Has Far to Go, 364
Toilet Training, 116
Tools, Equipment and Machinery adapted for the Vocational Education and Employment of Handicapped People, 133
Tools for Asssessibility, 425
The Total Care of Spinal Cord Injuries, 208, 233
Total Care of the Stroke Patient, 212, 232
Total Communication, 163, 193
Total Hip Prosthesis, 210, 239
Total Rehabilitation, 78, 105
Toward Independence, 109, 125
Toward Independent Living, 141
Toward Intimacy, 196, 304, 319
Toward Objective Mobility Evaluation, 41
Transportation Counseling for Handicapped Individuals, 19
Transportation for the Elderly and Handicapped, 373, 374, 392, 393
Travel Ability, 324, 342
Travel Agent Guidelines for Travel Planning for the
[Travel Planning for the] Physically Handicapped, 332
Travel in Adverse Weather Conditions, 51
Treatment of the Spinal Cord Injured, 208, 220

Understanding Aphasia, 213, 224
Understanding Arthritis and Rheumatism, 284
Understanding the Deaf/Blind Child, 33, 38, 349, 357
Understanding the Rights of the Handicapped, 267
Understanding those Feelings, 286
The Unexpected Minority, 348, 357
Union List of Audiovisuals in the Library Network of the Veterans Administration, 433
United States Code, 251
U.S. Housing Developments for the Elderly or Handicapped, 388
The Unseen Minority, 33, 43
The Upper Limb in Tetraplegia, 208, 230
Urinary Ostomies--A Guidebook for Patients, 285
The Urological Management of the Patient Following Spinal Cord Injury, 209, 233
User Groups and Site Selection, 389

VA Film Catalog, 432
The Value of Independent Living, 151
The Videolog, 433
Visual Communication of the Hard of Hearing, 158, 191
Visual Handicaps and Learning, 36

Visually Handicapped Children and Young People, 349, 353
Vital and Health Statistics. Series. 371, 374
Volta Review, 332, 420

Ward's Natural Sign Language Thesaurus of Useful Signs and Synonyms, 201
We Live with the WheelChair, 14
What can I do About the Part of Me I don't Like, 274, 278
What Do You Do When You See a Blind Person?, 422
What's the Difference? 85
Wheelchair Accessibility, 28
Wheelchair Bathrooms, 25
The Wheelchair Book, 19
Wheelchair Champions, 343
The Wheelchair Gourmet, 117
The Wheelchair in the Kitchen, 11
Wheelchair Selection, 26
The Wheelchair Traveler, 324, 327
Wheelchair Vagabond, 325, 340
When the Cook can't Look, 123
White Coat, White Cane, 33, 40

The White House Conference on Handicapped Individuals, 396
Who Are the Handicapped?, 95
Who Cares? 303
Why Section 504, 263
Within Reach, 304, 311
A Workbook in Auditory Training for Adults, 158, 198
Working with Parents of Handicapped Children, 281, 358
Workshop Materials, 246, 261
Workshop on Communication Systems for Persons with Impaired Hearing or Speech, 190

You can do it from a Wheelchair, 133
Your Child and Ileal Conduit Surgery, 289
Your Child's Hearing Aid, 157, 171
Your Child's Hearing and Speech, 159, 189
Your Future, 273, 282
Your Handicap--Don't Let it Handicap You, 291
Your Hearing Loss, 158, 180, 190
Youth Volunteers and the Disabled, 385

DATE DUE

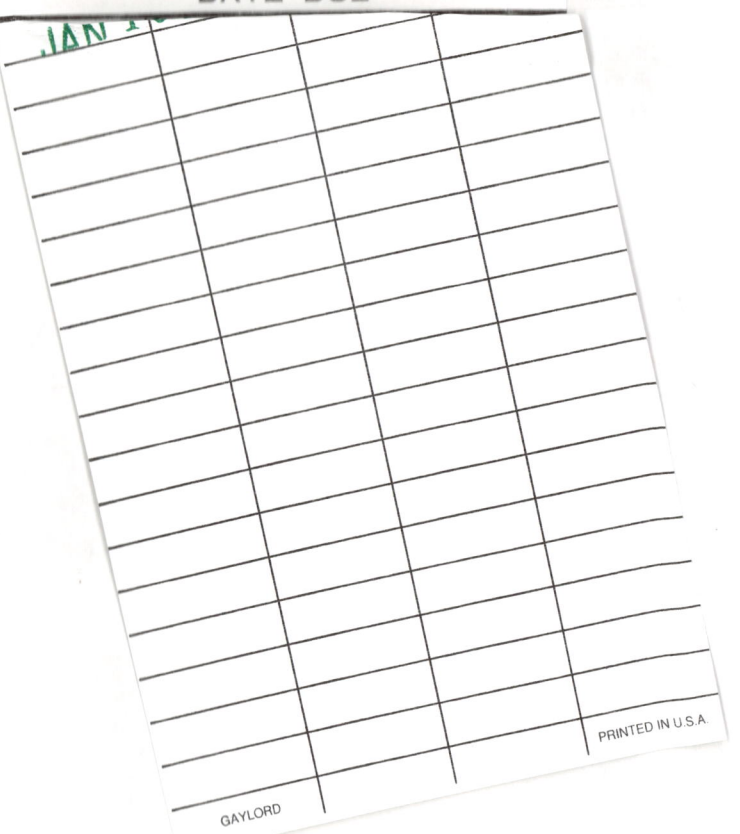

GAYLORD   PRINTED IN U.S.A.